Evidence-Based Interventional Pain Medicine

According to Clinical Diagnoses

Evidence-Based Interventional Pain Medicine

According to Clinical Diagnoses

EDITED BY

JAN VAN ZUNDERT MD, PhD, FIPP
Anesthesiologist
Department of Anesthesiology and Multidisciplinary Pain Centre
Ziekenhuis Oost-Limburg
Genk, Belgium

JACOB PATIJN MD, PhD
Neurologist
Department of Anesthesiology and Pain Management
Maastricht University Pain Centre
Maastricht, the Netherlands

CRAIG T. HARTRICK MD, DABPM, FIPP
Anesthesiologist
Departments of Anesthesiology, Biomedical Sciences, and Health Sciences
Oakland University William Beaumont School of Medicine
Rochester, MI, USA

ARNO LATASTER, MSc
Anatomist
Department of Anatomy and Embryology
Maastricht University
Maastricht, the Netherlands

FRANK J.P.M. HUYGEN MD, PhD, FIPP
Anesthesiologist
Department of Anesthesiology and Pain Management
Erasmus Medical Centre
Rotterdam, the Netherlands

NAGY MEKHAIL MD, PhD, FIPP
Carl E. Wasmuth Professor and Chair
Department of Pain Management
Cleveland Clinic
Cleveland, Ohio, USA

MAARTEN VAN KLEEF MD, PhD, FIPP
Anesthesiologist
Department of Anesthesiology and Pain Management
Maastricht University Medical Centre
Maastricht, the Netherlands

EDITORIAL COMMISSIONERS

ROGIER TROMPERT, Medical Illustrator

NICOLE VAN DEN HECKE, Coordinator

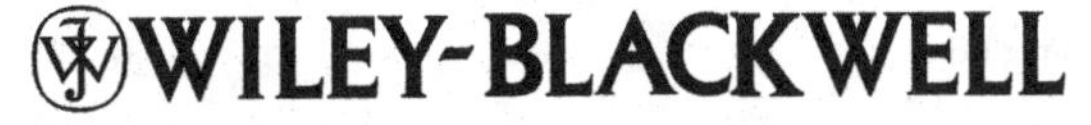

A John Wiley & Sons, Ltd., Publication

Wiley-Blackwell is an imprint of John Wiley & Sons, formed by the merger of Wiley's global Scientific, Technical and Medical business with Blackwell Publishing.

Registered office: John Wiley & Sons, Ltd, The Atrium, Southern Gate, Chichester, West Sussex, PO19 8SQ, UK

Editorial offices: 9600 Garsington Road, Oxford, OX4 2DQ, UK
The Atrium, Southern Gate, Chichester, West Sussex, PO19 8SQ, UK
111 River Street, Hoboken, NJ 07030-5774, USA

For details of our global editorial offices, for customer services and for information about how to apply for permission to reuse the copyright material in this book please see our website at www.wiley.com/wiley-blackwell

A catalogue record for this book is available from the British Library.

This book is published in the following electronic formats: ePDF 9781119968344; Wiley Online Library 9781119968375; ePub 9781119968351; mobi 9781119968368

Set in 9.25/12pt Minion by Toppan Best-set Premedia Limited, Hong Kong

1 2012

Contents

Contributor List

Honorio T. Benzon MD, FIPP
Department of Anesthesiology
Northwestern University Feinberg School of Medicine
Chicago, IL, USA

Kees Besse MD, FIPP
Department of Anesthesiology Pain and Palliative Medicine
Radboud University
Nijmegen Medical Centre
Nijmegen, the Netherlands

Allen W. Burton MD, FIPP
Department of Pain Medicine
UT MD Anderson Cancer Center
Houston, TX, USA

Jianguo Cheng MD, PhD
Department of Pain Management
Cleveland Clinic, Cleveland
OH, USA

Steven P. Cohen MD
Department of Anesthesiology & Critical Care Medicine
John Hopkins School of Medicine, Baltimore
Walter Reed Army Medical Center
Washington, DC, USA

Paul Cornelissen MD
Department of Anesthesiology and Pain Management
Jeroen Bosch Ziekenhuis's Hertogenbosch
the Netherlands

Miles Day MD, DABA FIPP, DABIPP
Professor
Medical Director
International Pain Centre Texas Tech
University HSC
Lubbock, Texas, USA

Jan De Witte MD
Department of Anesthesiology
Intensive Care Medicine, and Pain Management
OLV-Ziekenhuis, Aalst, Belgium

Richard Derby, MD, FIPP
Medical Director
Spinal Diagnostics and Treatment Center
Daly City, CA, USA

Jacques Devulder MD, PhD
Department of Anesthesiology and
Multidisciplinary Pain Centre
University Hospital Ghent
Ghent, Belgium

Sudhir Diwan, MD, DABIPP, FIPP
Executive Director
The Spine & Pain Institute of New York
Staten Island University Hospital
New York

Robert van Dongen MD, PhD, FIPP
Department of Anesthesiology, Pain and Palliative Medicine
Radboud University Nijmegen Medical Centre
Nijmegen, the Netherlands

Maarten van Eerd MD, FIPP
Department of Anesthesiology and Pain Management
Amphia Ziekenhuis, Breda
The Netherlands

Frank van Eijs MD
Department of Anesthesiology and Pain Management
St. Elisabeth Hospital
Tilburg, the Netherlands

Catharina G. Faber MD, PhD
Department of Neurology
Maastricht University Medical Centre
the Netherlands

Wilco E. van Genderen, MD
Department of Anesthesiology and Pain Management
Medical Centre Jan van Goyen
Amsterdam, the Netherlands

José W. Geurts, MSc
Department of Anesthesiology and Pain Management
Maastricht University Medical Centre
Maastricht, the Netherlands

Maurice J.M.M. Giezeman MD, PhD
Department of Anesthesiology and Pain Management
Diakonessenhuis, Utrecht
the Netherlands

Gerbrand J. Groen MD, PhD
Department of Anesthesiology & Pain Treatment,
University Medical Centre Groningen
University of Groningen, Groningen, the Netherlands

Craig T. Hartrick, MD, FIPP
Department of Anesthesiology, Biomedical Sciences, and Health Sciences
Oakland University William Beaumont School of Medicine
Rochester, MI, USA

Salim Hayek MD, PhD, FIPP
Division of Pain Medicine
University Hospitals
Cleveland, OH, USA

Marc Huntoon MD
Division of Pain Medicine
Chief
Professor of Anesthesiology
Vanderbilt University,
Nashville TN, USA

Frank Huygen MD, PhD, FIPP
Department of Anesthesiology and Pain Management
Erasmus University Medical Centre
Rotterdam

Markus Janssen MD, FIPP
Department of Anesthesiology and Pain Management
Maastricht University Medical Centre, Maastricht
The Netherlands

Jan Willem Kallewaard MD, FIPP
Department of Anesthesiology and Pain Management
Rijnstate Hospital
Arnhem, the Netherlands

Leonardo Kapural MD, PhD, FIPP
Department of Pain Management,
Cleveland Clinic
Cleveland, OH, USA

Yolande Keulemans, MD, PhD
Department of Gastroenterology
Maastricht University Medical Centre
Maastricht, the Netherlands

Maarten van Kleef, MD, PhD, FIPP
Department of Anesthesiology and Pain Management
Maastricht University Pain Centre
Maastricht, the Netherlands

Arno Lataster MSc
Department of Anatomy and Embryology
Maastricht University
Maastricht, the Netherlands

Robert Levy MD, PhD
Professor and Chairman
Department of Neurological Surgery and
Co-Director,
Shands Jacksonville Neuroscience Institute
University of Florida College of Medicine
Jacksonville, Fl, USA

Timothy R. Lubenow MD, FIPP
Department of Anesthesiology
Rush University Medical Center
Chicago, IL, USA

Nagy Mekhail, MD, PhD, FIPP
Department of Pain Management
Cleveland Clinic
Cleveland, OH, USA

Samer Narouze MD, MSc, FIPP
Centre For Pain Medicine
Summa Western Reserve Hospital
Cuyahoga Falls, Oh, USA

Turo J. Nurmikko MD, PhD
Pain Research Institute and
Faculty of Health and Life Sciences
University of Liverpool
Liverpool, UK

Nileshkumar Patel MD, MBA
Clinical Professor, Anesthesiology
Advanced Pain Management
Green Bay, WI, USA

Jacob Patijn, MD, PhD
Department of Anesthesiology and Pain Management
Maastricht University Pain Centre
Maastricht, the Netherlands

Dirk Peek MD
Department of Anesthesiology and Pain Medicine
St. Jans Gasthuis, Weert
The Netherlands

Wouter Pluijms MD
Department of Anesthesiology and Pain Management
Maastricht University Medical
Centre, Maastricht

Jason E. Pope, MD
Director of the Headache Center
Napa Pain Institute
Napa, CA
Assistant Professor of Anesthesiology
Vanderbilt University Medical Center
Nashville, TN

Martine Puylaert MD, FIPP
Department of Anesthesiology and
Multidisciplinary Pain Centre
Ziekenhuis Oost-Limburg
Genk, Belgium

Prithvi Raj, MD, FIPP
Department of Anesthesiology and Pain Medicine
Texas Tech University
Texas, TX, USA

Olav Rohof MD, PhD, FIPP
Orbis Medisch Centrum,
Pijnkliniek
Sittard Geleen
the Netherlands

Richard W. Rosenquist MD
Chairman of the Pain Management Department
Cleveland Clinic
Cleveland, OH, USA

Menno E. Sluijter MD, PhD, FIPP
Pain Unit, Swiss Paraplegic Centre
Nottwil, Switzerland

Peter Staats MD, FIPP
Department of Anesthesiology and Critical Care Medicine
John Hopkins University
Baltimore, MA, USA

Michael Stanton-Hicks MB; BS, Dr med, FIPP
Department of Pain Management
Cleveland Clinic, Cleveland
OH, USA

Robert Jan Stolker MD, PhD
Department of Anesthesiology and Pain Management
Erasmus University Medical Centre
Rotterdam the Netherlands

Hans van Suijlekom MD, PhD
Department of Anesthesiology and Pain Management
Catharina Ziekenhuis, Eindhoven
The Netherlands

Karolina Szadek MD
Department of Anesthesiology and Pain Management
Vrije Universiteit Amsterdam
Amsterdam, the Netherlands

Michel A. M. B. Terheggen MD
Department of Anesthesiology and Pain Management
Rijnstate Hospital
Arnhem, the Netherlands

Ricardo Vallejo MD, PhD, FIPP
Millennium Pain Center
Bloomington, IL, USA

Koen Van Boxem MD, FIPP
Department of Anesthesiology and Pain Management
Sint-Jozefkliniek, Bornem and Willebroek
Bornem, Belgium

Eric Vanduynhoven MD
Department of Anesthesiology and Pain Management
GZA, Campus Sint
Augustinus, Antwerp
Belgium

Pascal Vanelderen MD, FIPP
Department of Anesthesiology and
Multidisciplinary Pain Centre
Ziekenhuis Oost-Limburg, Genk, Belgium

Jan Van Zundert, MD, PhD, FIPP
Department of Anesthesiology and
Muitidisciplinary Pain Centre
Ziekenhuis Oost-Limburg, Genk, Belgium

Kris C. P. Vissers MD, PhD, FIPP
Department of Anesthesiology Pain and Palliative Medicine
Radboud University
Nijmegen Medical Centre
Nijmegen, the Netherlands

Michel Wagemans MD, PhD
Department of Anesthesiology and Pain Management
Renier de Graaf Groep
Delft, The Netherlands

Mark Wallace MD
Center for Pain Medicine
University of California
San Diego Medical Center
San Diego, CA, USA

Albert J. M. van Wijck MD, PhD
Department of Anesthesiology and Pain Management
University Medical Centre, Utrecht
the Netherlands

Andre Wolff MD, PhD
Department of Anesthesiology Pain and Palliative Medicine
Radboud University Nijmegen Medical Centre
Nijmegen, the Netherlands

Wouter Zuurmond MD, PhD
Department of Anesthesiology, Pain Therapy and Palliative Care
VU Medical Centre, Amsterdam
The Netherlands

Foreword

by Menno E. Sluijter MD, PhD, FIPP

Seeing this book makes me proud of my university city Maastricht, where I have left so many footsteps and where I still have many friends. It is a great honor for me to have been invited to write this foreword.

Besides accurately describing the various techniques in detail, this book has an accent on evidence-based medicine. This comes naturally for the Dutch since soberness and standing firmly on the ground belong to their prominent features. It makes the book into a solid and reliable guide for many pain practitioners.

My first footsteps in the world of invasive pain treatment date back to a very different period. My mentors and teachers were Jur Bouma in the Netherlands and legendary names, such as Sampson Lipton and Mark Mehta, who played such a pivotal role in their time. Those were the days when solitary observations easily sparked attention or even a trend. Epidural phenol at T12 has been recommended for anal pain for about a decade, one author copying it from another because it was so bizarre. Ondine's syndrome, as a complication of a cordotomy, received undue attention probably because of its romantic name. Evidence-based medicine was still a far cry.

This book therefore symbolizes for me how invasive pain treatment has become mature within a relatively short period. This process of growth has taken place despite a head wind that is specific for the subject. Many of the procedures are intricate, and success or failure may depend on seemingly trivial details, causing differences in results between researchers. Also pain is a subjective experience and this has various consequences. It makes it particularly difficult to translate results into numbers that are suitable for meaningful statistical analysis. It may even influence results. I firmly believe that a procedure that is performed by a friendly, interested doctor in a friendly environment has a greater chance of success than a procedure under less favorable circumstances. If this is placebo, so be it. It makes pain treatment different from putting a stent into a coronary artery or from removing a tumor under general anesthesia.

Maturity is a sign of growth and it has to be encouraged. Evidence-based medicine will be an indispensible and welcome element of invasive pain treatment in the time to come. It will save patients from getting useless treatments and it will convince insurers to follow up on reasonable demands. It will hopefully discourage those who seek financial gain from a vulnerable group of patients. It will also provide interventional pain treatment with the respected place in the medical community that it deserves.

But, on the other hand, maturity may also be taken as a sign of immanent old age. When reading this book the reader should also realize that all these procedures have once been done for the first time. This reflects a mixture of prudence and courage, but also alertness to observations and the urge to make it a better world for patients who could not be helped before. This process of growth and renewal must not be lost. It should be seen as a complement of evidence-based medicine rather than as a contradiction. After all, without ideas and innovation the need for evidence would soon dry up, and what good is a new procedure without evidence?

The book underscores the need for proper training. The prevalence of chronic pain is such that, despite the laudable efforts of World Institute of Pain, there is still a shortage of well trained doctors who can provide this type of treatment. This is a problem because reading even this book is not enough and practical training is costly in terms of material and manpower. It is to be hoped that the increasing number of potential trainers will gradually resolve the problem.

I recommend this book as a standard manual in the library of every interventionalist. Happy reading!

Foreword

by P. Prithvi Raj MD, FIPP

Jan Van Zundert, Jaap Patijn, Craig Hartrick, Arno Lataster, Frank Huygen, Nagy Mekhail, and Maarten van Kleef, all internationally renowned pain physicians, have embarked on writing "Evidence-Based Interventional Pain Medicine According to Clinical Diagnosis". They have devoted most of their lives to improving the pain management of patients globally. At their request, I am honored to write a Foreword for their new book.

To emphasize the importance of this book, I need to reiterate the statistics available to us on chronic pain today. Chronic pain prevails globally, the total number of persons living with this specific disease or condition with feeling of pain, ranges from 54% in Sweden to 13% in Japan. These studies show that in the rest of the developed countries, such as United States, United Kingdom and Australia, the incidence is somewhere in between. Studies also show that pain imposes a huge economic burden on all countries; for example, in the United States it was calculated that in 1991, the USA spent eighty-six billion dollars on chronic back pain management. Today, because the elderly are living longer, the prevalence of chronic pain is rising with age. Another problem one needs to recognize is that only one billion people in the developed countries have the luxury of utilizing the most advanced pain management techniques. The other five billion people, who have medium to low standards of living, are unable to receive the benefits of these new techniques of pain management.

The World Institute of Pain (WIP) and its members have been aware of this problem and the disparities between countries in terms of standard of care and practices of pain management. Since 1994, WIP's mission has been to train pain physicians and certify their competency in interventional pain management. By all accounts, this mission has become very successful globally.

Pain practice today is fortunate to have many physicians taking this practice as a professional part of their career. They come from all specialties and the book now has to reflect the advances in Pain Practice of all those specialties, not just those in Anesthesiology. The debate is still raging whether a single pain specialist can deliver better pain management than a group of specialists together. The cost of managing such multidisciplinary clinics has been called into question especially by the reimbursement agencies. A program developed by a multidisciplinary clinic is nowadays rejected outright by the reimbursement agencies, and even if it is approved, the efficacy of such programs is questionable. More and more the patients are referring themselves to the Pain Clinics where their pain will be relieved over the short-term rather than addressing the long-term goal of improving the patient's function and quality of life. That is why one finds a prolific growth of Interventional Pain Management Clinics and decrease in University-based Multidisciplinary Clinics. This is certainly the case in the USA and is also becoming common in other countries.

Pain Physicians have not tackled at all the discrepancy in pain practices between developed, developing and under developed countries. There is no factual account of the epidemiology of pain the world over; one cannot say for certain how many Pain Physicians are available per capita in any community. We certainly have made advances in understanding the new theories of pain, and in some pain syndromes, the longitudinal natural course, but we are far from having a reliable algorithm for any pain disorder. It is still hit and miss.

The challenge today is to train Pain Physicians in such a way that they have a standardized curriculum during their Residency and Pain Fellowship programs, followed by skilled practical training, either in Anesthesiology, Neurosurgery, Physical Medicine and Rehabilitation or Psychiatry. Once trained, they need to be examined and tested periodically for their competency. This will raise the standard of pain practice, not only in the USA, but all over the world.

Evidence-based medicine (EBM) or evidence-based practice (EBP) aims to apply the best available evidence gained from scientific methods to clinical decision making. It seeks to assess the strength of evidence of the risks and benefits of treatments (including lack of treatment) and diagnostic tests. Evidence quality can range from meta-analyses and systematic reviews of double-blind, placebo-controlled clinical trials at the top end, down to conventional wisdom at the bottom.

Let me explain the history of evidence-based medicine's origin. Traces of evidence-based medicine's origin can be found in ancient Greece. Although testing medical interventions for efficacy has existed since the time of Avicenna's The Canon of Medicine in the 11th century, it was only in the 20th century that this effort evolved to impact almost all fields of health care and policy. Professor Archie Cochrane, a Scottish Epidemiologist, through his book Effectiveness and Efficiency: Random Reflections on Health Services (1972) and subsequent advocacy caused increasing acceptance of the concepts behind evidence-based practice. Cochrane's work was honored through the naming of centers of evidence-based medical research—Cochrane Centers—and an international organization, the Cochrane Collaboration. The explicit methodologies used to determine "best evidence" were largely established by the McMaster University research group led by David Sackett and Gordon Guyatt. Guyatt later coined the term "evidence-based" in 1990. The term "evidence-based medicine" first appeared in the medical literature in 1992 in a paper by Guyatt et al. Relevant journals include the British Medical Journal's Clinical Evidence, the Journal of Evidence-Based Healthcare and Evidence-Based Health Policy. All of these were co-founded by Anna Donald, an Australian pioneer in the discipline.

There has been discussion of applying what has been learned from EBM to public policy. In his 1996 inaugural speech as President of the Royal Statistical Society, Adrian Smith held out evidence-based medicine as an exemplar for all public policy. He proposed that "evidence-based policy" should be established for education, prisons and policing policy, and all areas of government

This book "Evidence-Based Interventional Pain Medicine According to Clinical Diagnoses" fits the void where literature should conform to local necessities for information to be useful in that society. The format of the book is excellent; each chapter is consistent in describing an interventional technique in simple terms from history to complications and efficacy, stressing at all times the technique.

The reader who is interested in learning, training and practicing interventional pain medicine will find this book extremely useful and informative. It illustrates not only the usual common techniques but also the emerging techniques; this makes it unique and different from the usual text books on pain. I wholeheartedly recommend the interventional pain physician to have this book in their library.

Introduction

The use of interventional pain management techniques has gradually become integrated into the treatment plan of patients suffering from chronic pain. After a long period of empirical use, it is time to move on to the professionalization and standardization of this practice. Interventional pain management techniques are *target specific*. There is evidence that better patient selection increases the success ratio.[1] Therefore, a standard patient evaluation to "fine-tune" the clinical pain diagnosis is mandatory. A detailed description of the technical performance provides a guideline for the standardized interventional pain procedure.

The efficacy of these techniques has been described in randomized controlled trials, observational studies, retrospective studies, and case reports. Evidence-based practice guidelines provide a good review of the literature in a context that makes it accessible and useful to both the clinician and researcher.[2,3]

The available evidence is summarized by treatment option or technique. There are, however, several studies indicating that the chances for treatment success increase with better patient selection.[1,4–7] A wellformed management strategy starts with an accurate evaluation process to identify the pain diagnosis. It is of utmost importance to first check for the so-called red flags that may be indicative of an underlying primary pathology, which needs adequate treatment prior to symptomatic pain management techniques. The treatment relies on accurate use of conservative interventions, potentially in association with interventional pain management techniques. Consequently, evidence-based practice guidelines are of greater practical value when they are specific for each different pain diagnosis.

Guideline development

In daily practice the important goal of pain medicine is to use a specific treatment, conservative and/or interventional, for the right patient at the right moment. Therefore, treatment selection should be according to clinical diagnoses. To improve recognition and information retrieval, the articles have been organized according to a strict structure:

Introduction
Diagnosis
History
Physical examination
Additional tests
Differential diagnosis
Treatment
Conservative management
Interventional management
Complications of interventional treatment
Evidence for interventional management
Recommendations
Treatment algorithm
Techniques
Summary

Although the scientific literature is predominantly Anglo-Saxon and most doctors use the English denominations of anatomical structures, in this series, anatomical structures were indicated with the Latin denomination (Terminologia Anatomica) and the English denomination was, where appropriate, added between brackets.[8] This option was specifically chosen to help people around the world to use the correct denomination when expressing themselves in a language other than English.

This series has focused on interventional pain management techniques, because they have undergone a rapid evolution in recent decades with additional well-conducted research being published regularly. The use of these techniques for the right indication may improve the quality of life of carefully selected patients. Moreover, for correct application of interventional pain management techniques, both good theoretical knowledge and practical experience are mandatory. These skills can only be acquired through training and continuing education.

The strict rules used to establish EBM guidelines may lead to exclusion of relatively new treatments that are only supported by noncontrolled trials. For the interventional pain management techniques covered in this series, in-depth literature searches on efficacy, side effects, and complications have been performed. The incidence of side effects and complications was largely derived from three reviews that specifically address the complications of interventional pain management techniques.[2,9,10] Disease and diagnosis related information was retrieved from high-quality review articles.

Guideline rationale

To make informed recommendations, the available evidence must be assigned "weight." When scoring the evidence of interventional pain management techniques, perhaps even more than for any other treatment modality, the principle "*Primo non nocere*" holds true. The "weighted" rating must consider the evidence for effect and balance this evidence against the incidence and severity of side effects and complications. The scoring system that best observed these considerations was published by Guyatt et al.,[11] "Grading strength of recommendations and quality of evidence in clinical guidelines." The method was then adapted specifically for interventional pain management techniques.[12]

First, a determination was made as to whether the potential benefits outweigh the risk and/or burden. The benefit/risk assessment was assigned a *numerical value* of 1 if the benefit because of the effectiveness of the treatment was greater than the risk and burden of potential complications. A value of 2 was given when the benefit of the effect was closely balanced with the risk and burden of possible side effects.

The *grade* of the evidence was then indicated by a letter: A, B, or C. Following this system, a value of A indicates the highest level of evidence (various randomized controlled trials [RCTs] of good quality), B represents evidence derived from RCTs with methodological limitations or large observational studies, and C is assigned when the evidence is limited to observational studies or case series. Additionally, a score of "0" is given for techniques that are only described in case reports. Finally, the evidence was interpreted for outcome, indicated as follows: positive outcome (+), negative outcome (−), or, when both positive and negative studies were included, (±) was used.

The grading and subsequent implications are summarized in Table 1.

In the recommendations, the practical *implication* "study related" is used for treatment options currently having low-level evidence as determined by systematic recording of the following:

- Patient characteristics
- Diagnostic process
- Treatment including the details of the technique concerned
- Evaluation of the result (preferably Global Perceived effect, VAS, EuroQol, and a complaint-specific scale at 3, 6, and if necessary at 12 months)
- Side effects and complications

Systematic reporting of results can help to accumulate information that further enables estimation of the "value" of a technique when it has been applied to a larger number of patients. This information may form the motivation for a prospective randomized study.

Certain pain management techniques require an extensive expertise and specialized materials and equipment. Therefore, it is appropriate that those specific techniques should be performed in specialized pain centers.

Table 1. Summary of Evidence Scores and Implications for Recommendation.

Score	Description	Implication
1 A +	Effectiveness demonstrated in various RCTs of good quality. The benefits clearly outweigh risk and burdens	Positive recommendation
1 B +	One RCT or more RCTs with methodological weaknesses, demonstrate effectiveness. The benefits clearly outweigh risk and burdens	
2 B +	One or more RCTs with methodological weaknesses, demonstrate effectiveness. Benefits closely balanced with risk and burdens	
2 B ±	Multiple RCTs, with methodological weaknesses, yield contradictory results better or worse than the control treatment. Benefits closely balanced with risk and burdens, or uncertainty in the estimates of benefits, risk and burdens.	Considered, preferably study-related
2 C +	Effectiveness only demonstrated in observational studies. Given that there is no conclusive evidence of the effect, benefits closely balanced with risk and burdens	
0	There is no literature or there are case reports available, but these are insufficient to prove effectiveness and/or safety. These treatments should only be applied in relation to studies.	Only study-related
2 C −	Observational studies indicate no or too short-lived effectiveness. Given that there is no positive clinical effect, risk and burdens outweigh the benefit	Negative recommendation
2 B −	One or more RCTs with methodological weaknesses, or large observational studies that do not indicate any superiority to the control treatment. Given that there is no positive clinical effect, risk and burdens outweigh the benefit	

Each diagnostic process has been well described and the evidence for management options reviewed within the context of a specific diagnosis. For recommended interventional techniques, a detailed description for performance is provided. Other common treatment options are beyond the scope in this series. Importantly, the literature for the pharmacological treatment is not covered in depth and little attention is paid to the multidisciplinary management and the role of cognitive behavioral treatment in this series.

This book was initially based on practice guidelines written by Dutch and Flemish (Belgian) experts that are assembled in a handbook for the Dutch-speaking pain physicians. After translation, the articles were updated and edited in cooperation with U.S./International pain specialists. Because this updating process and the sequential publication of articles, the latest literature update varies from one article to another. Sixty authors, each expert in their field, have contributed to this series.

The validation of the guidelines was carried out in a process of peer review in two stages.

The first edition of the guidelines in Dutch was submitted to the members of the Associations of anesthesiologists with special interest for pain management from the Netherlands (Nederlandse Vereniging voor Anesthesiologie sectie Pijngeneeskunde [NVAsP]) and the Dutch-speaking part of Belgium (Vlaamse Anesthesiologische Vereniging voor Pijnbestrijding [VAVP]). During the review process, more than 200 remarks and questions were raised by the members and treated by the authors. In this way, the guidelines were accepted by means of a broad consensus.

Secondly, as part of the publications of this series in Pain Practice, each translated and updated chapter was reviewed and updated by minimum two U.S. coauthors and each article underwent the journal's peer review.

The evidence rating of the interventional techniques is summarized in Table 2.

Table 2. Summary of the Evidence Rating Per Diagnosis.

Trigeminal neuralgia		
Radiofrequency (RF) treatment of the Gasserian ganglion	2 B+	Recommended
Pulsed RF treatment of the Gasserian ganglion	2 B−	Negative recommendation
Cluster headache		
RF treatment of the pterygopalatine ganglion (sphenopalatinum)	2 C+	To be considered
Occipital nerve stimulation	2 C+	To be considered in specialized centers and study related
Persistant idiopathic facial pain		
Pulsed RF treatment of the ganglion pterygopalatinum (sphenopalatinum)	2 C+	To be considered
Cervical radicular pain		
Interlaminar epidural corticosteroid administration	2 B+	Recommended
Transforaminal epidural corticosteroid administration	2 B−	Negative recommendation
RF treatment adjacent to the cervical ganglion spinale (DRG)	2 B+	Recommended
Pulsed RF treatment adjacent to the cervical ganglion spinale (DRG)	1 B+	Recommended
Spinal cord stimulation	0	Study related in specialized centers
Cervical facet pain		
Intra-articular injections	0	Study related
Therapeutic (repetitive) cervical ramus medialis (medial branch) of the ramus dorsalis block (local anesthetic with or without corticosteroid)	2 B+	Recommended
RF treatment of the cervical ramus medialis (medial branch) of the ramus dorsalis	2 C+	To be considered
Cervicogenic headache		
Injection of nervus occipitalis major with corticosteroid + local anesthetic	1 B+	Recommended
Injection of atlanto-axial joint with corticosteroid + local anesthetic	2 C−	Negative recommendation
RF treatment of the cervical ramus medialis (medial branch) of the ramus dorsalis	2 B±	To be considered
Pulsed RF treatment of the cervical ganglion spinale (DRG) (C2–C3)	0	Study related
Whiplash-associated disorders		
Botulinum toxin type A	2 B−	Negative recommendation
Intra-articular corticosteroid injection	2 C−	Negative recommendation
RF treatment of the cervical ramus medialis (medial branch) of the ramus dorsalis	2 B+	Recommended

Continued

Table 2. Continued.

Occipital neuralgia		
Single infiltration of the nervi occipitales with local anesthetic and corticosteroids	2 C+	To be considered
Pulsed RF treatment of the nervi occipitales	2 C+	To be considered
Pulsed RF treatment of the cervical ganglion spinale (DRG)	0	Study related
Subcutaneous stimulation of the nervi occipitales	2 C+	To be considered in specialized centres
Botulinum toxin A injection	2 C±	Only study related
Painful shoulder complaints		
Corticosteroid injections	2 B±	To be considered
Continuous cervical epidural infusion	2 C+	To be considered
Pulsed RF treatment of the nervus suprascapularis	2 C+	To be considered
Thoracic pain		
Intercostal block	0	Study related
RF treatment of thoracic ganglion spinale (DRG)	2 C+	To be considered
Pulsed RF treatment of thoracic ganglion spinale (DRG)	2 C+	To be considered
Lumbosacral radicular pain		
Interlaminar epidural corticosteroid administration	2 B±	To be considered
Transforaminal epidural corticosteroid administration in "contained herniation"	2 B+	Recommended
Transforaminal epidural corticosteroid administration in "extruded herniation"	2 B−	Negative recommendation
RF lesioning adjacent to the lumbar ganglion spinale (DRG)	2 A−	Negative recommendation
Pulsed RF treatment adjacent to the lumbar ganglion spinale (DRG)	2 C+	To be considered
Spinal cord stimulation (FBSS only)	2 A+	Recommended in specialized centers
Adhesiolysis—epiduroscopy	2 B±	To be considered in specialized centers
Pain originating from the lumbar facet joints		
Intra-articular corticosteroid injections	2 B±	To be considered
RF treatment of the lumbar rami mediales (medial branches) of the dorsal ramus	1 B+	Recommended
Sacroiliac joint pain		
Therapeutic intra-articular injections with corticosteroids and local anesthetic	1 B+	Recommended
RF treatment of rami dorsales and rami laterales	2 C+	To be considered
Pulsed RF treatment of rami dorsales and rami laterales	2 C+	To be considered
Cooled / RF treatment of the rami laterales	2 B+	Recommended
Coccygodynia		
Local injections corticosteroids/local anesthetic	2 C+	To be considered
Intradiscal corticosteroid injections, ganglion impar block, RF ganglion impar, caudal block	0	Study related
Neurostimulation	0	Study related
Discogenic low back pain		
Intradiscal corticosteroid administration	2 B−	Negative recommendation
RF treatment of the discus intervertebralis	2 B±	To be considered
Intradiscal electrothermal therapy	2 B±	To be considered
Biacuplasty	0	Study related
Disctrode	0	Study related
RF of the ramus communicans	2 B+	Recommended
Complex regional pain syndrome		
Intravenous regional block guanethidine	2 A−	Negative recommendation
Ganglion stellatum (stellate ganglion) block	2 B+	Recommended
Lumbar sympathetic block	2 B+	Recommended
Plexus brachialis block	2 C+	To be considered
Epidural infusion analgesia	2 C+	To be considered
Spinal cord stimulation	2 B+	Recommended in specialized centers
Peripheral nerve stimulation	2 C+	To be considered in specialized centers
Herpes zoster and post-herpetic neuralgia		
Interventional pain treatment of acute herpes zoster		
Epidural corticosteroid injections	2 B+	Recommended
Sympathetic nerve block	2 C+	To be considered

Table 2. Continued.

Prevention of PHN		
One-time epidural corticosteroid injection	2 B –	Negative recommendation
Repeated paravertebral injections	2 C +	To be considered
Sympathetic nerve block	2 C +	To be considered
Treatment of PHN		
Epidural corticosteroid injections	0	Study related
Sympathetic nerve block	2 C +	To be considered
Intrathecal injection	?	
Spinal cord stimulation	2 C +	To be considered in specialized centers
Painful diabetic polyneuropathy		
Spinal cord stimulation	2 C +	To be considered in specialized centers
Carpal tunnel syndrome		
Local injections with corticosteroids	1 B +	Recommended
Pulsed RF treatment median nerve	0	Study related
Meralgia paresthetica		
Lateral femoral cutaneous nerve (LFCN) infiltration with local anesthetic ± corticosteroid	2 C +	To be considered
Pulsed RF treatment of LFCN	0	Study related
Spinal cord stimulation	0	Study related in specialized centers
Phantom pain		
Pulsed RF treatment of the stump neuroma	0	Study related
Pulsed RF treatment adjacent to the spinal ganglion (DRG)	0	Study related
Spinal cord stimulation	0	Study related in specialized centers
Traumatic plexus lesion		
Spinal cord stimulation	0	Study related in specialized centers
Pain in patients with cancer		
Epidural and intrathecal administration of analgesics		
Intrathecal medication delivery	2 B +	Recommended
Epidural medication delivery	2 C +	To be considered
Unilateral oncologic pains below the shoulder or dermatome C5		
Cervical cordotomy	2 C +	To be considered in specialized centers
Upper abdominal pain due to cancer of the pancreas/stomach		
Neurolytic plexus coeliacus block	2 A +	To be considered
Neurolytic nervus splanchnicus block	2 B +	Recommended
Visceral pain due to pelvic tumors		
Neurolytic plexus hypogastricus block	2 C +	Recommended
Perineal pain due to pelvic tumors		
Intrathecal phenolization of lower sacral roots of cauda equina	0	Study related
Spinal pain due to vertebral compression fractures		
Vertebroplasty	2 B +	Recommended
Kyphoplasty	2 B +	Recommended
Chronic refractory angina pectoris		
Spinal cord stimulation	2 B +	Recommended in specialized centers
Ischemic pain in the extremities and Raynaud's phenomenon		
Ischemic vascular disease		
Sympathectomy	2 B ±	To be considered
Spinal cord stimulation	2 B ±	To be considered in specialized centers
Raynaud's phenomenon		
Sympathectomy	2 C +	To be considered
Pain in chronic pancreatitis		
RF nervus splanchnicus block	2 C +	To be considered
Spinal cord stimulation	2 C +	To be considered in specialized centers

Future guidelines

Thanks to the continual development of more specific diagnostic tools and to the improved understanding of the pathophysiology, and consequently the mechanism of action of the different treatment options; it is believed that treatment selection for chronic pain syndromes will become more mechanism based. Careful attention to this evolution is warranted and, when necessary, an update of the guidelines should be made.

This book on interventional pain management. can be considered an ongoing project. The methodology for literature retrieval and selection of the publications to be withheld, as well as the method for evidence scoring, should evolve with each update.

A treatment can only be recommended when the effect is proven in well-designed trials. Randomized controlled trials provide the highest level of evidence. With interventional pain management techniques, however, blinding patients and investigators can be problematic. The most important obstacle encountered during the conduct of a double-blind randomized sham-controlled trial is the patient inclusion. When explaining that there is a chance for a sham or placebo treatment, patients frequently refuse to give informed consent, and even when they are included in the study, they may withdraw, opting to go *medical shopping*. Therefore, the methodology for randomized clinical trials on interventional pain management techniques should be revisited.

The *prerandomization* design may form a solution for the inclusion problem, because patients are randomized to the interventional group or to the conservative treatment group prior to requesting consent. Patients in the control group are asked to fill out questionnaires relative to their health at regular time points, because it is the objective to carefully evaluate the treatment effect.[1]

The editors want to express their special gratitude to all the co-authors of the different articles and especially Arno Lataster for reviewing each paper as to the correct use of the anatomical terminology, Rogier Trompert for the anatomical illustrations and Nicole Van den Hecke for coordination of the entire project.

The entire project was supported by the World Institute of Pain (WIP), and the Dutch and Flemish association of pain anesthesiologists (NVA and VAVP).

Supporting information

Please note: Wiley–Blackwell are not responsible for the content or functionality of any supporting information supplied by the authors. Any queries (other than missing material) should be directed to the corresponding author for the article.

References

1. Van Zundert J, Van Boxem K, Joosten EA, Kessels A. Clinical trials in interventional pain management: optimizing chances for success? *Pain.* 2010;151:571–574.
2. Boswell MV, Trescot AM, Datta S, et al. Interventional techniques: evidence-based practice guidelines in the management of chronic spinal pain. *Pain Physician.* 2007;10:7–111.
3. Practice guidelines for chronic pain management: an updated report by the American Society of Anesthesiologists Task Force on Chronic Pain Management and the American Society of Regional Anesthesia and Pain Medicine. *Anesthesiology.* 2010;112: 810–833.
4. Karppinen J, Ohinmaa A, Malmivaara A, et al. Cost effectiveness of periradicular infiltration for sciatica: subgroup analysis of a randomized controlled trial. *Spine.* 2001;26:2587–2595.
5. Karppinen J, Malmivaara A, Kurunlahti M, et al. Periradicular infiltration for sciatica: a randomized controlled trial. *Spine.* 2001;26: 1059–1067.
6. Lord SM, Barnsley L, Wallis BJ. Percutaneous radiofrequency neurotomy in the treatment of cervical zygapophyseal joint pain. *N Engl J Med.* 1996;335:1721–1726.
7. van Kleef M, Barendse GA, Kessels F, Voets HM, Weber WE, de Lange S. Randomized trial of radiofrequency lumbar facet denervation for chronic low back pain. *Spine.* 1999;24:1937–1942.
8. *Federative Committee on Anatomical Terminology. Terminologia Anatomica.* Stutgart: Georg Thieme Verlag; 1998.
9. Rathmell JP, Lake T, Ramundo MB. Infectious risks of chronic pain treatments: injection therapy, surgical implants, and intradiscal techniques. *Reg Anesth Pain Med.* 2006;31:346–352.
10. Deer T, Sitzman T. Complications and risk management for interventional spinal therapies. *Pain Med.* 2008;9:S1–S141.
11. Guyatt G, Gutterman D, Baumann MH, et al. Grading strength of recommendations and quality of evidence in clinical guidelines: report from an american college of chest physicians task force. *Chest.* 2006;129:174–181.
12. van Kleef M, Mekhail N, van Zundert J. Evidencebased guidelines for interventional pain medicine according to clinical diagnoses. *Pain Pract.* 2009;9:247–251.

Search strategy and evidence rating

For the non-interventional treatments, reviews of the most recent information was retrieved. For the interventional treatment options, it was the objective to have the most accurate information.

We searched PubMed with the following search strategy:

("Indication/epidemiology"[Mesh] OR "Indication/etiology"[Mesh] OR "Indication/pathology"[Mesh] OR "Indication/physio pathology"[Mesh] OR "Indication/therapy"[Mesh])

The search for the first chapter of this book was finished in November 2008 and for the last article in October 2010.

A research associate selected all the abstracts that reported on: injection therapy, epidural steroid injection, radiofrequency, pulsed radiofrequency, neurostimulation/neuromodulation and other interventional pain therapy.

The full publications of the selected abstracts were retrieved and the reference list of those articles and important review articles were hand-searched for additional information.

The authors were experts in the field of the specific indication and well-aware of the most up-to-date information, including abstracts and posters presented at congresses, which were excluded from the evaluation.

Two independent reviewers (MvK and JVZ) assessed the studies and proposed an evidence rating based on the rating described in above (Table 1).

Afterwards two other editors, one anesthesiologist and one neurologist, validated or adapted the proposed rating (FH, JP).

All articles were submitted for review and comments to the entire Dutch speaking anesthesiologists pain physicians community (Netherlands and Flemish part of Belgium). After one month all questions and remarks were discussed at the annual national meeting and a broad consensus was reached. In the second stage at least two key opinion leaders of the US have reviewed, updated and finally validated the content and the evidence rating for each article.

The last phase consisted of submission for publication in the peer reviewed journal *Pain Practice*.

1 Trigeminal Neuralgia

Maarten van Kleef, Wilco E. van Genderen, Samer Narouze, Turo J. Nurmikko, Jan Van Zundert, José W. Geurts and Nagy Mekhail

Introduction

"Trigeminal Neuralgia is the worst pain in the world," declared Peter J. Jannetta, MD in "*Striking Back!*", a layman's guide for facial pain patients.[1] Trigeminal neuralgia, or "Tic Douloureux", is a painful condition of the face. This pain has been known since ancient times; there are descriptions of facial pain by Ibn Sina (980–1073) in an Arabic text. An example of early interventional treatment is that by Locke in 1677, who applied sulphuric acid to the face of the Duchess of Northumberland in an attempt to treat her trigeminal neuralgia.

A survey conducted in 6 European countries indicated that trigeminal neuralgia significantly impacted the quality of life and the socioeconomic functioning of affected patients.[2] Trigeminal neuralgia is the most common form of facial pain in people older than 50 years of age. Various epidemiological studies have shown the annual incidence to be about 4–5 new patients per 100,000. The highest incidence occurs in the ages between 50 and 70 years; in 90% of the cases the symptoms begin after the age of 40 years. Trigeminal neuralgia is more prevalent in women than men with a ratio of 1.5:1.[3]

The pathophysiology is unclear. Based on clinical observations, compression of the nervus trigeminus near the origin of the brain stem, the so-called root entry zone, by blood vessels or tumor, may cause trigeminal neuralgia. Local pressure causes demyelination that leads to abnormal depolarization resulting in ectopic impulses.

Symptoms

Trigeminal neuralgia is recognized by unilateral short-lived, strong, sharp, shooting pains in 1 or more branches of the fifth cranial nerve. The description of the pain is very important; it must be sharp, shooting, lancinating, and "electric shock". The pain can be brought on by ordinary stimuli, such as eating, washing, shaving, cold, warmth, and draught. The distribution of the pain in the various branches of the nervus trigeminus is given in Table 1.1.

In the case history, 6 questions should be asked:

1 Does the pain occur in attacks?
2 Are most of the attacks of short duration (seconds to minutes)?
3 Do you sometimes have extremely short attacks?
4 Are the attacks unilateral?
5 Do the attacks occur in the region of the nervus trigeminus?
6 Are there unilateral autonomic symptoms?

In this way, a differential diagnosis can be made relatively quickly and an impression can be formed of whether it is essential trigeminal neuralgia.

Physical examination

Neurological examination seldom reveals any abnormalities in patients with idiopathic trigeminal neuralgia, but all cranial nerves do need to be tested. Patients who have neurological disorders often have a so-called secondary trigeminal neuralgia whereby the trigeminal neuralgia is a symptom of another disease, e.g., tumor of the angulus pontocerebellaris or multiple sclerosis.

Additional test

When the diagnosis of trigeminal neuralgia is made, the patient needs to undergo an magnetic resonance imaging (MRI) scan to exclude specific pathologies such as a tumor or multiple sclerosis, which could cause a secondary trigeminal neuralgia. The

Evidence-Based Interventional Pain Medicine: According to Clinical Diagnoses, First Edition. Edited by Jan Van Zundert, Jacob Patijn, Craig T. Hartrick, Arno Lataster, Frank J.P.M Huygen, Nagy Mekhail, Maarten van Kleef.

Table 1.1. Pain distribution in the various nerve branches in trigeminal neuralgia.

V1 only	4%
V2 only	17%
V3 only	15%
V2 + V3	32%
V1 + V2	14%
V1 + V2 + V3	17%

See Rozen.[3]

MRI scan can also be used if there is a suspected compression of the nervus trigeminus in the fossa cranialis posterior. Sometimes the MRI scan is sensitive enough to detect blood vessels that have come in contact with the nervus trigeminus. The role of venous compression in the pathogenesis of trigeminal neuralgia is controversial.[4,5] Notably, on MRI scanning, compressing blood vessels are seen in one-third of asymptomatic patients. A recent evidence-based review concluded that there is insufficient evidence to support or deny the usefulness of MRI to identify neurovascular compression.[6]

Table 1.2. Trigeminal neuralgia: clinical diagnostic criteria.

Characteristic	Description
Character	Shooting, like an electric shock, stabbing, superficial
Seriousness	Moderate to very intense
Duration	Each pain attack lasts seconds but a number of different attacks can occur simultaneously after which there is a pain free interval
Periodicity	Periods of weeks to months without pain
Location	Distribution of T. neuralgia, mainly unilateral
Emanation	Within the area of the trigeminal nerve
Trigger factors	Light touching, such as when eating, talking or washing
Alleviating factors	Frequent sleep, anti-epileptics
Accompanying characteristics	Trigger zones, weight loss, poor quality of life, depression

Differential diagnosis

Less frequently trigeminal neuralgia is seen in younger patients. It is important that multiple sclerosis always be considered in the differential diagnosis, especially in bilateral cases. The International Headache Society described the following criteria for essential trigeminal neuralgia.[7]

A Paroxysmal pain that lasts from a fraction of a second to 2 minutes, occurring in 1 or more branches of the nervus trigeminus, and fulfilling criteria B and C.
B The pain has at least one of the following characteristics:
  1 intense, sharp, superficial or stabbing.
  2 precipitated from trigger areas or by trigger factors.
C The attacks are stereotypically described by the patient.
D There are no signs of neurological disorders.
E The attacks are not caused by other disorders.

The International Headache Society have suggested their own diagnostic criteria for trigeminal neuralgia (Table 1.2).[8] The differential diagnosis of essential trigeminal neuralgia is extensive and involves all unilateral pain in the pathway of the nervus trigeminus. The most important differential diagnostic considerations are specific facial pain, nonspecific facial pain, temporomandibular arthrosis, dental disorders, and vascular migraine. A detailed overview of the differential diagnosis of facial pain can be found in Table 1.3.[9]

Treatment options

Conservative treatments

The selection of the pharmacological treatment is based on a systematic review of data of relatively older studies[10] or on a more up-to-date Cochrane database.[11] The medication of choice is carbamazepine. From an observational study, it appears that carbamazepine can reduce the pain symptoms in about 70% of the cases. Oxcarbazepine has shown similar efficacy.[6] Other medications that can be tried, although there is no clinical evidence for their efficacy, are gabapentin, pregabalin, and baclofen. Rozen summarized the recommendations for the medical treatment of trigeminal neuralgia in Table 1.4.[3]

Interventional treatments

If the medical treatment is unsuccessful or has too many side effects, an invasive treatment can be carried out. In this case, there are currently 5 clinically appropriate possibilities:

1 Surgical microvascular decompression (MVD).[12]
2 Stereotactic radiation therapy, Gamma knife.[13]
3 Percutaneous balloon microcompression.[14]
4 Percutaneous glycerol rhizolysis.[15]
5 Percutaneous radiofrequency (RF) treatment of the Gasserian ganglion.[16]
6 Gasserian ganglion stimulation/neuromodulation (*experimental*).[17]

Surgical MVD

During MVD, the vessels that are in contact with the root entry zone are coagulated and arteries are separated from the nerve using an inert sponge or felt.[18]

Stereotactic radiation therapy, Gamma knife

The Gamma knife, a stereotactic radio therapeutic method, entails high dose irradiation of a small section of the nervus trigeminus. This results in nonselective damage to Gasserian ganglion. The advantage is that this is a noninvasive treatment that

Table 1.3. Differential diagnosis of trigeminal neuralgia.

Indicate answer with a ✓ for the following afflictions	Does the pain occur in attacks?	Are most of the attacks of a short duration (seconds to minutes)?	Do you sometimes have ultra short attacks?	Are the attacks unilateral?	Do the attacks occur in the region of the nervus trigeminus?	Are there unilateral autonomous symptoms?
	No	No	No	No	No	Yes
• Musculoskeletal	✓	✓	✓	✓	✓	✓
• Dentoalveolar	✓	✓	✓	✓	✓	✓
• Ear, Nose and Throat	✓	✓	✓	✓	✓	✓
• Giant cell arthritis	✓	✓	✓	✓	✓	✓
• Glaucoma		✓	✓	✓	✓	✓
• Cluster headaches		✓	✓	✓	✓	✓
• Atypical migraine		✓	✓	✓	✓	✓
• Chronic paroxysmal hemicrania		✓	✓	✓	✓	✓
• Temporomandibular joint syndrome			✓	✓	✓	✓
• Cracked tooth syndrome			✓	✓	✓	✓
• Idiopathic stabbing headache				✓	✓	✓
• Glossopharyngeal neuralgia					✓	✓
• Nervus Intermedius neuralgia					✓	✓
• SUNCT						✓
• Trigeminal neuropathy						
• Atypical trigeminal neuralgia						
• Typical trigeminal neuralgia						

See Nurmikko.[32]

Table 1.4. Medical treatments for trigeminal neuralgia.

Medication	Dosage	Time to pain relief
Carbamazepine	400–800 mg/day	24–48 h
Phenytoin	300–500 mg/day	24–48 h
Baclofen	40–80 mg/day	?
Clonazepam	1,5–8 mg/day	?
Valproate	500–1500 mg/day	Weeks
Lamotrigine	150–400 mg	24 h
Pimozide	4–12 mg	?
Gabapentin	900–2400 mg/day	1 week
Oxcarbazepine	900–1800 mg/day	24–72 h

See Rozen.[3]

can be applied under local anesthetic and light sedation. At the moment, while there are an increasing number of efficacy studies being carried out on this treatment, the initial efficacy appears to be limited; between 60% and 70% indicate a reduction in pain. The long-term effects are not yet known.[13]

Percutaneous balloon microcompression

In microcompression of Gasserian ganglion, the nervus trigeminus is compressed by a small balloon, which is percutaneously introduced into Meckel's cavity using a needle. The effect of this technique relies on ischemic damage of the ganglion cells. Although there are insufficient good qualitative data, this technique, with regard to efficacy, appears to be comparable with percutaneous RF treatment of Gasserian ganglion. The advantage of this technique is that it is also suitable for treatment of trigeminal neuralgia of the first branch, allowing the corneal reflex to remain intact.[14,19]

Percutaneous glycerol rhizolysis

During percutaneous glycerol rhizolysis, a needle is introduced into the cisterna trigemini, visualized using fluoroscopy. In a seated patient, with the head flexed, a contrast dye can be injected to determine the size of the cisterna. Then, after the contrast dye is aspirated, an equal volume of glycerol is injected.[15]

Percutaneous RF treatment of the Gasserian ganglion

RF treatment of Gasserian ganglion should be considered in the elderly patient.[14] The outcome of treatment of Gasserian ganglion is reportedly less favorable than with open operation (MVD) but it is less invasive and has lower morbidity and mortality rates.[20]

Gasserian ganglion stimulation/neuromodulation (experimental)

Gasserian ganglion electric stimulation was first described by Shelden et al. in 3 patients with trigeminal neuralgia.[17] Meyerson and Hakansson reported Gasserian ganglion stimulation via a subtemporal craniotomy in 5 patients suffering atypical trigeminal neuralgia.[21] Later, a percutaneous approach was described by Meglio, however, lead migration presented a technical challenge.[22] More recently, Machado et al. reported percutaneous Gasserian ganglion stimulation in 8 patients with trigeminal neuropathic pain. Only 3 patients continued to have >50% pain improvement after 1 year of treatment.[23] They concluded that lead mobility due to difficulty anchoring the lead remains a significant barrier to achievement of optimal results and called for innovative lead designs.

For patients with trigeminal neuralgia refractory to medical therapy Gasserian ganglion percutaneous technique, Gamma knife, and MVD may be considered, although strong evidence on the efficacy of these interventions is lacking.[6] More research is needed to establish the value of these interventions.

Generally, it is accepted that the first choice of treatment in younger patients would be MVD. There are several systematic reviews available that compare the most appropriate techniques in the treatment of trigeminal neuralgia.[20,24–27] Given the most recent studies, MVD treatment remains the best therapeutic option with regard to improvement in the quality of life of the trigeminal neuralgia patient, and also when considering the long-term pain relief experienced after operation. The other 3 minimally invasive therapies score less well because they have more risk of pain relapse after treatment. However, the differences are very small. Medication therapy scores the least well in the reviews. This is mainly because the pain relief frequently comes at the cost of severe side effects associated with chronic medication use.

For the elderly patient, treatment using RF treatment of Gasserian ganglion is often preferred over MVD. This is due to the increased morbidity and mortality that are associated with the MVD operation. However, one publication stated that in otherwise healthy people over the age of 70, MVD poses no appreciable increase in risk.[28] MVD is more effective than the Gamma knife treatment. About 60% of the treated patients are painfree for at least 60 months, if the treatment is correctly given. Zakrzewska has indicated that in about 50% of patients, there is sensory loss in the treated branches of the nervus trigeminus.[29] As such, this technique should not be used in secondary trigeminal neuralgia, as seen in postherpetic neuralgia. The only current exception is secondary trigeminal neuralgia due to multiple sclerosis. While pulsed RF treatment would seem to be a reasonable alternative to RF, in the only randomized controlled trial comparing these techniques in the treatment of trigeminal neuralgia, PRF failed to demonstrate efficacy.[30]

Complications

The percutaneous RF procedure has a very low morbidity and virtually no mortality. The most prevalent complications are sensory loss in the treated branch or paralysis of the musculus masseter. In the long term, anesthesia dolorosa, corneal hypoesthesia and keratitis, and temporary paralysis of the third and fourth cranial nerves can occur. A more frequent and less serious complication is hematoma of the cheek, which generally disappears after a few days.

Kanpolat et al. reported the results of 25 years experience with 1,600 patients.[31] The above-mentioned complications are: decreased corneal reflex (5.7%), weakness and paralysis of the musculus masseter (4.1%), dysesthesia (1%), anesthesia dolorosa (0.8%), keratitis (0.6%), and temporary paralysis of the third and fourth cranial nerves (0.8%).

Table 1.5. Summary of evidence for interventional management of trigeminal neuralgia.

Technique	Assessment
Radiofrequency treatment of Gasserian ganglion	2 B+
Pulsed radiofrequency treatment of Gasserian ganglion	2 B–

See van Kleef et al.[33]

Evidence for interventional pain treatment

The evidence for interventional pain treatment is summarized in Table 1.5.

Recommendations

The treatment of a patient with essential trigeminal neuralgia should be multidisciplinary and the various treatment options (MVD, Gamma knife, and RF treatment of Gasserian ganglion) and their risks should be discussed with the patient. These related therapies have never been compared with one another in prospective randomized studies. Recommendations are, therefore, relative. With regard to the elderly patient with comorbidities, RF treatment of Gasserian ganglion can be recommended. In younger patients, an MVD according to Jannetta could be considered.[18]

Clinical practice algorithm

An algorithm for clinical assessment and treatment is illustrated in Figure 1.1.

The technique of RF treatment of Gasserian ganglion

The Gasserian ganglion is named after Johann Lorenz Gasser, a Viennese anatomist. The ganglion lies in Meckel's cavity of the cranium close to the os petrosum, a part of the os temporale. The Gasserian ganglion is surrounded medially by the sinus cavernosus, superiorly by the underside of the lobus temporalis and posteriorly by the brainstem. From top to bottom the ganglion has 3 branches: the first branch is the nervus ophtalmicus, the second branch is the nervus maxillaris, and the third branch is the nervus mandibularis. The Gasserian ganglion has a somatotopic arrangement, in that the nervus ophtalmicus is the most craniomedial and the nervus mandibularis lies the most lateral.

The procedure is performed using fluoroscopy whereby the patient lies supine on the table and the C-arm is rotated to obtain a submental view, then slowly tilted obliquely toward the affected side until the foramen ovale is well visualized medially with respect to the processus mandibularis, and lateral to the maxilla. The C-arm position is then adjusted such that the foramen is seen as

Clinical Practice Algorithm

Intense paroxysmal unilateral facial pain

↓

MRI scan

↓

Differential diagnosis by means of 6 questions

↓

Medication treatment gives insufficient pain relief and/or side effects are intolerable

↓

Young patient → Microvascular decompression

Elderly patient → Radiofrequency treatment of Gasserian ganglion

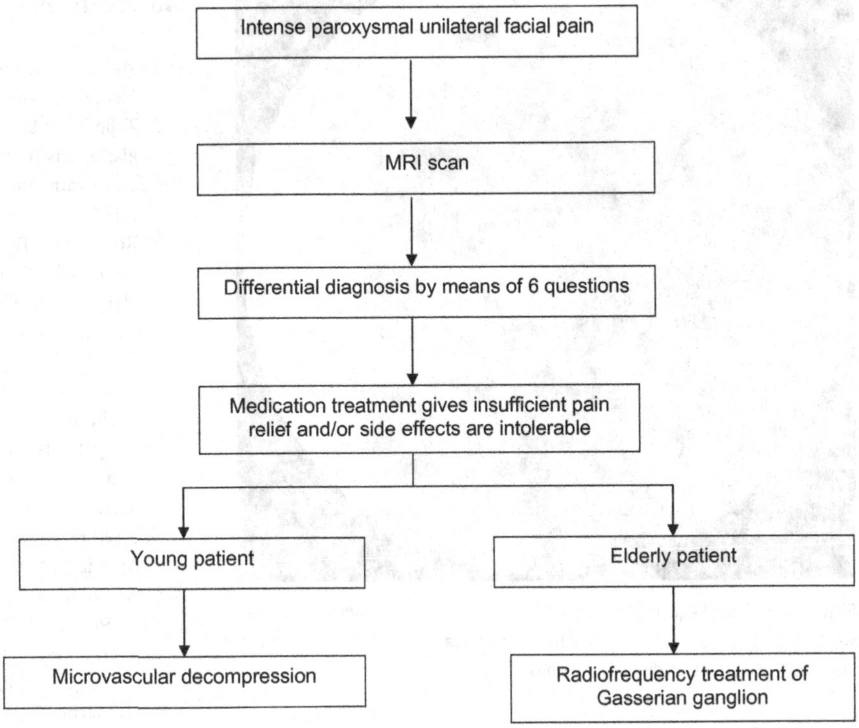

Figure 1.1. Clinical practice algorithm for the treatment of trigeminal neuralgia.

an oval. If one wishes to treat the maxillary branch and the mandibular branch, the entry point of the needle is 2 cm lateral to the corner of the mouth on the ipsilateral side of the lesion. The needle is aimed at the middle of the foramen. If one only wants to treat the mandibular branch, the entry point of the needle is 1 cm lateral to the corner of the mouth and one aims the needle at the lateral part of the foramen ovale. If one only wants to treat the ophthalmic branch, the entry point of the needle lies 3 cm lateral to the corner of the mouth and one aims the needle at the medial part of the foramen ovale.

For this treatment, we use an Sluijter-Mehta-Kanula cannula, 10 cm 22 G with a 2 mm active tip. Once the anatomical landmarks have been identified, an intravenous sedative dose of propofol or similar agent is given. The Sluijter-Mehta-Kanula needle is then advanced toward the foramen ovale (tunnel-view) (see Figures 1.2 and 1.3). It is important to place a finger in the mouth to be certain that there is no penetration of the oral mucosa. Once the needle is through the foramen ovale into Meckel's cavity, stimulation can take place. The stimulation parameters are as follows: first the motor functions are tested, whereby there should be little or no contraction of the musculus masseter, preferably above a threshold of 0.6 V. With motor stimulation, the needle needs to be advanced carefully approximately 2 mm. Then the patient is allowed to awaken, by discontinuing the propofol sedation, and sensory stimulation can be carried out at 50 Hz. Paresthesia should be felt between 0.05 and 0.2 V in the area corresponding to

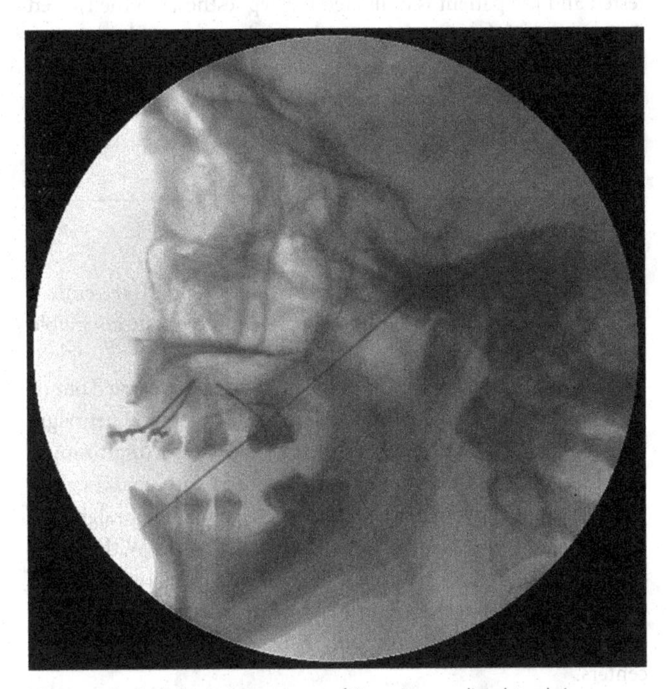

Figure 1.2. Radiofrequency treatment of Gasserian ganglion: lateral view. Needle is positioned through the base (foramen ovale) of the skull. Note the sella turcica and clivus.

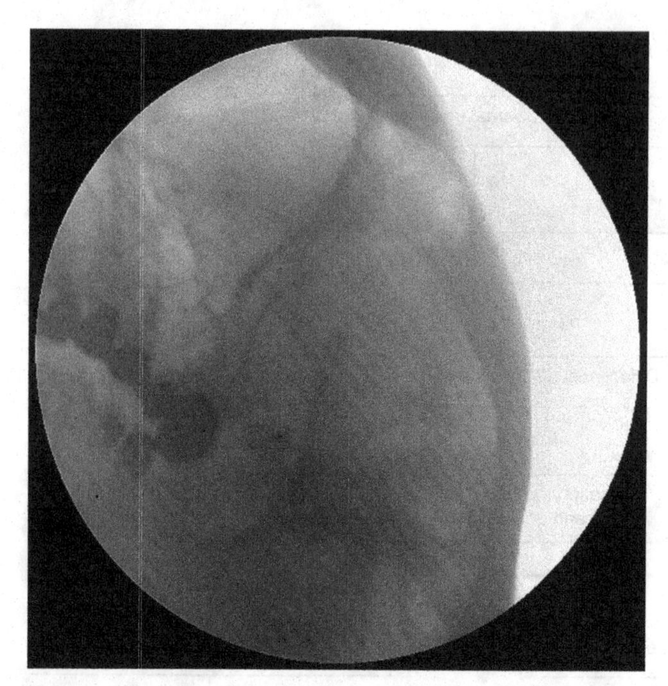

Figure 1.3. Radiofrequency treatment of Gasserian ganglion: oblique submental view. Electrode aimed at the middle of the foramen ovale. On the lateral side the mandibula and on the medial side the sinus maxillaris.

the patient's pain. After appropriate paresthesia, a 60°C RF treatment can be done for 60 seconds. After this, the corneal reflex is tested and the patient is evaluated for hypoesthesia in the treated dermatome. If there is no hypoesthesia, then a second treatment is done at 65°C for 60 seconds, and if there is still no hypoesthesia then a third RF treatment can be done at 70°C for another 60 seconds.

Summary

As suggested by T. Nurmikko, classical (essential) trigeminal neuralgia can be diagnosed by asking 6 simple questions (Table 1.3).[9,32]

It is important that an MRI of the brain has been carried out in each patient, in order to exclude a secondary trigeminal neuralgia that requires a more causal treatment, before resorting to invasive therapy. The first treatment of choice is carbamazepine or oxcarbazepine. In younger patients with trigeminal neuralgia, the first choice of invasive treatment is probably MVD. With regard to elderly patients, RF treatment of Gasserian ganglion is recommended even though there is a lack of prospective comparative data. This treatment should only be carried out in specialized centers.

There is not enough data at this time to support the widespread use of trigeminal neuromodulation and these modalities of treatment should only be reserved for selected patients with intractable trigeminal neuropathic pain who failed to improve with other more conservative options.

References

1. Weigel G, Kenneth F, Casey M. *Striking Back!* Gainsville: Trigeminal Neuralgia Association; 2000.
2. Tolle T, Dukes E, Sadosky A. Patient burden of trigeminal neuralgia: results from a cross-sectional survey of health state impairment and treatment patterns in six European countries. *Pain Pract.* 2006; 6:153–160.
3. Rozen TD. Trigeminal neuralgia and glossopharyngeal neuralgia. *Neurol Clin.* 2004;22:185–206.
4. Hamlyn PJ, King TT. Neurovascular compression in trigeminal neuralgia: a clinical and anatomical study. *J Neurosurg.* 1992;76: 948–954.
5. Klun B. Microvascular decompression and partial sensory rhizotomy in the treatment of trigeminal neuralgia: personal experience with 220 patients. *Neurosurgery.* 1992;30:49–52.
6. Gronseth G, Cruccu G, Alksne J, et al. Practice parameter: the diagnostic evaluation and treatment of trigeminal neuralgia (an evidence-based review): report of the Quality Standards Subcommittee of the American Academy of Neurology and the European Federation of Neurological Societies. *Neurology.* 2008;71:1183–1190.
7. International Headache Society Classification Subcommittee. The international classification of headache disorders: 2nd edition. *Cephalgia.* 2004;24:9–160.
8. Headache Classification Committee of the International Headache Society. Classification and diagnostic criteria for headache disorders, cranial neuralgias and facial pain. *Cephalalgia.* 1988; 8(supple 7):1–96.
9. Nurmikko T. Trigeminal neuralgia. *Int J Pain Med Pall Care.* 2003; 3:2–11.
10. McQuay H, Carroll D, Jadad AR, Wiffen P, Moore A. Anticonvulsant drugs for management of pain: a systematic review. *BMJ.* 1995;311:1047–1052.
11. Wiffen P, Collins S, McQuay H, Carroll D, Jadad A, Moore A. Anticonvulsant drugs for acute and chronic pain. *Cochrane Database Syst Rev.* 2000;CD001133.
12. Janetta P. Trigeminal neuralgia: treatment by microvascular decompression. In: Wilkins R, Regachary S, eds. *Neurosurgery.* New York: McGrawy-Hill; 1996:3961–3968.
13. Young RF, Vermulen S, Posewitz A. Gamma knife radiosurgery for the treatment of trigeminal neuralgia. *Stereotact Funct Neurosurg.* 1998;70(suppl 1):192–199.
14. Mullan S, Lichtor T. Percutaneous microcompression of the trigeminal ganglion for trigeminal neuralgia. *J Neurosurg.* 1983;59: 1007–1012.
15. Hakanson S. Trigeminal neuralgia treated by the injection of glycerol into the trigeminal cistern. *Neurosurgery.* 1981;9:638–646.
16. Sweet WH, Wepsic JG. Controlled thermocoagulation of trigeminal ganglion and root for differential destruction of pain fibers. Part I: trigeminal neuralgia. *J Neurosurg.* 1974;39:143–156.
17. Shelden CH, Pudenz RH, Doyle J. Electrical control of facial pain. *Am J Surg.* 1967;114:209–212.
18. Jannetta PJ, McLaughlin MR, Casey KF. Technique of microvascular decompression. Technical note. *Neurosurg Focus.* 2005;18:E5.
19. Belber CJ, Rak RA. Balloon compression rhizolysis in the surgical management of trigeminal neuralgia. *Neurosurgery.* 1987;20: 908–913.

20. Lopez BC, Hamlyn PJ, Zakrzewska JM. Systematic review of ablative neurosurgical techniques for the treatment of trigeminal neuralgia. *Neurosurgery*. 2004;54:973–982; discussion 982–973.
21. Meyerson BA, Hakansson S. Alleviation of atypical trigeminal pain by stimulation of the gasserian ganglion via an implanted electrode. *Acta Neurochir Suppl (Wien)*. 1980;30:303–309.
22. Meglio M. Percutaneous implantable chronic electrode for radiofrequency stimulation of the gasserian ganglion: a perspective in the management of trigeminal pain. *Acta Neurochir (Wien)*. 1984;33: 521–525.
23. Machado A, Ogrin M, Rosenow JM, Henderson JM. A 12-month prospective study of gasserian ganglion stimulation for trigeminal neuropathic pain. *Stereotact Funct Neurosurg*. 2007;85:216–224.
24. Lopez BC, Hamlyn PJ, Zakrzewska JM. Stereotactic radiosurgery for primary trigeminal neuralgia: state of the evidence and recommendations for future reports. *J Neurol Neurosurg Psychiatry*. 2004;75:1019–1024.
25. Zakrzewska JM, Thomas DG. Patient's assessment of outcome after three surgical procedures for the management of trigeminal neuralgia. *Acta Neurochir (Wien)*. 1993; 122:225–230.
26. Spatz AL, Zakrzewska JM, Kay EJ. Decision analysis of medical and surgical treatments for trigeminal neuralgia: how patient evaluations of benefits and risks affect the utility of treatment decisions. *Pain*. 2007;131:302–310.
27. Tatli M, Satici O, Kanpolat Y, Sindou M. Various surgical modalities for trigeminal neuralgia: literature study of respective long-term outcomes. *Acta Neurochir (Wien)*. 2008;150:243–255.
28. Javadpour M, Eldridge PR, Varma TR, Miles JB, Nurmikko TJ. Microvascular decompression for trigeminal neuralgia in patients over 70 years of age. *Neurology*. 2003;60:520.
29. Zakrzewska JM, Jassim S, Bulman JS. A prospective, longitudinal study on patients with trigeminal neuralgia who underwent radiofrequency thermocoagulation of the gasserian ganglion. *Pain*. 1999;79:51–58.
30. Erdine S, Ozyalcin NS, Cimen A, Celik M, Talu GK, Disci R. Comparison of pulsed radiofrequency with conventional radiofrequency in the treatment of idiopathic trigeminal neuralgia. *Eur J Pain*. 2007;11:309–313.
31. Kanpolat Y, Savas A, Bekar A, Berk C. Percutaneous controlled radiofrequency trigeminal rhizotomy for the treatment of idiopathic trigeminal neuralgia: 25-year experience with 1,600 patients. *Neurosurgery*. 2001;48:524–532; discussion 532–524.
32. Nurmikko T. Trigeminal neuralgia and other facial neuralgias. In: Cervero F, Jensen TS, eds. *Handbook of Clinical Neurology*, Vol. 81 (3rd Series. Vol. 3), *Pain*. New York: Elsevier; 2006:573–596.
33. van Kleef M, Mekhail N, Van Zundert J. Editorial; Evidence based guidelines for interventional pain medicine according to clinical diagnoses. *Pain Pract*. 2009;9:247–251.

2 Cluster Headache

Maarten van Kleef, Arno Lataster, Samer Narouze, Nagy Mekhail, José W. Geurts and Jan Van Zundert

Introduction

Cluster headache is a primary neurovascular headache. It is a strictly unilateral headache that is associated with ipsilateral cranial autonomic symptoms and usually has circadian and circannual patterns. A cluster headache is characterized by the clustered nature of the attacks. The attacks can be provoked by vasodilators such as alcohol and nitroglycerine. Despite the low prevalence of cluster headaches, it has been shown that this affliction has a large socioeconomic impact. Almost 80% of the patients report restrictions in daily activities, which, in 13%, were even present outside of attack periods.[1] Noticeably, patients with cluster headaches have often endured a long course prior to diagnosis. Sometimes, they have even undergone operations on the sinus maxillaris/septum nasi or had their teeth removed. The prevalence of cluster headaches can be estimated at approximately 0.5 to 1.0/1,000.[2] The first attacks appear between the ages of 20 and 40 years. In contrast with migraine, cluster headaches affect mainly men in a ratio of 5:1.[3] There are indications that the risk for cluster headache is notably higher in patients with a family history of cluster headaches.[4]

Diagnosis

History

The attacks consist of a strictly unilateral, strong, piercing pain around or behind the eye. The pain often occurs simultaneously with ipsilateral signs of autonomic dysregulation, whereby a red watering eye, nasal congestion and/or rhinorrhea, and even miosis and/or ptosis can occur. The autonomic characteristics of cluster headache are given in Table 2.1.[4] Apart from miosis and/or ptosis, which may persist between attacks, autonomic features tend to cease with the pain.[5]

During attacks, there is a high degree of restlessness, and the patient often moves around, unable to remain quiescent . The attacks are often of short (15 minutes) or sometimes long duration (3 hours) and, strangely enough, usually occur at night. The attacks appear to be associated with REM sleep.

In the most typical form, there will be periods of episodic headaches (clusters), lasting from a few weeks to months, whereby the attack frequency can vary from one every 2 days to eight per day. After such a period, a patient may often experience one or more attack-free years before a new attack period occurs. In a small number of patients, the attack pattern changes from episodic to chronic, wherein daily attacks occur for years and years. The chronic form of headache occurs in about 15% of the patients with cluster headache and is therefore relatively rare.

Physical examination

The neurological examination usually does not reveal any peculiarities in these patients.

Additional tests

The diagnosis of cluster headache is made based on the patient's case history. Additional tests, blood tests, or X-rays to exclude other causes of the headache are seldom necessary because cluster headache is distinctive.

Differential diagnosis

The International Headache Society's International Classification of Headache Disorders 2nd Edition (ICHD-II) has stated diagnostic criteria for cluster headache and classified them into two forms: episodic and chronic (Tables 2.2 and 2.3).[6]

Episodic cluster headaches occur in periods lasting from 7 days to 1 year and are separated by at least a 1-month pain-free interval. The attacks in the chronic form occur for more than 1 year without remission periods or with remission periods lasting less than 1 month.

Evidence-Based Interventional Pain Medicine: According to Clinical Diagnoses, First Edition. Edited by Jan Van Zundert, Jacob Patijn, Craig T. Hartrick, Arno Lataster, Frank J.P.M Huygen, Nagy Mekhail, Maarten van Kleef.

Table 2.1. Autonomic characteristics of cluster headache.

Ipsilateral to site of pain
Lacrimation or conjunctival injection
Rhinorrhea or nasal congestion
Cranial and/or facial sweating
Miosis and/or ptosis
Edema of the eyelid or orofacial tissues (including the gingiva and palate)
Facial flushing or pallor
Swelling around the eye and orofacial tissues (including the mouth)
Thermography determined "cold spot" at the site of pain (usually supraorbital)
Systemic
Bradycardia
Vertigo and ataxia
Syncope
Hypertension
Increased gastrointestinal acid production

From Balasubramaniam and Klasser.[4]

Table 2.2. Diagnostic criteria for cluster headache.

A. At least five attacks fulfilling B through D
B. Severe or very severe unilateral orbital, supraorbital and/or temporal pain lasting 15 to 180 minutes if untreated
C. Headache is accompanied by at least one of the following:
1. Ipsilateral conjunctival injection and/or lacrimation
2. Ipsilateral nasal congestion and/or rhinorrhea
3. Ipsilateral eyelid edema
4. Ipsilateral forehead and facial sweating
5. Ipsilateral miosis and/or ptosis
6. A sense of restlessness or agitation
D. Attacks have a frequency from one every other day to eight per day.
E. Not attributed to another disorder

Table 2.3. International classification of headache disorders 2nd edition criteria for episodic and chronic cluster headache.

Episodic cluster headache
A. All fulfilling criteria A through E of Table 2.2
B. At least two cluster periods lasting from 7 to 365 days and separated by pain free remissions of >1 month.
Chronic cluster headache
A. All fulfilling criteria A through E of Table 2.2
B. Attacks recur for >1 year without remission periods or with remission periods lasting <1 month

The clinical picture of cluster headache is very specific. Yet, attention must be paid to the possible underlying head and neck pathology that causes symptomatic cluster headache such as nasopharyngeal carcinoma, sphenoidal meningioma, carotid artery dissection, vertebral artery dissection, pituitary adenoma, or aneurysm.[4] Balasubramaniam and Klasser discuss "red flags," which should be taken into account. These encompass a chronic unremitting headache, a lasting residual headache of a low intensity after cessation of the cluster headache attack, minimal response to standard treatment, the presence of abnormal physical findings such as vital signs, and abnormal cranial nerve examination with the exception of miosis and ptosis.[4]

Treatment options

Conservative management

As with migraine, the therapy for cluster headache consists of symptomatic/abortive treatment to alleviate symptoms and shorten the duration of the attacks, and preventative/prophylactic treatment to prevent the attacks and reduce their number. Ergotamines and sumatriptan injections are effective abortives for cluster headache, as for migraine. It is important to realize that cluster headache attacks are usually episodic, and prophylactic medications like verapamil must be rapidly administered. Those treatments should be stopped once the cluster period is over. Although some prophylactic medications, such as, carbamazepine, and propanolol, have no effect on cluster headache, they are frequently prescribed nonetheless.

Symptomatic/abortive therapy

Abortive therapy of cluster headache that consists of oxygen inhalation, 100% oxygen 7 L/minute via a facial mask, is one of the most effective methods and, by far, the safest. In about 70% of cases, the attack is halted within 15 to 30 minutes. A recent Cochrane review found limited evidence for this therapy.[7]

The effectiveness of subcutaneous sumatriptan on cluster headache has been demonstrated in a doubleblind, placebo-controlled study. In 70% of the patients treated with subcutaneous sumatriptan, 6 mg, the headache disappeared within 15 minutes compared with 26% treated with placebo.[8]

The third abortive therapy is 2 to 4 mg of sublingual ergotamine tartrate. Tablets of ergotamine are not, or insufficiently, effective most likely because of limited absorption. Subcutaneous or intravenous administration is probably more effective. Currently, there are no randomized studies investigating the effects of this medication.

Preventative/prophylactic therapy

Verapamil, 120 to 480 mg per day, is an effective and the safest prophylactic. The efficacy of verapamil is known from clinical practice, but there are few controlled studies. In an open-label study, 69% of patients reported an improvement after the administration of verapamil.[4]

It is claimed that prednisone has a favorable effect on cluster headache. Yet there is actually little evidence to support this. Most of the studies are open label, some studies are retrospective, and, at the moment, few reasons exist to prescribe prednisone for cluster headaches.[4]

In open-label trials, a favorable effect is reported for lithium by 80% of the patients. This effect has been confirmed in a double-blind, placebo-controlled study.[9]

Interventional management

The role of radiofrequency (RF) treatment of the ganglion pterygopalatinum (PPG)

When pharmacological and oxygen therapies are ineffective, an interventional treatment can be carried out (Figure 2.3). This interventional treatment involves blocking the ganglion pterygopalatinum (PPG, previously: sphenopalatinum) and should preferably be carried out at the beginning of a cluster period.

The PPG is located in the fossa pterygopalatina, which is a small "upside-down" pyramidal space, 2 cm high and 1 cm wide. The fossa pterygopalatina is located behind the posterior wall of the sinus maxillaris and is bordered posteriorly by the medial plate of the processus pterygoideus, superiorly by the sinus sphenoidalis, and medially by the perpendicular plate of the os palatinum, and laterally communicates with the fossa infratemporalis.[10,11] Superolaterally lies the foramen rotundum with the exiting nervus maxillaris, and inferomedially there is the vidian nerve (nervus petrosus major and nervus petrosus profundus) within the canalis pterygoideus. The fossa pterygopalatina contains the arteria maxillaris interna and its branches, the nervus maxillaris, and the PPG and its afferent and efferent branches. The PPG is located posterior to the concha nasalis media (middle turbinate) and is few millimeters deep to the lateral nasal mucosa. It is suspended from the nervus maxillaris by the nervi pterygopalatini; inferiorly, it is connected to the nervus palatinus major and minor, and posteriorly, it is connected to the vidian nerve. Efferent branches of the PPG form the three rami nasales posteriores ganglii pterygopalatini (posterior nasal branches of the PPG) and the nervus pharyngeus[11,12] (Figures 2.1 and 2.2).

The rationale for the RF treatment of the PPG in cluster headache is influenced by the parasympathetic symptoms during the attack and perhaps by vasoactive substances such as calcitonin gene-related peptide.[13]

In a retrospective analysis of patients with refractory cluster headache treated by RF treatment of the PPG, 56 patients with episodic and 10 patients with chronic cluster headache were followed up over a period of 12 to 70 months. In the group with episodic cluster headache, 60.7% experienced complete pain relief, while only 3 out of 10 patients with chronic cluster headache had the same result.[11] The above report showed that RF treatment of the PPG may improve episodic cluster headache but not chronic cluster headache. However, recently, Narouze et al. reported favorable outcome after intractable chronic cluster headache as well. In this retrospective study of 15 patients, they reported significant improvement in both mean attack intensity and mean attack frequency for up to 18 months.[14]

After RF treatment of the PPG, postoperative epistaxis, bleeding in the jaw and unintentional partial lesion of the nervus maxillaris were observed. In one report, one out of the 19 patients experienced hypesthesia of the palatum.[15]

Occipital nerve stimulation (ONS)

ONS in patients with refractory cluster headache has been described in few case series.[16–19] One systematic review of ONS for chronic headache (including cluster headache) has been found.[20] This treatment appears to mainly decrease the intensity of the attacks. Noticeably, there is a relatively long (2 months or more)

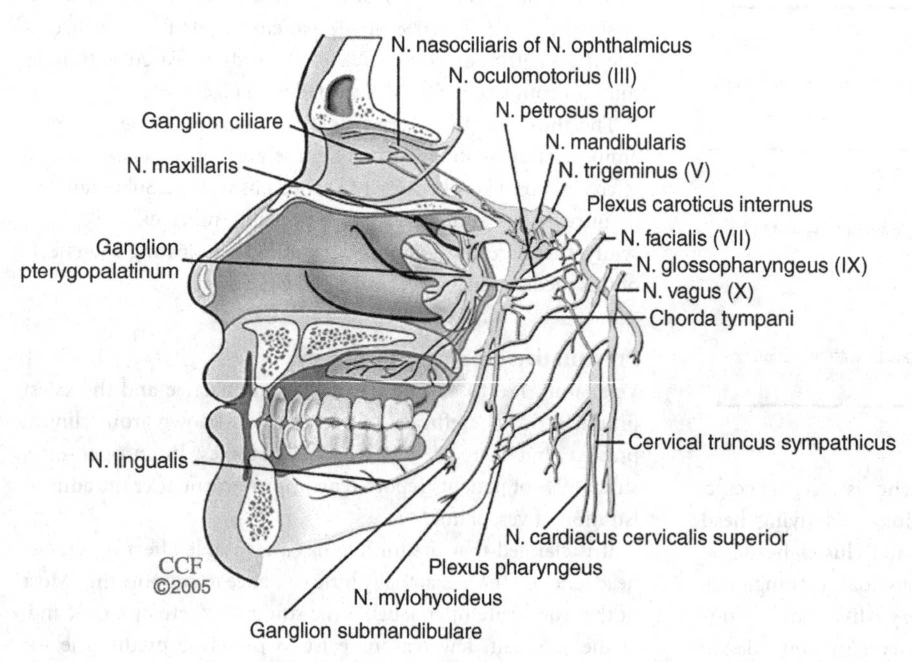

Figure 2.1. Anatomy of the ganglion pterygopalatinum (ganglion sphenopalatinum) within the fossa pterygopalatina.

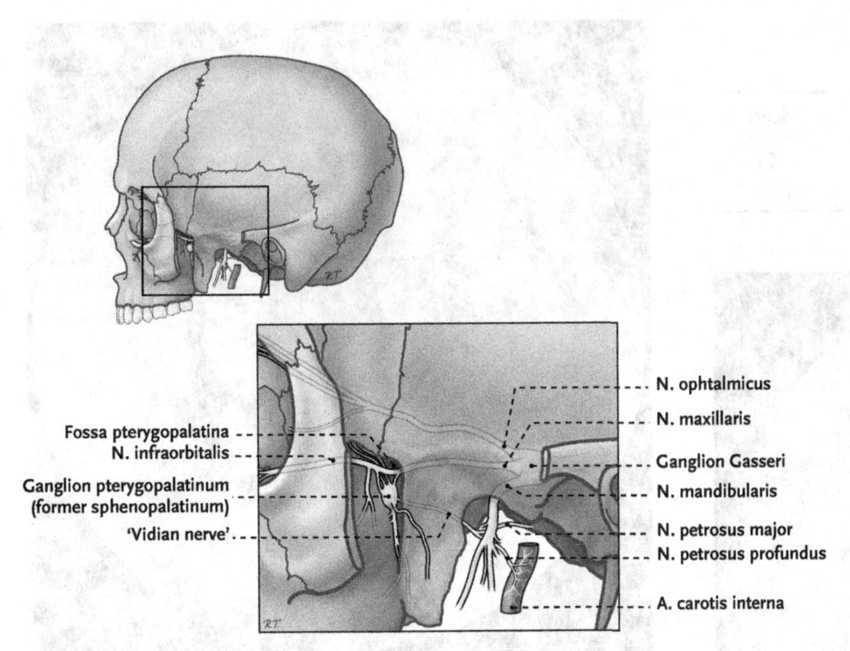

Figure 2.2. Anatomy of the ganglion pterygopalatinum. Illustration: Roger Trompert, Medical Art, www.medical-art.nl.

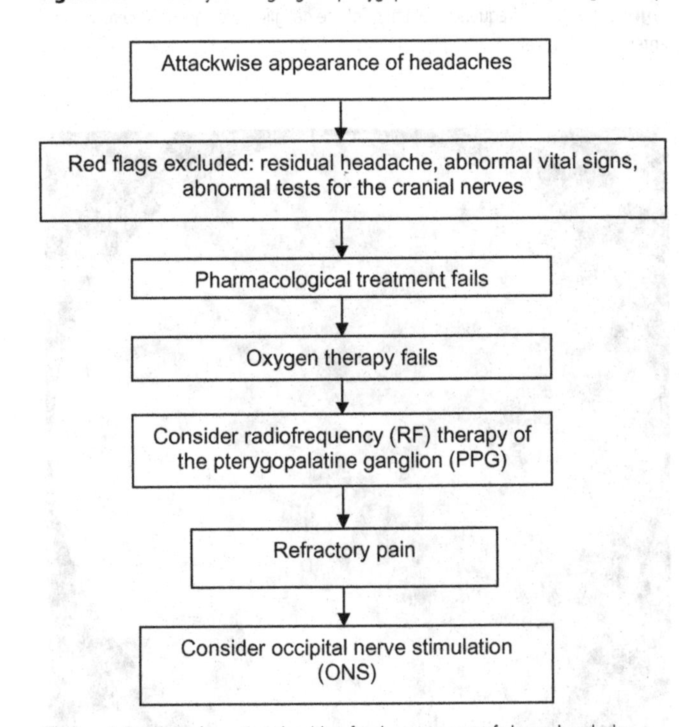

Figure 2.3. Clinical practice algorithm for the treatment of cluster headache.

period of latency between the implantation of the electrode and a clinical effect.

Complications of interventional management

Total destruction of the PPG could result in dryness of the eyes. However, under normal conditions, the RF treatment only aims at a partial lesion of the ganglion. A possible complication is hypesthesia of the palatum molle, which generally disappears after 6 to 8 weeks. Another complication is nosebleeding and swelling of the cheek as the result of a hematoma. A bothersome complication is the accidental lesion of the nervus maxillaris, which can occur when the technique is not properly carried out. A thorough understanding of the anatomy allows the clinician to predict correct needle placement during RF treatment, according to the result of the stimulation, and hence can reduce the incidence of complications (Table 2.4).[21]

Table 2.4. Different possible scenarios of stimulation before applying radiofrequency treatment of the ganglion pterygopalatinum[21].

Location of paresthesia	Nerves stimulated	Location of needle tip	Action needed
Upper teeth and gums	Rami alveolares superiores	Superolateral	Redirect the needle; caudally and medially.
Hard palate	Nervus palatinus major and nervi palatini minores	Anterior, lateral, caudal	Redirect the needle; posteromedially and cephalad.
Root of the nose	PPG efferents, Rami nasales posteriores	Correct needle placement	None

PPG, ganglion pterygopalatinum.

Evidence for interventional management

A summary of the available evidence is given in Table 2.5.

Recommendations

In patients with therapy-resistant cluster headache, study-related RF treatment of the PPG can be considered. With cluster headache, which is refractory to other treatment options, ONS

Table 2.5. Summary of evidence for interventional pain management of cluster headache.

Technique	Score
Radiofrequency treatment of the ganglion pterygopalatinum	2 C+
Occipital nerve stimulation	2 C+

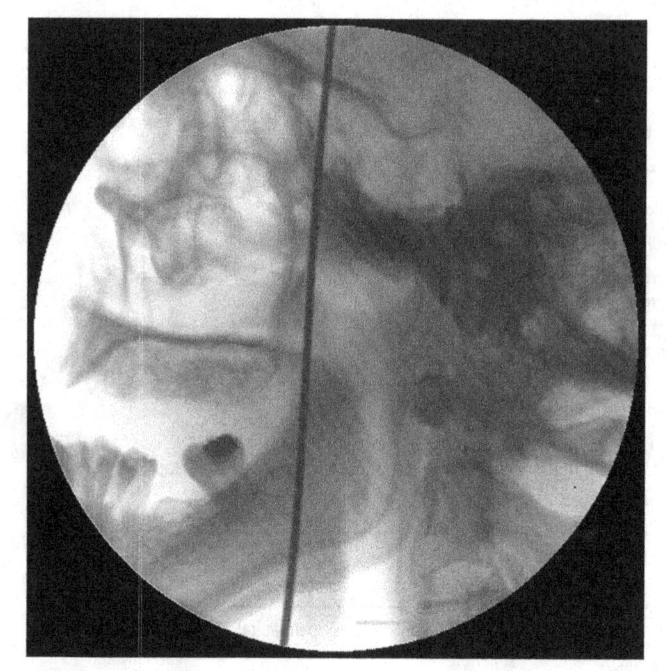

Figure 2.4. Radiofrequency treatment of the ganglion pterygopalatinum: lateral view projection of the metal bar indicates the line over the fossa pterygopalatina.

may be considered, preferably in the context of a study in specialized centers (Table 2.5).

Clinical practice algorithm

Techniques

The practice algorithm for the management of cluster headache is given in figure 2.3.

The RF treatment of the PPG procedure

The patient is positioned lying on the back and the fossa pterygopalatina is identified by using lateral fluoroscopy. A line is drawn on the skin over the fossa and the introduction point is chosen just below the arcus zygomaticus (Figure 2.4). The skin is anesthetized and a 100-mm radiofrequency electrode with a 2-mm active tip is slowly introduced. This needle is carefully inserted in a superior and anterior direction using lateral fluoroscopy toward the anterosuperior point of the fossa pterygopalatina (Figures 2.5 and 2.6). The C-arm is now placed in an anteroposterior position; the tip of the canula should be lying just lateral to the nasal wall. The stylet is removed, and a thermocouple RF-probe is placed. The position of the electrode is confirmed by electrostimulation using 50 Hz. It is important to use a 2-mm active tip, otherwise damage can occur to the nervus maxillaris during the lesion. Generally, the patient feels paresthesia on the lateral side and back of the nose at a threshold of 0.4 V. There should be no paresthesia felt in the soft palate or the upper jaw because this

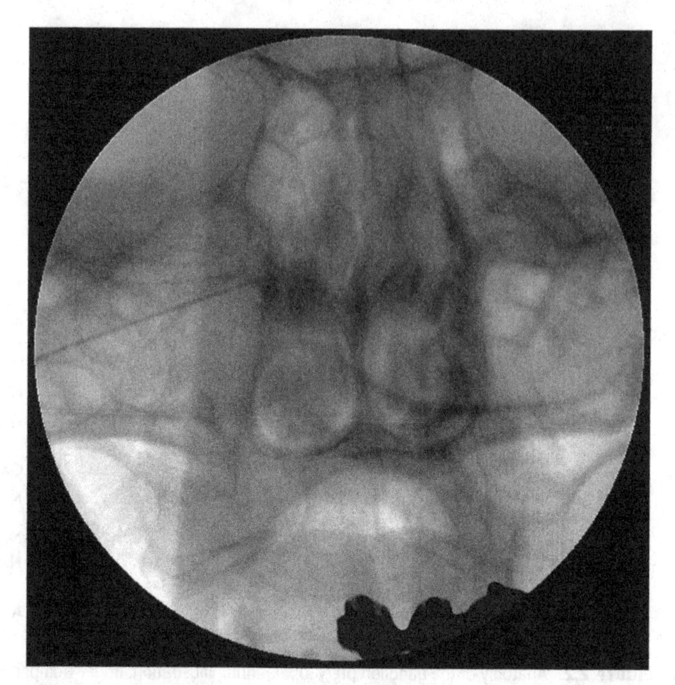

Figure 2.5. Radiofrequency treatment of the ganglion pterygopalatinum: anteroposterior view.

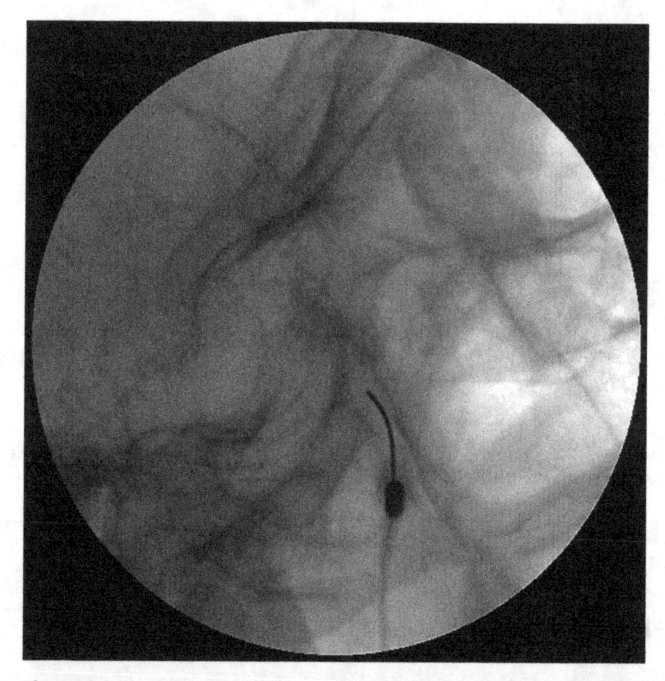

Figure 2.6. Radiofrequency treatment of the ganglion pterygopalatinum: lateral view. Needle high in the fossa pterygopalatina.

indicates the stimulation of the nervus maxillaris or its branches (Table 2.4).

After a limited amount of local anesthesia (maximum of 1 mL), a lesion is carried out for 60 s at 80°C, and this lesion is repeated twice whereby the electrode is inserted further.

Summary

The diagnosis of cluster headache is based on the case history and indications from the physical examination. The primary treatment is medication, but, in patients who are therapy resistant, RF treatment of the PPG can be considered. This treatment should be carried out at the beginning of a cluster period. In patients with cluster headache refractory to all other treatments, ONS may be considered, preferably within a clinical study in specialized centers.

References

1. Jensen RM, Lyngberg A, Jensen RH. Burden of cluster headache. *Cephalalgia*. 2007;27:535–541.
2. Leroux E, Ducros A. Cluster headache. *Orphanet J Rare Dis*. 2008;3:20.
3. Sjaastad O, Bakketeig LS. Cluster headache prevalence. Vaga study of headache epidemiology. *Cephalalgia*. 2003;23:528–533.
4. Balasubramaniam R, Klasser GD. Trigeminal autonomic cephalalgias. Part 1: cluster headache. *Oral Surg Oral Med Oral Pathol Oral Radiol Endod*. 2007;104:345–358.
5. Lance JW, Anthony M. Migrainous neuralgia or cluster headache? *J Neurol Sci*. 1971;13:401–414.
6. Silberstein SD, Olesen J, Bousser MG, et al. The international classification of headache disorders. 2nd ed. (ichd-ii)—revision of criteria for 8.2 medication-overuse headache. [erratum appears in cephalalgia. 2006 mar;26(3):360]. *Cephalalgia*. 2005;25:460–465.
7. Schnabel A, Bennet M, Schuster F, et al. Hyperbzw. Normobare sauerstofftherapie zur behandlung von migrane und clusterkopfschmerzen (hyper- or normobaric oxygen therapy to treat migraine and cluster headache pain). Cochrane review. *Schmerz*. 2008;22:129–132, 134–126.
8. Group TSCHS. Treatment of acute cluster headache with sumatriptan. *N Engl J Med*. 1991;325:322–326.
9. Steiner TJ, Hering R, Couturier EG, et al. Doubleblind placebo-controlled trial of lithium in episodic cluster headache. *Cephalalgia*. 1997;17:673–675.
10. Salar G, Ori C, Iob I, et al. Percutaneous thermocoagulation for sphenopalatine ganglion neuralgia. *Acta Neurochir (Wien)*. 1987; 84:24–28.
11. Sanders M, Zuurmond WW. Efficacy of sphenopalatine ganglion blockade in 66 patients suffering from cluster headache: a 12- to 70-month follow-up evaluation. *J Neurosurg*. 1997;87:876–880.
12. Day M. Neurolysis of the trigeminal and sphenopalatine ganglions. *Pain Pract*. 2001;1:171–182.
13. Edvinsson L. Blockade of CGRP receptors in the intracranial vasculature: a new target in the treatment of headache. *Cephalalgia*. 2004;24:611–622.
14. Narouze S, Kapural L, Casanova J, et al. Sphenopalatine ganglion radiofrequency ablation for the management of chronic cluster headache. *Headache*. 2009;49:571–577.
15. Filippini-de Moor G, Barendse G, van Kleef M, et al. Retrospective analysis of radiofrequency lesions of the sphenopalatine ganglion in the treatment of 19 cluster headache patients. *Pain Clin*. 1999;11: 285–292.
16. Magis D, Allena M, Bolla M, et al. Occipital nerve stimulation for drug-resistant chronic cluster headache: a prospective pilot study. *Lancet Neurol*. 2007;6:314–321.
17. Schwedt TJ, Dodick DW, Trentman TL, et al. Occipital nerve stimulation for chronic cluster headache and hemicrania continua: pain relief and persistence of autonomic features. *Cephalalgia*. 2006;26: 1025–1027.
18. Burns B, Watkins L, Goadsby PJ. Treatment of medically intractable cluster headache by occipital nerve stimulation: long-term follow-up of eight patients. [see comment]. *Lancet*. 2007;369 :1099–1106.
19. Burns B, Watkins L, Goadsby PJ. Treatment of intractable chronic cluster headache by occipital nerve stimulation in 14 patients. *Neurology*. 2009;72:341–345.
20. Jasper JF, Hayek SM. Implanted occipital nerve stimulators. *Pain Physician*. 2008;11:187–200.
21. Narouze S. Complications of head and neck procedures. *Tech Reg Anesth Pain Manag*. 2007;11:171–177.

3 Persistent Idiopathic Facial Pain

Paul Cornelissen, Maarten van Kleef, Nagy Mekhail, Miles Day and Jan Van Zundert

Introduction

Persistent Idiopathic Facial Pain (PIFP) is a general term under which various painful syndromes of the face and mouth are classified. PIFP is a poorly understood affliction. The diagnosis and treatment are therefore often difficult. The etiology of this pain syndrome is so controversial that some doctors in the past often denied its existence and discounted it as a mainly psychological problem.[1] The International Headache Society (HIS) released the second edition of the *International Classification of Headache Disorders* in 2004. PIFP, previously known as atypical facial pain, is described as a persistent facial pain that does not have the classical characteristics of cranial neuralgias and for which there is no obvious cause (code 13.18.4).[2] According to these criteria, a diagnosis of PIFP is possible if the facial pain is localized, present daily, and throughout all or most of the day.

The precise incidence of PIFP is unknown, but it is assumed that it is an affliction of older people.[3] The affliction is seen primarily in older adults and rarely in children.[4,5]

The pathophysiology of PIFP is unknown. In PIFP, there is no abnormal processing of somatosensory stimuli in the pain area or facial area of the primary somatosensory cortex of the brain. PIFP cannot be related to a psychiatric disorder. It is likely that PIFP is brought about by isolated neurophysiological mechanisms in the brain or through abnormal psychological mechanisms that have yet to be classified.[6]

Osteoporosis, appearing after menopause, can induce neuralgias as a result of osteonecrosis of cavities. Sinus or dental infections are possible contributory risk factors but are unlikely solitary causes of PIFP. Odontogenic pains such as pulpitis, pericoronitis, and alveolitis should, however, be excluded. In addition to (or as a result of) odontogenic causes, neuralgias can also develop. Hormonal influences such as estrogen levels have been suggested, but, as yet, no causal link has been established.

Diagnosis

History

PIFP often starts in the nasolabial fold or side of the chin and spreads out to the upper or lower jaw or a large part of the neck. The pain has a chronic character, which is daily and usually present throughout the whole day. In the beginning, the pain is often localized at one side of the face but can later affect both sides. The pain is usually 'deep' and does not stay within the usual anatomical boundaries.[2]

Physical examination

A patient with inexplicable facial pain should be carefully examined. Neurological and physical examination findings in PIFP, by definition, should be normal.

Additional tests

Every patient with PIFP should be extensively evaluated and, if indicated, should be examined by an oral/maxillofacial surgeon and neurologist mainly to exclude underlying pathology. However, there is no specification as to which additional tests or medical imaging should be applied. In some cases, a magnetic resonance image of the skull should be considered.

Differential diagnosis

The diagnostic process for PIFP is not easy and follows a process of elimination of other causes of facial pain: a diagnosis of exclusion. In some cases, a nasopharyngeal tumor can cause facial pain, and the diagnosis can only be made once there is a neurological consequence. Other rare causes are lung tumors that, via referred pain probably by the tenth cranial nerve nerrvus (vagus), cause facial pain.[7,8] The pain in this circumstance is usually unilateral and localized near the ear, the jaws, and the temporal region.[9]

Evidence-Based Interventional Pain Medicine: According to Clinical Diagnoses, First Edition. Edited by Jan Van Zundert, Jacob Patijn, Craig T. Hartrick, Arno Lataster, Frank J.P.M Huygen, Nagy Mekhail, Maarten van Kleef.

Hidden dental problems, such as infections of the sinus maxillares or jaws after previous tooth extractions, can also be the cause of facial pain complaints.[10]

PIFP does not have clear criteria for diagnosis. The IHS has put forward the following diagnostic criteria.[2]

A Pain in the face is present daily and persistent for all or most of the day, fulfilling criteria B and C.
B Pain is confined at onset to a limited area on one side of the face and is deep and poorly localized.
C Pain is not associated with sensory loss or other physical signs.
D Investigations including X-ray of the face and jaws do not demonstrate any relevant abnormality.

The following diagnoses should be excluded, according to the IHS, before the diagnosis of PIFP can be made:

- Pain due to bone disorders of the skull
- Cervicogenic headache
- Acute glaucoma, refraction anomalies, strabismus
- Ear disorders
- Sinusitis
- Disorders of the jaw, teeth, and related structures
- Disorders of the temporomandibular joint
- Disorders of the cranial nerves such as trigeminal compression, optical neuritis, diabetic ocular neuritis, herpes zoster and post-herpetic neuralgia, Tolosa–Hunt syndrome, neck–tongue syndrome
- Trigeminal neuralgia
- Glossopharyngeal neuralgia
- Neuralgia of the intermediate nerve
- Superior laryngeal neuralgia
- Nasociliary neuralgia
- Supraorbital neuralgia
- Terminal branch neuralgias
- External compression headaches
- Headache caused by an external application of a cold stimulus
- Headache caused by the inhalation or ingestion of a cold stimulus
- Constant pain caused by compression, irritation of the cranial nerves or upper cervical roots by structural lesions
- Ophthalmic migraine
- Anesthesia dolorosa
- Central poststroke pain

Rare neuralgias of the face

The differential diagnosis is fully discussed in the chapter on trigeminal neuralgia. The following six structured questions can be used to lead to a definite diagnosis (Table 3.1, also Table 3.2 in the chapter "1. Trigeminal Neuralgia").[11]

Table 3.1. Six questions to determine the differential diagnosis.

1. Does the pain occur in attacks?
2. Are most of the attacks of a short duration (seconds to minutes)?
3. Do you sometimes have extremely short attacks?
4. Are the attacks unilateral?
5. Do the attacks occur in the distribution of the trigeminal nerve?
6. Are there unilateral autonomous symptoms?

Table 3.2. Summary of evidence for interventional management of persistent idiopathic facial pain.

Technique	Score
Pulsed radiofrequency treatment of the ganglion pterygopalatinum (sphenopalatinum)	2 C+

Painful opthalmoplegia

In the description of painful ophthalmoplegia, a clinical picture that consists of a unilateral pain in the orbits, in combination with palsies of the third, fourth, and/or sixth cranial nerves, is drawn. Other terms for this affliction include Tolosa–Hunt syndrome, superior orbital fissure syndrome, orbital-apex syndrome, and cavernous sinus syndrome. Extensive additional tests need to be carried out in order to demonstrate a treatable cause.

Neck–tongue

The neck–tongue syndrome is a rare affliction. Children or young adults notice, with a sudden rotation of the neck, a sharp pain in the back of the head and neck that is accompanied by tingling and a numb feeling in the ipsilateral half of the tongue.

SUNCT syndrome

Another recently identified unilateral syndrome characterized by neuralgiform pain of short duration is SUNCT-syndrome. This is mainly found in men, and the pain is mainly localized in the area of the frontal nerve. It differs from cluster headache in that the attacks are of short duration and high frequency. The pain is refractory to medication that is usually effective for cluster headache.

Anesthesia dolorosa

Anesthesia dolorosa can also occur in the face after lesioning of a peripheral nerve. It can be a complication of a neurosurgical procedure or neurodestructive nerve block in the treatment of trigeminal neuralgia. A de-afferentation pain then occurs in the area of the decreased sensibility.

Central facial pain

The International Association for the Study of Pain (IASP) has defined central facial pain as pain that is caused by a lesion or dysfunction in the central nervous system. Regarding facial pain, one may consider multiple sclerotic foci, syringomyelia and syringobulbia, and thalamic pain caused by a CVA, tumors, and others, as examples of central pain. Central pain is usually chronic, persisting for many years.

Treatment options

Conservative management

Pharmacological treatment with tricyclic antidepressants and anti-epileptic drugs can be tried.[12] Amytryptiline is the primary choice, with a dosage of 25 to 100 mg per day.[13–15] Positive results have also been reported with venlafaxine[16] and fluoxetine.[17]

Interventional management

The pulsed radiofrequency (PRF) treatment of the ganglion pterygopalatinum (sphenopalatinum) in patients with facial pain, including atypical facial pain, was described in a retrospective study.[18] Of the treated patients, 21% reported complete pain relief, and 65% experienced a good to moderate improvement.

Surgical and invasive treatments

Invasive therapy appears to be of little use. Surgical treatments, including trigeminal vascular decompression, are not effective.[19] In one study, deep-brain stimulation of the hypothalamus was described for three patients with PIFP. This treatment was not successful.[20] The treatment of PIFP is difficult and often requires a multidisciplinary approach. The most important part of the treatment is psychological counseling and pharmacological therapy.[3]

Complications of interventional management

Until now, no complications have been reported with PRF treatment. With conventional radiofrequency treatment of the ganglion pterygopalatinum, transient bradycardia was reported.[21]

Evidence for interventional management

A summary of the available evidence is given in Table 3.2.

Recommendations

In patients with chronic atypical facial pain refractory to conservative therapy, PRF treatment of the ganglion pterygopalatinum can be considered.

Clinical practice algorithm

The practice algorithm for the management of PIFP is represented in figure 3.1.

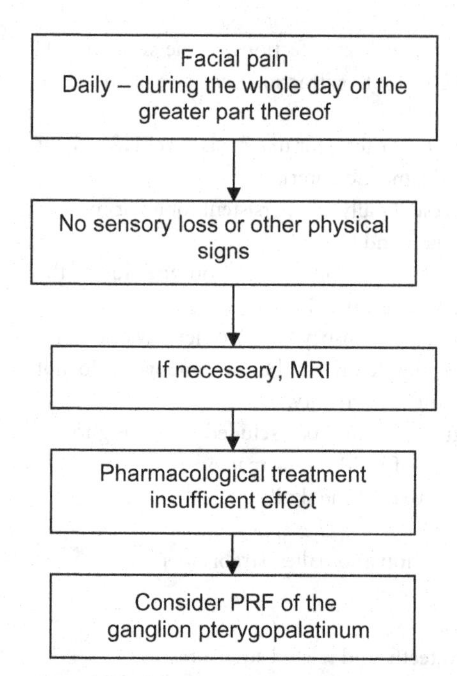

Figure 3.1. Clinical practice algorithm for the treatment of atypical facial pain. MRI, magnetic resonance imaging; PRF, pulsed radiofrequency.

Techniques

The radiofrequency treatment of the ganglion pterygopalatinum is described in the article on cluster headache in this issue[22] (see page 12).

PRF current of 45 V with a maximal temperature of 42°C is applied one or more times during a period of 120 seconds.

Summary

The diagnosis of chronic atypical facial pain is made mainly through a process of elimination of other causes. Therefore, a multidisciplinary examination and consultation are often required.

Pharmacological treatment with tricyclic antidepressants and anti-epileptic drugs can be tried. The conservative pharmacological treatment with amitryptiline is the primary choice. Venlafaxine and fluoxetine can also be considered.

When the pharmacological therapy fails, PRF treatment of the ganglion pterygopalatinum (sphenopalatinum) can be considered.

References

1. Gayford JJ. The aetiology of atypical facial pain and its relation to prognosis and treatment. *Br J Oral Surg.* 1970;7:202–207.
2. IHC IHSCS. International Classification of headache disorders, 2nd ed. *Cephalalgia.* 2004;24:1–160.
3. Madland G, Feinmann C. Chronic facial pain: a multidisciplinary problem. *J Neurol Neurosurg Psychiatry.* 2001;71:716–719.
4. Kavuk I, Yavuz A, Cetindere U, et al. Epidemiology of chronic daily headache. *Eur J Med Res.* 2003;8:236–240.
5. Sardella A, Demarosi F, Barbieri C, et al. An up-to-date view on persistent idiopathic facial pain. *Minerva Stomatol.* 2009;58:289–299.
6. Lang E, Kaltenhauser M, Seidler S, et al. Persistent idiopathic facial pain exists independent of somatosensory input from the painful region: findings from quantitative sensory functions and somatotopy of the primary somatosensory cortex. *Pain.* 2005;118:80–91.
7. Capobianco DJ. Facial pain as a symptom of non-metastatic lung cancer. *Headache.* 1995;35:581–585.

8. Sarlani E, Schwartz AH, Greenspan JD, et al. Facial pain as first manifestation of lung cancer: a case of lung cancer-related cluster headache and a review of the literature. *J Orofac Pain.* 2003;17:262–267.
9. Agostoni E, Frigerio R, Santoro P. Atypical facial pain: clinical considerations and differential diagnosis. *Neurol Sci.* 2005;26(suppl 2):s71–s74.
10. Ratner EJ, Person P, Kleinman DJ, et al. Jawbone cavities and trigeminal and atypical facial neuralgias. *Oral Surg Oral Med Oral Pathol.* 1979;48:3–20.
11. Kleef Mv G WEv, Narouze S, et al. 1. Trigeminal neuralgia. *Pain Pract.* 2009;9:252–259.
12. Sommer C. Patientenkarrieren, gesichtsschmerz und neuralgien. *Schmerz.* 2004;18:385–391.
13. Sharav Y, Singer E, Schmidt E, et al. The analgesic effect of amitriptyline on chronic facial pain. *Pain.* 1987;31:199–209.
14. List T, Axelsson S, Leijon G. Pharmacologic interventions in the treatment of temporomandibular disorders, atypical facial pain, and burning mouth syndrome. A qualitative systematic review. *J Orofac Pain.* 2003;17:301–310.
15. Pettengill CA, Reisner-Keller L. The use of tricyclic antidepressants for the control of chronic orofacial pain. *Cranio.* 1997;15:53–56.
16. Forssell H, Tasmuth T, Tenovuo O, et al. Venlafaxine in the treatment of atypical facial pain: a randomized controlled trial. *J Orofac Pain.* 2004;18:131–137.
17. Harrison S, Glover L, Maslin L, Feinmann C, Pearce S, Harris M. A comparison of antidepressant medication alone and in conjunction with cognitive behavioural therapy for chronic idiopathic facial pain. In: Jensen G, Turner JA, Weisenfeld-Hallin Z, eds. *Proceedings of the 8th World Congress on Pain: Progress in Pain Research and Management*, Vol. 8. Seattle, WA: IASP Press; 1997:663–672.
18. Bayer E, Racz GB, Miles D, et al. Sphenopalatine ganglion pulsed radiofrequency treatment in 30 patients suffering from chronic face and head pain. *Pain Pract.* 2005;5:223–227.
19. Evans RW, Agostoni E. Persistent idiopathic facial pain. *Headache.* 2006;46:1298–1300.
20. Broggi G, Franzini A, Leone M, et al. Update on neurosurgical treatment of chronic trigeminal autonomic cephalalgias and atypical facial pain with deep brain stimulation of posterior hypothalamus: results and comments. *Neurol Sci.* 2007;28(Suppl 2):S138–S145.
21. Konen A. Unexpected effects due to radiofrequency thermocoagulation of the sphenopalatine ganglion: 2 case reports. *Pain Dig.* 2000;10:30–33.
22. van Kleef M, Lataster A, Narouze S, Mekhail N, Geurts JW, van Zundert J. 2. Cluster headache. *Pain Pract.* 2009;9:435–442.

4 Cervical Radicular Pain

Jan Van Zundert, Marc Huntoon, Jacob Patijn, Arno Lataster, Nagy Mekhail and Maarten van Kleef

Introduction

Cervical radicular pain is pain perceived in the upper limb, shooting or electric in quality, caused by irritation and or injury of a cervical spinal nerve.[1,2] In the classification of the International Association for the Study of Pain,[3] cervical radicular pain is defined as pain perceived as arising in the upper limb caused by ectopic activation of nociceptive afferent fibers in a spinal nerve or its roots or other neuropathic mechanisms. This is, however, a problematic definition, as the presence of ectopic activation has rarely, if ever, been demonstrated in a clinical setting.[4]

Cervical radicular pain must be distinguished from cervical radiculopathy. In the latter disorder there is an objective loss of sensory and/or motor function. Radicular pain and radiculopathy are not synonymous even though in the literature these terms are used inter-changeably. Radicular pain is a symptom that is caused by ectopic impulse formation, while radiculopathy also includes neurologic signs such as sensory or motor changes. Still these two disorders may occur simultaneously. Moreover, they may be caused by the same clinical entities; for example, narrowing of the foramen intervertebralis, discus intervertebralis herniation, and radiculitis due to arthritis, infection, or inflammatory exudates.[3] Both syndromes can form a continuum whereby radiculopathy may advance from initial radicular pain when the underlying disorder progresses.[4]

The natural history of cervical radicular pain or radiculopathy is not described in detail in the literature. Data on incidence and prevalence are scarce. The most frequently used epidemiologic data are from Rochester, MN, USA (1976 to 1990), where the incidence is calculated based on the information from the computerized medical record linkage system for the Mayo Clinic and its two affiliated hospitals. The authors claim that their database is essentially an enumeration of the Rochester population. They found in a population between 13 and 91 years an annual incidence of cervical radiculopathy of 83 per 100,000.[5] Although the authors classified the patients as suffering from radiculopathy, the described population most probably included cervical radicular pain, because sensory changes were only reported in 33% and weakness in 64%. The average age-adjusted incidence rates per 100,000 people were 107 for males and 64 for females. The highest incidence was found in the age group between 50 and 54 years with an average of 203 per 100,000 people. In 15% of the patients, a history of physical exertion or trauma preceded the onset of symptoms, and 41% of the patients had a previous history of lumbar radiculopathy. According to this study, the most frequently involved level was C7 in 45% to 60% of the cases. Another study indicated that level C6 represents approximately 20% to 25% and levels C5 and C8 each represent approximately 10% of the cases.[6]

Diagnosis

History

Cervical radicular pain is characterized by pain in the neck that radiates over the posterior shoulder into the arm and sometimes into the hand. The radiation follows a segment-specific pattern. Pain originating from C4 is confined to the neck and suprascapular region. Pain originating from C5 radiates up to the upper arm, and pain from C6 and C7 radiates from the neck to the shoulder, the forearm, and the hand. The pain covers the posterolateral side of the upper arm, but the pain from C7 extends more dorsally.[2,7]

Pain from various dermatomes can overlap and there is no specific region of the arm, which is characteristic for a particular segment. Radicular pain is not limited to a particular dermatome and can be perceived in all structures that are innervated by the affected nerve roots such as muscles, joints, ligaments, and the skin.[2]

Evidence-Based Interventional Pain Medicine: According to Clinical Diagnoses, First Edition. Edited by Jan Van Zundert, Jacob Patijn, Craig T. Hartrick, Arno Lataster, Frank J.P.M Huygen, Nagy Mekhail, Maarten van Kleef.

Physical examination

As with other types of spinal pain, there is no gold standard for the diagnosis of cervical radicular pain. For this reason a diagnosis is made based on a combination of history, clinical examination, and additional tests.[4]

Classical neurologic examination includes testing sensation, strength, and tendon reflexes.[8] Specific clinical tests have been described for the diagnosis of cervical radicular pain, including the neck compression test (Spurling test), the shoulder abduction test, and the axial manual traction test.[4] A description of these tests can be found in Table 4.1.

The validity of these three tests in the diagnosis of root compression in cervical disk disease was investigated regarding radicular pain, neurologic signs, and root compression signs in myelography. All of these tests have a high specificity (81% to 100%) but a low sensitivity. The Spurling test was similarly evaluated using electromyography as the reference test. The results were comparable: sensitivity 30%, specificity 93%. These three examinations are considered valuable aids in the clinical diagnosis of a patient with neck and arm pain. The neurologic characteristics of cervical radicular pain[9] are given in Table 4.2.

Additional tests

The three most frequently requested types of additional tests are medical imaging techniques, electrophysiologic tests, and diagnostic selective nerve root blocks.

Table 4.1. Clinical tests for the diagnosis of cervical radicular pain.

Test	Description
Spurling test	Neck extended with head rotated to affected shoulder while axially loaded. Reproduction of the patient's shoulder or arm pain indicates possible cervical spinal nerve root compression
Shoulder abduction test	The patient lifts a hand above his or her head. A positive result is the decrease or disappearance of the radicular symptom.
Axial manual traction test	In supine position an axial traction force corresponding to 10 to 15 kg is applied. A positive finding is the decrease or disappearance of the radicular symptom.

From: Van Zundert et al.[4] With permission of the publisher.

Table 4.2. Neurologic characteristics of cervical radicular pain.

Disc level	Root	Pain distribution	Muscle weakness	Sensory loss	Reflex loss
C4 to C5	C5	Margo medialis scapulae, lateral upper arm to elbow	M. deltoideus, m. supraspinatus, m. infraspinatus	Lateral upper arm	Supinator reflex
C5 to C6	C6	Lateral forearm, thumb and index finger	M. biceps brachii, m. brachioradialis, wrist extensors	Thumb and index finger	Biceps reflex
C6 to C7	C7	Medial scapula, posterior arm, dorsum of forearm, third finger	M. triceps brachii, wrist flexors, finger extensors	Posterior forearm, third finger	Triceps reflex
C7 to T1	C8	Shoulder, ulnar side of forearm, fifth finger	Thumb flexors, abductors, intrinsic hand muscles	Fifth finger	–

Adapted from Carette S. and Fehlings MG.[9] with Permission of the Publisher.

Medical imaging

Medical imaging is mainly used to exclude primary pathologies, the so-called "red flags" (e.g., tumor, infection, and fractures). Computed tomography (CT) provides good imaging of the cortical bone structures. CT scans are able to reproduce the changes in bone structure more sensitively than nuclear magnetic resonance images (MRI), but they have limitations in detecting soft tissue lesions. MRI is better suited to demonstrate changes in the disci intervertebrales, the spinal cord, the nerve roots, and the surrounding soft tissue.

MRI is currently regarded as the most suitable medical imaging technique for patients with cervical radicular pain. There are no data available regarding the sensitivity and specificity of the various imaging techniques, given that there is no "gold standard" for the diagnosis of cervical radicular pain.[4] A direct link between the pain syndrome and the results of medical imaging does not exist. Prospective studies have shown abnormal MRI images in 19% to 28% of asymptomatic patients.[10,11]

Electrophysiologic tests

Of the various electrodiagnostic studies, needle electromyography and nerve conduction tests are considered useful if the physical examination and case history do not enable differentiation between cervical radicular pain and other neurologic causes of pain in the arm and neck. Approximately 3 weeks after nerve compression, one sees typical abnormal insertion activity, with positive sharp wave potentials and vibration potentials in the arm muscles.[9]

Electrophysiologic tests can be requested when nerve damage is suspected but will not provide any information about the pain. For this reason, in recent years, Quantitative Sensory Testing (QST) has been recommended in the literature as an electrophysiologic test that can provide more specific information about pain. A QST study in patients with cervical radicular symptoms showed an increased detection threshold for light touch and allodynia (touch-induced pain), which differed significantly from that in healthy subjects. QST confirmed the level of involvement identified by means of diagnostic selective nerve root blocks.[12]

Diagnostic selective nerve root blocks

Radiologic images depict the morphologic characteristics of the pathology. In patients with chronic pain in general, and in particular cervical radicular pain, it is extremely difficult to determine with certainty which discus intervertebralis or nerve root is causing the pain. For this reason, one or more diagnostic selective nerve root blocks are applied to determine the probable pain-generating nerve root level. The diagnostic blocks are applied in separate sessions per level. Under radiological visualization using a contrast dye (fluoroscopy), a small amount of local anesthetic is injected (0.5 mL).[13] During a period of 30 to 60 minutes after injection, the pain score is evaluated at regular time intervals. When there is at least a 50% decrease in pain, further treatment at this nerve root level is indicated.

Differential diagnosis

Given that there is no gold standard for the diagnosis of cervical radicular pain, clinical practice relies upon extensive history and clinical examinations and, if indicated, medical imaging and/or electrophysiologic tests. Finally, there is confirmation of the likely pain-generating nerve root level using diagnostic selective nerve root blocks.

The differential diagnosis will initially aim to exclude any "red flags" such as infections, vascular disorders, and tumors. One of the most frequently occurring tumors that need to be excluded is the Pancoast tumor: a tumor of the pulmonary apex that can cause compression of the arteria subclavia, the nervus phrenicus, the plexus brachialis, and compression of the sympathetic ganglion, resulting in a range of symptoms that are known as Horner's syndrome. If the radicular pain is associated with strongly expressed spinal complaints, the differential diagnosis needs to exclude primary spinal tumors as well as metastases. Other less frequent tumors of the spinal nerves include neurofibroma. Pain resulting from carpal tunnel syndrome can also ascend to the neck and may be more intense at night.[14]

Clinical examination is very important in the differential diagnosis of brachialgia based upon shoulder pathology or pain originating from the facet joints. With shoulder pain there is usually limited movement of the shoulder joint, whereas with pain originating from the facet joints, there is usually limited rotation of the cervical spinal column. There is a paravertebral pressure that is not associated with a radicular distribution pattern but sometimes is associated with a pseudoradicular distribution to include the occipital and/or shoulder region. For detailed diagnostics, please refer to other related chapters.

Treatment options

Conservative management

Nonsteroidal anti-inflammatory medications are primarily recommended for short-term treatment because of the balance between efficacy and side effects. The anticonvulsants, such as carbamazepine, oxcarbamazepine, gabapentin, and pregabalin, are frequently used to treat neuropathic pain but they have not been studied in the treatment of cervical radicular pain.[4]

A Cochrane review evaluating the evidence for patient education for neck pain with or without radiculopathy concluded that the available evidence does not show effectiveness for educational interventions for various disorders and time intervals, including recommendations to activate, use of stress coping skills, and "neck school."[15]

Another Cochrane review assessed the potential value of mechanical traction for neck pain with or without radiculopathy and found no evidence to support or refute the efficacy or effectiveness of continuous or intermittent traction for pain reduction, improved function or global perceived effect when compared to placebo traction, or heat or other conservative treatments in patients with chronic neck disorders.[16]

Multidisciplinary rehabilitation with physiotherapy is recommended.[17]

Interventional management

Epidural corticosteroid administration

The principle of epidural administration of corticosteroids relies on the anti-inflammatory response induced by inhibition of the phospholipase A2-initiated arachidonic acid cascade. There are two possible administration routes: the interlaminar and transforaminal routes (Figure 4.1). There are no direct comparisons available between interlaminar and transforaminal administration at a cervical level.

Interlaminar administration: efficacy

A systematic review[18] found two controlled studies involving the cervical interlaminar administration of corticosteroids. An earlier randomized study comparing interlaminar and intramuscular corticosteroid administration found that 68% of the patients treated using the interlaminar method had significant pain relief lasting at least 1 year compared to 12% in the group treated intramuscularly.[19]

A second study examined the effect of co-administration of epidural morphine with corticosteroid and local anesthetic vs. corticosteroid and local anesthetic. Despite a better transient improvement the first day after the intervention in the group receiving additional morphine, long-term results did not differ between groups.[20] The update from the Cochrane systematic review only included the first study.[21]

A recently published systematic review[22] on the effectiveness of cervical interlaminar epidural steroid injections in the management of chronic neck pain included 3 randomized control trials (RCTs): the two studies mentioned above and a study comparing the efficacy of single injections with continuous infusion.[23] Patients were divided into 4 groups based on the duration of their pain, within each group of 40 patients half were randomized to receive up to 9 epidural injections with 4 to 5 days interval or administration of local anesthetic + corticosteroid via an epidural catheter followed by administration of local anesthetic every 6,

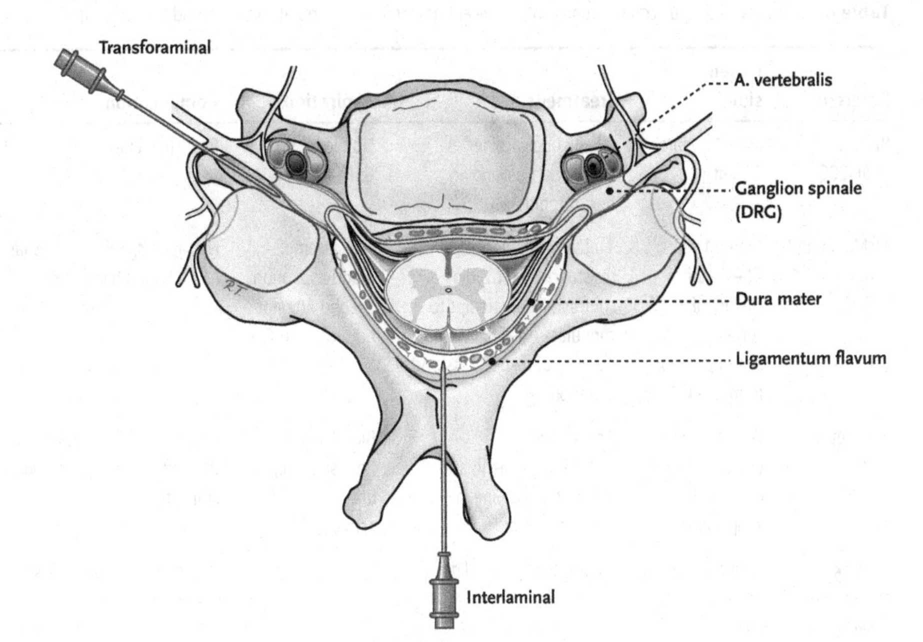

Figure 4.1. Interlaminar and transforaminal administration in the epidural space. Illustration: Rogier Trompert, Medical Art, www.medical-art.nl.

12, or 24 hours along with corticosteroid every 4 to 5 days for a total period of 30 days. The continuous administration provided better pain relief than the single injection in patients with cervical radicular pain lasting longer than 6 months, but no difference was observed in patients with complaints of shorter duration. The systematic review also included 5 observational studies of variable quality.[24–27] The global conclusion of this systematic review is that interlaminar cervical epidural corticosteroid injections provide a significant effect on cervical radicular pain.[22]

Interlaminar administration: complications

Interlaminar cervical corticosteroid administration is described in one review as relatively safe.[28] A systematic review of the literature found only two studies that specifically looked at the complications of cervical corticosteroid administration. One study showed a <1% complication rate while the other reported a rate of 16.8%. This difference is mainly due to the time when the complications were noted and the method by which they were registered. Minor complications that spontaneously disappeared, often within 24 hours, include, among others: increasing axial neck pain, posture-independent headache, facial flushing, and vasovagal episodes. Major complications mentioned included epidural hematoma and accidental subdural injection with, as a result, hypoventilation and hypotension. Accidental subdural injection-induced hypoventilation must be distinguished from the apnea and acute cardiovascular collapse that may result from an intrathecal injection. Paresthesia has been described after root damage. There were two reports of permanent damage to the spinal cord in patients who were sedated and possibly unable to report warning symptoms during the procedure. Intravascular uptake of the contrast dye has also been reported, although this occurs less frequently in interlaminar administration compared to the transforaminal route. When the interlaminar corticosteroid administration is correctly carried out, in a cooperative patient, using fluoroscopy and contrast medium, the incidence of complications is low.[28]

Transforaminal administration: efficacy

The transforaminal administration route rapidly gained in popularity because of the more accurate administration of the active product at the level of the affected nerve root. The first randomized, controlled study by Anderberg et al.[29] studied 40 successive patients with cervical radicular pain. They were randomly given a transforaminal epidural injection of either corticosteroid with a local anesthetic or saline with a local anesthetic. Three weeks postinjection there were no differences in the subjective effects between the treatments. Earlier reports from prospective, noncontrolled studies, however, reported a positive outcome that could not be confirmed by the RCT.

Transforaminal administration: complications

There have been various instances of serious complications reported in the literature, and this is without doubt just the tip of the iceberg. In a recently published anonymous survey by pain specialists, members of the American Pain Society, 287 respondents mentioned 78 complications, mainly neurologic in character, of which 15 were fatal.[30]

The reported complications following transforaminal cervical corticosteroid injections were summarized in the comprehensive review of Malhotra et al.[31], though this group already identified 14 case reports an additional case was reported since their last literature update.[32] A summary of those complications is given in Table 4.3.

Except for the case reported by J.H. Lee et al. in 2008, which concerns direct lesion of the spinal cord due to inadvertent air and contrast injection in the cervical cord,[32] and the case reported by J.Y. Lee et al.,[33] which is a spinal cord compression due to epidural hematoma, the cases can be divided into lesions of the spinal cord

Table 4.3. Review of serious complications with cervical transforaminal epidural corticosteroid administration.

Reference	Patient/level/ side	Treatment	Aspiration	Complication	Onset of complication	Outcome
Brouwers et al. 2001[34]	Man 48 years, C6 left	0.5 mL bupivacaine 0.5% and tramcinolon-hexacetonide 2%	No blood, no CSF	Paralytic below C3	±1 minute	Died after 1 month due to stomach perforation
McMillan and Crumpton 2003[37]	Man 54 years, C5–C6 left History of surgery for decompression from C3–C7	1 mL air with "loss of resistance" 2 mL radio contrast. Final attempt to cannulate C4–C5 aborted because of restlessness and agitation	First attempt blood aspiration. Second attempt no blood, no CSF.	Nystagmus, agitation, aphasia, and bilateral blindness	45 minutes after initial injection of air and radio contrast without other medication	After 30 days discharged with moderate disturbance of short term memory right sided hemianopsy
Rozin et al. 2003[38]	Woman 44 years, C7 left. History of whiplash injury	3 mL (80 mg) methylprednisolone and 0.75% bupivacaine in aliquots of 1 mL	Blood aspiration. Repositioning until no blood aspiration	Loss of consciousness. CT scan showed hemorraghia around brain stem	Immediately after injection of the 3rd mL aliquot	Died one day after injection
Karasek and Bogduk 2004[49]	Woman 55 years, C6–C7 right	bolus 0.8 mL of 2% lidocaine	No information	feeling unwell, weakness in four limbs	1 minute after injection	Symptoms resolved after 20 minutes
Tiso et al. 2004[39]	Woman 48 years, C6 right	0.25% bupivacaine 2 mL and 80 mg triamcinolone	No aspirations	Unresponsive, comatose. Transferred to ICU, awoke 1 hour later	upon self transfer from C-arm table to stretcher	Died next day
Rosenkranz et al. 2004[35]	Man 44 years, C7 left	1 mL mepivacaine 1% and 0.5 mL triamcinolone acetonide (20 mg)	No information given	Anterior spinal artery syndrome	3 minutes after injection	After 3 months spontaneous respiration, no improvement in neurological function. Discharged with serious neurological complications after infarction of the arteria spinalis anterior
Ludwig and Burns 2005[36]	Man 53 years, C6 left	0.75 mL of 0.75% bupivacaine and 0.75 mL triamcinolone	No blood aspiration	Weakness in left arm an bilateral lower limbs	10 minutes	Incomplete tetraplegia
Beckman et al. 2006[40]	Man 31 years, C7-T1 left	60 mg methylprednisolone and 0.75 mL 1% lidocaine. Stopped before completion because of patient complaints of neck pain and nonspecific headache	No aspiration	Headache and nausea, vomiting while sitting up. Cerebral infarction and infarction of the brain stem	Shortly after procedure The evening of the procedure	Survived with diplopia and disturbances of the short term memory
Ziai et al. 2006[41]	Man 41 years, C5–C6 left	3 epidural injections one week apart, 40 mg methylprednisolone acetate and 1 mL saline	No arterial flashback	Nausea, vomiting and headache Became disoriented ±7.5 hours post injection. Brain stem and thalamus infarction and signs of hydrocephalus	During third procedure within minutes of injection	Died shortly after the procedure. Obduction showed bleeding around the arteria vertebralis at the left side at C5
Suresh et al. 2007[42]	Man 60 years, C5 right	1 mL (40 mg) triamcinolone	No blood aspiration	Patient became disoriented and hypertensive. After 8 hrs situation worsened.	Immediately post procedure	Could leave hospital after 1 month with diplopia, speech and equilibrium disturbances
Muro et al. 2007[44]	Woman 72 years, C5–C6 and C6–C7 left	40 mg methylprednisolone acetate and 0.7 mL of 0.5% bupivacaine	No vascular uptake of contrast	Low extremity weakness Examination: paretic in upper extremities and plegic in lower extremities	30 minutes after procedure	No improvement of motor function transfer to rehabilitation

Table 4.3. Continued.

Reference	Patient/level/ side	Treatment	Aspiration	Complication	Onset of complication	Outcome
JY Lee et al. 2007[33]	Woman 38 years, C7-T1 right	3 transforaminal injections. No information on drugs	No information	Severe upper thoracic back pain and progressive loss of sensation in lower extremities MRI heterogeneous mass compressing spinal cord from T1 to T5 Surgery revealed a thick layer of coagulated blood compressing the dura and epidural veins	4 days after last injection	After surgical emergey decompression of spinal canal, regain of function as of day 3. At 6 months full recovery of strength and sensation
JH Lee et al. 2008[32]	Man 55, C7 left	Contrast injection patient reported shock-like pain radiating into left hand. Procedure was terminated	No information	Patient developed incomplete tetraplegia.	2 to 3 minutes	After 1 year still weakness of the left hand grip strength. A claw hand deformity and refractory pain.
Ruppen et al. 2008[43]	Man 45 years, C7	40 mg triamcinolone and 1.5 mL saline	Repeatedly negative	Numbness in right leg, progressed to loss of sensation and plegia of the right leg	30 seconds	1 hour post injection: aspirin 300 mg, heparin 15,000 units daily and nifedipine 20 mg. Full recovery

CSF, cerebro spinal fluid; CT, computed tomography; ICU, intensive care unit; MRI, magnetic resonance imaging.

caused by the anterior spinal artery syndrome,[34–36] and effects on the central nervous system involving brain stem and cerebellum related to inadvertent injection of the arteria vertebralis.[37–44]

Though the mechanisms behind these serious complications are not fully understood, two main considerations must be highlighted: anatomic and pharmacologic.

Anatomical considerations

The normal vascular supply to the cervical spinal cord has been described by Gillilan and others in the human fetus.[45] Branches from the arteria subclavia include the arteria vertebralis, which is usually the first and largest branch. The second and third branches from the arteria subclavia (truncus thyrocervicalis and truncus costocervicalis) eventually give rise to the arteria cervicalis ascendens, medially continuing as inferior thyroidal artery and the arteria cervicalis profunda, respectively.

The arteria vertebralis may be subdivided into V1, V2, and V3 segments. The V1 segment represents the distance from the origin on the arteria subclavia to its entrance in the foramen transversum. The V2 segment includes the area from entrance of the foramen transversum to C2, and the V3 segment includes its course through the C1 foramen transversum, after which it turns medially and dorsally through the sulcus arteriae vertebralis on the upper surface of C1: arcus posterior to penetrate the membrana atlantooccipitalis posterior and dura and pass through the foramen magnum into the cranial cavity. The arteriae vertebrales eventually come together to form the arteria basilaris on the ventral surface of the medulla, but prior to this each of them gives rise to a branch. These branches fuse to form the arteria spinalis anterior that runs in the fissura mediana anterior of the spinal cord. The longitudinal arteria spinalis anterior must be reinforced by segmental arteriae radiculares (medullary arteries) that are primarily from the V2 segment of the arteria vertebralis, but also come from the arteria cervicalis ascendens and arteria cervicalis profunda.

The V2 and V3 segments of the arteria vertebralis are prone to significant variability in their course. A recent study of 500 arteriae vertebrales on 200 MRIs and 50 contrast-enhanced CT scans is illustrative of these variations.[46] The authors found that in only 93% of cases did the arteria vertebralis enter the foramen transversarium at C6. The vast majority of these anomalies saw the V2 segment begin at C5, but the arteria vertebralis was noted to enter the foramen transversarium at C3, C4, or C7 as well. When the arteria vertebralis entered the foramen transversarium at an aberrant level, the unfilled foramina transversaria appeared much smaller on CT than the contralateral side. In addition, in 2% of all specimens the arteria vertebralis formed a medial loop, whose inside border was medial to the uncovertebral joint or into the foramen intervertebrale.

A recent anatomic study of human cadavers[47] noted several other potential variations in normal anatomy: (1) there were instances of several arteriae cervicales profundae arising from the arteria subclavia directly, or from a very short truncus costocervicalis (Figure 4.2). These arteriae cervicales profundae often enter the foramen intervertebrale in its aspect near sites of recommended transforaminal needle placement (Figure 4.3); (2) a single arteria cervicalis ascendens was noted to enter the foramen intervertebrale at C4 and eventually supply the arteria spinalis anterior; (3) a large

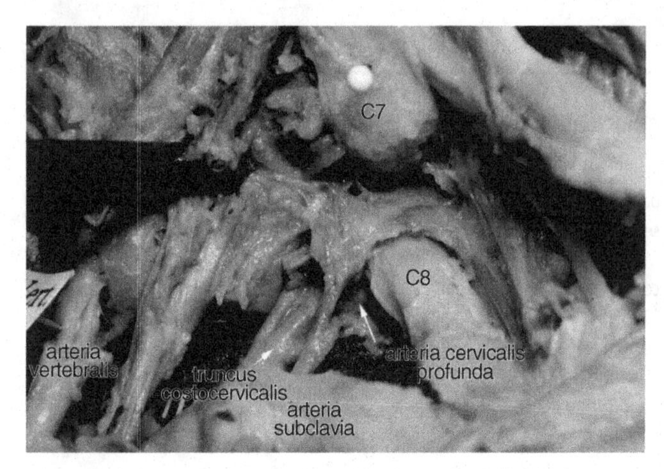

Figure 4.2. The three branches from the arteria subclavia are shown. Most medially (left lower) the arteria vertebralis is seen, then the truncus thyrocervicalis in the forceps, followed more laterally by the truncus costocervicalis. One of the arteriae cervicales profundae branches from the truncus costovertebralis passes posterior to the C8 ramus ventralis.

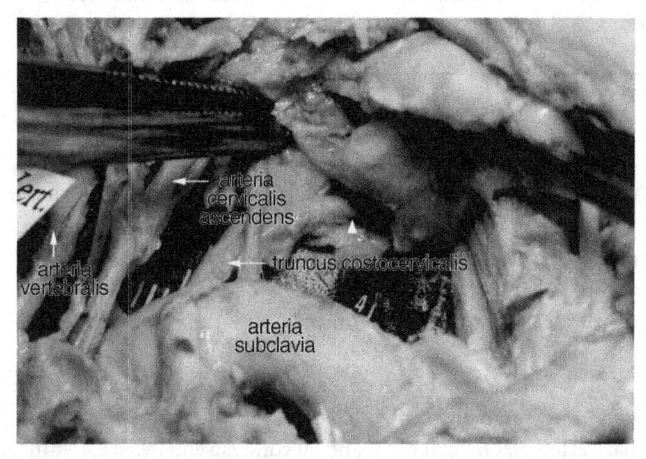

Figure 4.3. In this figure, the detail of the arteria cervicalis profunda (arrowhead) continuing from the truncus costocervicalis profunda can be seen as it enters the posterior aspect of the foramen intervertebrale to the C8 ventral ramus. This is the area of ideal needle pathway for transforaminal epidural injection.

segmental medullary contributing artery was noted to be the main supplier to the arteria spinalis anterior when the ipsilateral arteria vertebralis entered the spine at C5 instead of C6; (4) several anastomoses were noted between all three main supply arteries in several cadavers, suggesting a great potential for communication; and (5) in general, if the arteria cervicalis profunda tended to enter the foramina intervertebralia it was at either C7/T1 or C6/C7, and the arteria cervicalis ascendens tended to enter the foramina intervertebralia at C5/C6 or higher. A recent study utilizing ultrasound guidance for cervical transforaminal injections[48] noted a remarkably similar percentage of arterial vessels in the posterior aspect of the foramina intervertebralia (20%) as the cadaver study noted above. Cumulatively, these anatomic features suggest that there is no specific "safe zone" for needle placements in the posterior cervical foramina intervertebralia. It is unclear whether hypoplastic or aberrant arteriae vertebrales or other arterial variants described above absolutely increase the risks of transforaminal epidural injections, but certainly vessel vulnerability warrants greater care in the performance of these procedures.

Pharmacologic considerations

The case report of Karasek and Bogduk[49] reporting transient quadriplegia after injection of only local anesthetic, suggest inadvertent puncture of a cervical arteria radicularis and transient anesthesia of the spinal cord. However, when a spinal cord infarction is demonstrated, after the injection of depot corticosteroid, only partial recovery of the motor function occurs[35,36] and one case had a fatal outcome due to complications.[34]

It has been postulated that upon inadvertent injection into the cervical arteria radicularis, the particulate steroids may act as an embolus and cause spinal cord infarction and permanent impairment. Particle size of different corticosteroid preparations were studied undiluted and diluted in saline or local anesthetic. The results of this in-depth research illustrated that differences in the percentage of large particles exist between compounded and commercially available preparations. Because the specifications of corticosteroid preparations commercially available in different countries may be different, it is difficult to draw conclusions for clinical practice.[50]

A recent study in a swine model underscores the potential for catastrophic outcomes from particulate steroids injected intra-arterially. Okubadejo and colleagues[51] instrumented the arteriae vertebrales in 11 pigs and intentionally injected them with either particulate (methylprednisolone) or nonparticulate steroid (dexamethasone). Interestingly, the animals that received particulate steroid could not be removed from life support. Each of these 4 particulate steroid-receiving animals had evidence on histologic examination of severe tissue edema, ischemic changes, and other pathologies. None of the animals receiving nonparticulate steroid had any issues. These animal cases appear to be functionally similar to the case described by Beckman et al.[40] The study by Dreyfuss et al.[52] comparing triamcinolone to dexamethasone (nonparticulate) for cervical epidural injections was quite small, but certainly their efficacy data combined with the animal study described above seem to suggest that nonparticulate steroid may be a good alternative for those physicians who continue to perform transforaminal injections.

When patients demonstrate central symptoms such as nystagmus, confusion, and coma, it is less obvious to indicate an embolus caused by particulate steroids. In the McMillan and Crumpton[37] case, no steroid was injected. Moreover, there are two cases where the patient developed symptoms of brain stem infarction several hours after the injection as opposed to the almost immediate effect seen in others.[40,41] In his comments on the case reported by Beckman et al.,[40] de Leon-Casasola remarks that the late onset of symptoms indicates that steroid embolism was not responsible for the complication. It clearly depicts the clinical course of arteria vertebralis dissection.[53] Dissection of the arteria vertebralis and disruption of the blood brain barrier causes ischemia and brain death due to acute intracranial hypertension. This mechanism is probably involved in the case described by Rosenkranz et al.[35]

These serious and up till now inexplicable complications provide good reason to be extremely cautious about performing transforaminal cervical epidural injections with depot corticosteroids. In a letter to the editor following the review of the complications,[31] we strongly recommended curtailing use of transforaminal cervical epidural corticosteroid administration until the mechanisms of those serious complications and the methods to prevent them have been better elucidated.[54]

Practical recommendations

Direct comparisons between interlaminar and transforaminal corticosteroid injections in the cervical epidural space are not available. The positive RCT for interlaminar administration and, moreover, the quick succession of reports of serious complications after transforaminal cervical epidural corticosteroid injections supports the preference for interlaminar administration.

There are no studies which have investigated the effectiveness of the various depot corticosteroids, so no distinction can be confirmed between them. The particle size of the depot corticosteroid is possibly related to the reported neurologic complications, but also on this topic the literature is inconclusive.[50] Currently there is no evidence that a higher dose of corticosteroids will result in a better clinical effect.[55] On the other hand the risk of endocrine side effects is notably higher.[56]

In the randomized clinical trial, 1 to 3 epidural doses administered at intervals of 2 weeks were described.[19] Shortening the interval between two corticosteroid administrations may result in higher plasma levels and thus increase the risk for endocrine and other systemic side effects.

(Pulsed) radiofrequency treatment

Radiofrequency treatment: efficacy

The efficacy of radiofrequency (RF) treatment adjacent to the ganglion spinale (dorsal root ganglion (DRG)) was reported in two randomized clinical studies.[57,58]

The first study compared RF adjacent to the cervical ganglion spinale (DRG) with a sham intervention. In the actively treated group, 8 weeks postintervention the Number Needed to Treat, i.e., the number of patients that need to be treated in order to have at least one patient who has at least a 50% reduction in pain, was 1.4.[57]

The second study compared RF with an electrode tip temperature of 40°C with RF at 67°C.[58] At 6 weeks and at 3 months after treatment there was a significant decrease in the visual analog scale pain score in both groups. There was no significant difference in outcome between the two groups.

Radiofrequency treatment: complications

In the above-mentioned studies, transient neuritis and/or a burning sensation in the treated spinal nerve were reported. Additionally, a slight loss of muscular strength in the hand and arm of the treated side was reported.

Pulsed radiofrequency treatment: efficacy

Currently preference is given to pulsed radiofrequency treatment (PRF) where the tip temperature of the electrode does not exceed the critical threshold of 42°C and consequently there is minimal neuro-destruction. In an RCT, PRF appeared to be more effective than placebo 3 months post-treatment. Also 6 months post-treatment there was a positive trend in the PRF treatment but in this study the outcome fell short of statistical significance.[59]

Pulsed radiofrequency treatment: complications

Up until now there have been no reported complications associated with PRF.[60]

Surgical treatment

Surgical treatment can provide pain relief in patients whose symptoms seem to be refractory to all other treatments. Surgical treatment is indicated in cervical radiculopathy with spinal cord compression (myelomalacia) because of the risk for possibly irreversible neurologic deficiency.

In a randomized study where surgical treatment was compared with conservative treatment a significant improvement in pain relief was noted 3 months after the intervention. A year post-treatment however there was no difference between the two groups.[61] A small, randomized study indicated no differences in neurologic outcome between patients who were surgically or conservatively treated.[62]

Spinal cord stimulation

Spinal cord stimulation (SCS) consists of percutaneously applying an electrode at the level of the involved segment of the spinal cord. These are then connected to a generator that delivers electric shocks in order to stimulate the painful dermatome and introduce an altered pain pathway. The mechanism behind SCS rests on the gate control theory of pain.[63]

Up until now there is no literature on the outcome of SCS in the treatment of cervical radicular pain.

SCS can be considered in clinical practice for chronic cervical radicular pain in well-selected patients when other types of treatment have failed, given that the efficacy has been demonstrated in other comparable neuropathic pain syndromes.

Evidence for interventional management

A summary of the available evidence is given in Table 4.4.

Recommendations

Based on the available evidence regarding efficacy and complications, the following treatments are recommended for cervical radicular pain:

Table 4.4. Summary of evidence for interventional management of cervical radicular pain.

Technique	Score
Interlaminar corticosteroid administration	2B+
Transforaminal corticosteroid administration	2B–
Radiofrequency treatment adjacent to the ganglion spinale (dorsal root ganglion (DRG))	2B+
Pulsed radiofrequency treatment adjacent to the ganglion spinale (dorsal root ganglion (DRG))	1B+
Spinal cord stimulation	0

1 In the subacute phase, an interlaminar epidural administration of local anesthetic and corticosteroids is recommended. The cervical transforaminal epidural corticosteroid retained a negative recommendation.
2 For chronic cervical radicular pain, PRF adjacent to the cervical DRG is the first line recommended interventional pain management technique, because there are up till now no reports of neurologic complications with PRF. In the event that this has a poor or short-term effect an RF treatment adjacent to the cervical DRG is recommended.
3 If the symptoms persist then study-related SCS can be considered after extensive multidisciplinary evaluation. Spinal cord stimulation should be performed in specialized centers.

Clinical practice algorithm

A suggested clinical practice algorithm is shown in Figure 4.4.

Technique(s)

Interlaminar cervical epidural steroid administration

During the planning of cervical epidural infiltrations, review of a preprocedural MRI should be strongly considered. The procedure should be performed under fluoroscopy. Correlation of fluoroscopic images with the MRI may avert potential complications in cases of large disk protrusions mechanically deforming the posterior epidural space.[64]

Cervical epidural infiltrations are preferably carried out with the patient in a sitting position. The cervical spinal column is bent forwards. The skin is disinfected. For positions C5 to C6 or C6 to C7, the anesthetist places his middle and index fingers on both sides of the processus spinosi.[65] After a midline needle placement "down the barrel," with the needle firmly fixed, the operator can switch to a lateral view and very slowly advance the needle as it approaches the base of the processus spinosi, while concomitantly using a glass syringe loss of resistance or alternatively using hanging drop technique under fluoroscopic guidance.[65] (Figures 4.5)

A small amount of contrast dye can be injected in order to ensure the correct epidural placement of the needle using fluoroscopy (Figures 4.6). When the needle is correctly inserted, a syringe containing the administration solution is attached. Aspiration is carefully carried out in order to identify cerebrospinal fluid or blood.

Larkin et al.[66] described another technique, using a styletted catheter that is placed in the potentially safer area of the T2 to T4 epidural space and advanced toward the desired cervical root with continuous fluoroscopy.

An important warning was recently published by Racz and Heavner about the risks of generating high pressure in the epidural space if the flow is obstructed. They stress the need for ensuring transforaminal outlet flow and recommend immediately flexing and rotating the patient's head upon the first signs of spinal cord ischemia.[67]

(Pulsed) radiofrequency treatment[59]

Diagnostic blocks

After the clinical diagnosis of cervical radicular pain is made, confirmation of the most affected segment is carried out using diagnostic selective nerve root blocks. The patient is placed in supine position on a translucent operation table. The C-arm of the fluoroscope is placed such that the beam is parallel to the axis of the foramen intervertebrale. The axis points 25 to 35° oblique and 10° caudally. In this way, the entry point is determined by the projection of a metal ruler over the caudal part of the foramen intervertebrale. A 60-mm 24G neuroradiography needle is introduced parallel to the beam (tunnel view) (Figure 4.7). Then the beam direction is changed to the anteroposterior position and the introducer needle is further introduced until the tip is projected just laterally to the facet column. When the segmental nerve is identified using 0.4 mL iohexol contrast dye, 0.5 to 1.0 mL lidocaine is slowly injected around the nerve. Overflow into the epidural space is avoided by "real time" observation of the radio-opaque mixture. The pain relief is observed for 30 minutes after the infiltration. A positive diagnostic block provides at least 50% pain relief.

PRF technique—placement of the electrode

The entry point is determined in the same way as for diagnostic blocks, by projecting a metal ruler over the caudal and posterior part of the foramen intervertebrale. The cannula (22G SMK-C5 needle 54 mm with 4 mm active tip. Cotop International B.V., Amsterdam, the Netherlands) is introduced parallel to the beam and if required the direction is corrected while the cannula is still in the uppermost subcutaneous layers. The correct position is reached when the cannula is projected as a point on the screen. This point must lie just above the dorsal part of the foramen intervertebrale. This is the transition between the middle and most caudal third part of the foramen intervertebrale. This position is chosen in order to avoid possible damage to the arteria vertebralis that runs anterior to the foramen intervertebrale. The direction of the beam is then changed to anteroposterior position and the cannula is moved up further until the tip is projected over the middle of the facetal column (Figures 4.8).

CLINICAL PRACTICE ALGORITHM

Cervical radicular pain

Red flags excluded?

Yes

Conservative treatment was adequately carried out without satisfactory results (VAS>4)

Yes

Subacute pain

Interlaminar corticosteroid administration

Chronic pain

Confirmation of the presumed causative level with a selective diagnostic block

Pulsed radiofrequency treatment adjacent to the cervical ganglion spinale (dorsal root ganglion (DRG))

Poor or short lasting result

Conventional radiofrequency adjacent to the cervical ganglion spinale (dorsal root ganglion (DRG))

Poor result

Consider study-related SCS

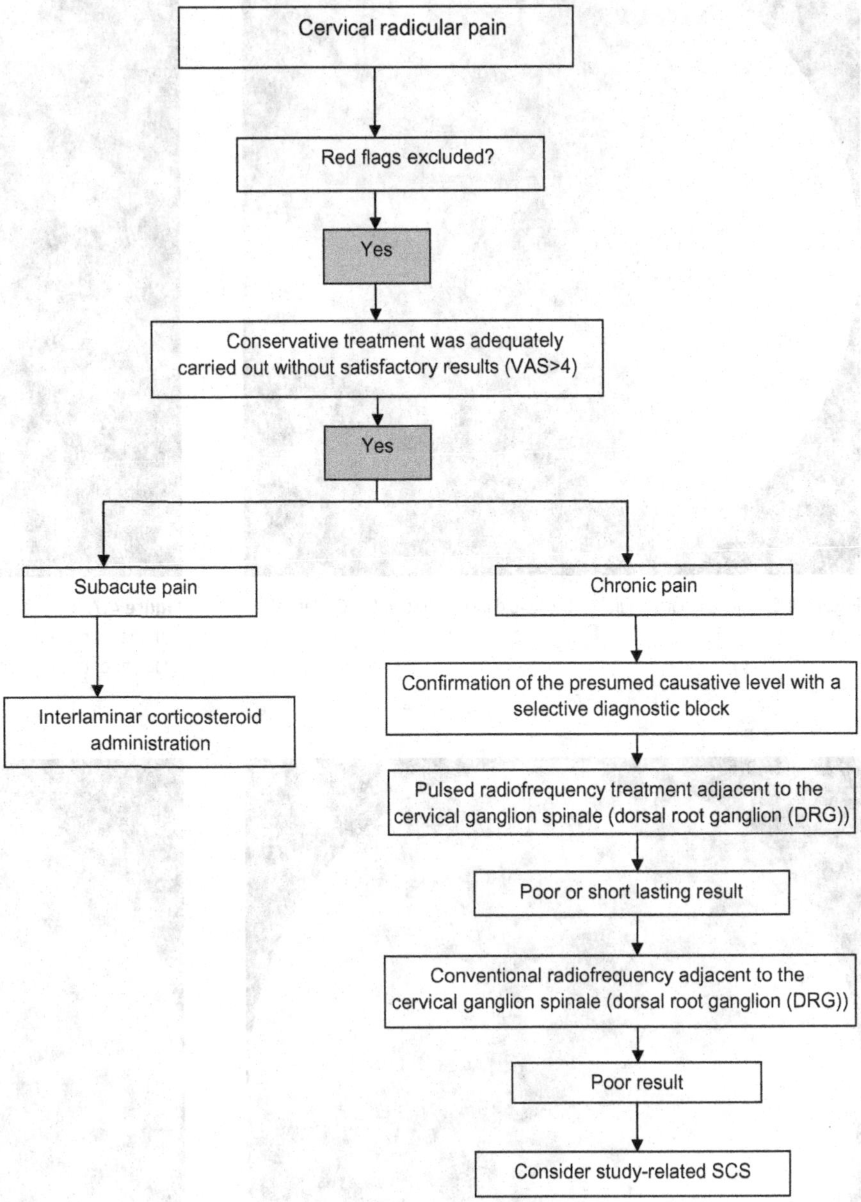

Figure 4.4. Clinical practice algorithm for the treatment of cervical radicular pain.

The stylet is then exchanged for an RF electrode. The impedance is measured in order to check if a closed electrical circuit is present. Then stimulation is started at 50 Hz in order to determine the sensory stimulation threshold. The patient must feel a tingling at less than 0.5 V. This indicates that the tip is in close proximity to the DRG.

Pulsed radiofrequency treatment

The RF current is delivered in small bursts at 45 V; this output can always be adjusted if the temperature rises above 42°C. Forty-two degrees is the maximum temperature, but not the obligatory temperature to be reached. The pulsed current is delivered for 120 seconds.

Summary

1 There is no gold standard for the diagnosis of cervical radicular pain.

2 Case history and clinical examination form the cornerstones of the diagnostic process.

3 Medical imaging, with a slight preference for MRI, is indicated when specific pathologies and/or abnormal neurologic symptoms are suspected.

4 The suspected level can be confirmed using diagnostic selective nerve root blocks.

5 Whenever conservative treatments fail:

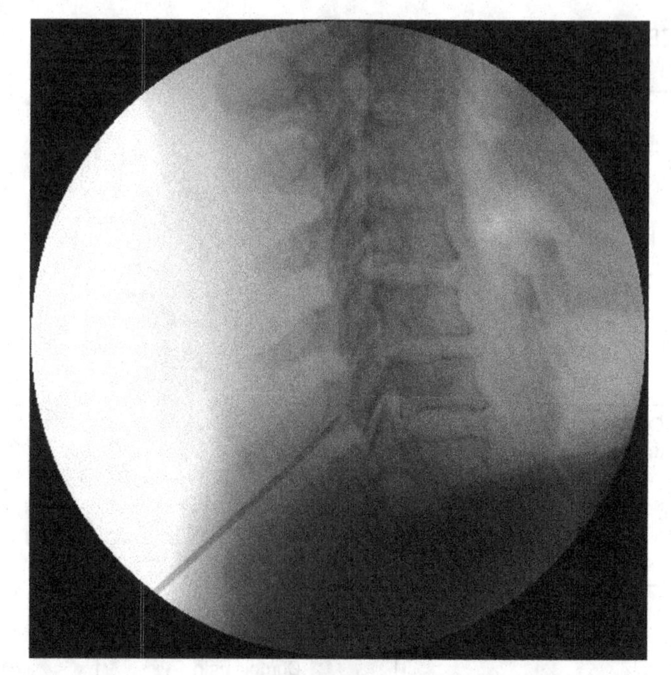

Figure 4.5. Interlaminar epidural corticosteroid administration C6–C7, lateral view.

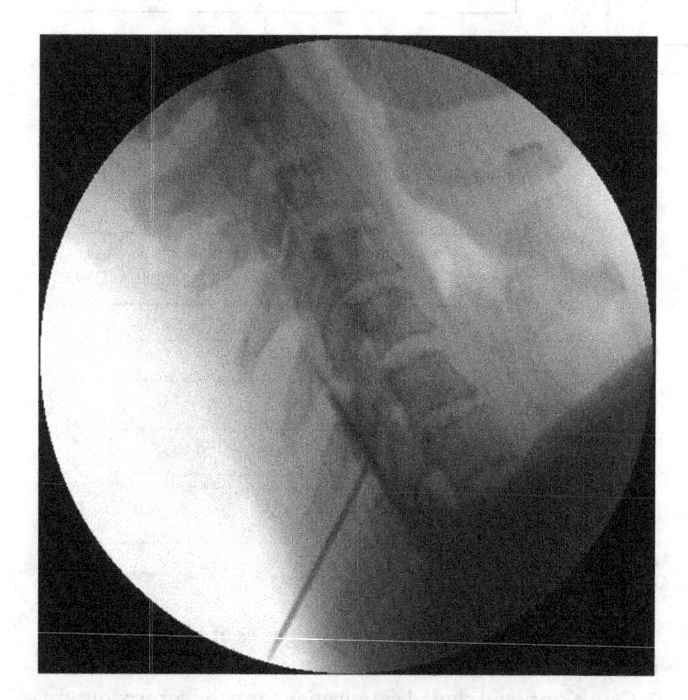

Figure 4.6. Interlaminar epidural corticosteroid administration C6-C7: lateral view. The needle and the spread of the contrast dye.

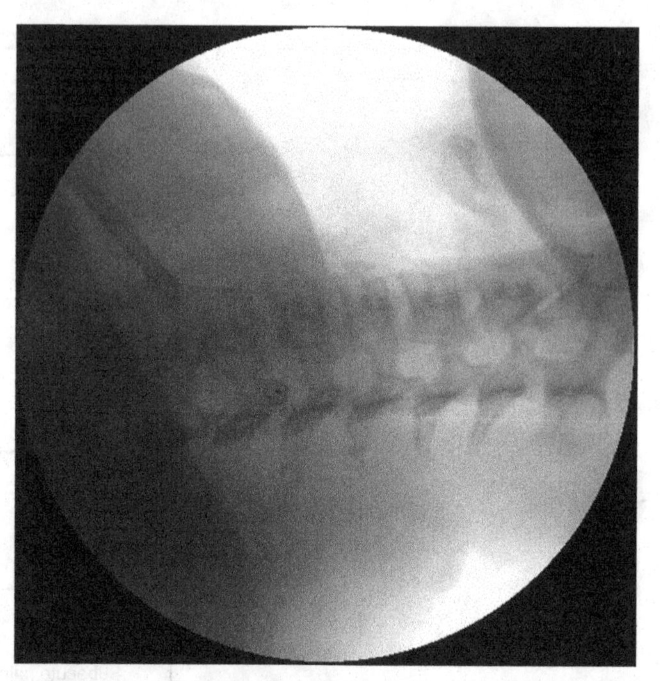

Figure 4.7. Cervical ganglion spinale (DRG) (pulsed) radiofrequency treatment. with the C-arm in the lateral oblique position. The needle in the posterior caudal quadrant of the foramen intervertebrale.

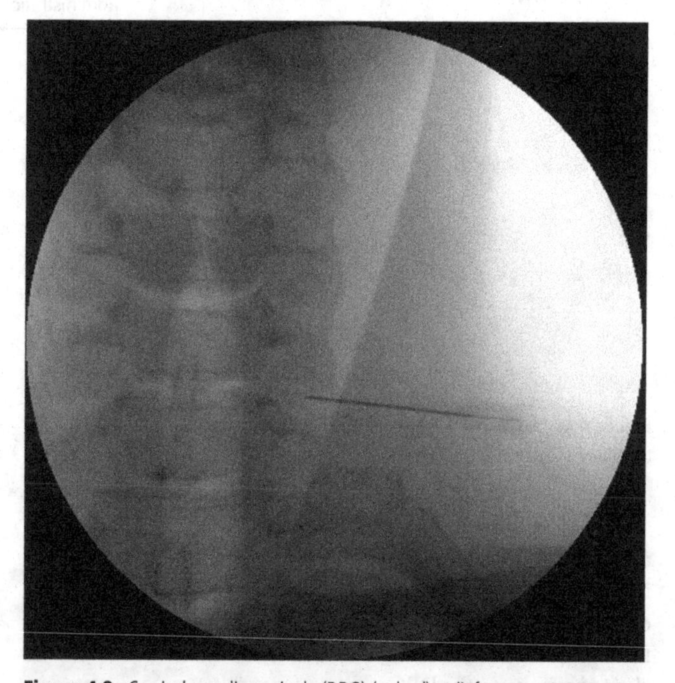

Figure 4.8. Cervical ganglion spinale (DRG) (pulsed) radiofrequency treatment: needle is in the middle of the facetal column in AP view.

• With (sub)acute cervical radicular pain, interlaminar corticosteroid administration is recommended

• With chronic cervical radicular pain, PRF adjacent to the DRG is recommended.

6 If these therapies fail, study-related spinal cord stimulation can be considered in specialized centers.

References

1. Rathmell JP, Aprill C, Bogduk N. Cervical transforaminal injection of steroids. *Anesthesiology.* 2004;100:1595–1600.
2. Bogduk N. *Medical Management of Acute Cervical Radicular Pain: and Evidence-based Approach.* 1st ed. Newcastle, Australia: The Newcastle Bone and Joint Institute; 1999.
3. Merskey H, Bogduk N. *Classification Descriptions of Chronic Pain Syndromes and Definitions of Pain Terms.* 2nd ed. Seattle, WA: IASP Press; 1994.
4. Van Zundert J, Harney D, Joosten EA, et al. The role of the dorsal root ganglion in cervical radicular pain: diagnosis, pathophysiology, and rationale for treatment. *Reg Anesth Pain Med.* 2006;31:152–167.
5. Radhakrishnan K, Litchy WJ, O'Fallon WM, Kurland LT. Epidemiology of cervical radiculopathy. A population-based study from Rochester, Minnesota, 1976 through 1990. *Brain.* 1994;117(Pt 2): 325–335.
6. Sluijter ME. *Radiofrequency Part I.* Meggen, Switzerland: Flivopress. 2001.
7. Slipman CW, Plastaras CT, Palmitier RA, Huston CW, Sterenfeld EB. Symptom provocation of fluoroscopically guided cervical nerve root stimulation. Are dynatomal maps identical to dermatomal maps? *Spine.* 1998;23:2235–2242.
8. Fager CA. Identification and management of radiculopathy. *Neurosurg Clin N Am.* 1993;4:1–12.
9. Carette S, Fehlings MG. Clinical practice. Cervical radiculopathy. *N Engl J Med.* 2005;353:392–399.
10. Boden SD, McCowin PR, Davis DO, Dina TS, Mark AS, Wiesel S. Abnormal magnetic-resonance scans of the cervical spine in asymptomatic subjects. A prospective investigation. *J Bone Joint Surg Am.* 1990;72:1178–1184.
11. Teresi LM, Lufkin RB, Reicher MA, et al. Asymptomatic degenerative disk disease and spondylosis of the cervical spine: MR imaging. *Radiology.* 1987;164:83–88.
12. Voerman VF, van Egmond J, Crul BJ. Elevated detection thresholds for mechanical stimuli in chronic pain patients: support for a central mechanism. *Arch Phys Med Rehabil.* 2000;81:430–435.
13. Anderberg L, Saveland H, Annertz M. Distribution patterns of transforaminal injections in the cervical spine evaluated by multi-slice computed tomography. *Eur Spine J.* 2006;15:1465–1471.
14. Mumenthaler M, Mattle H. Intervertabral disk disease as a cause of radicular syndromes. In: Mumenthaler M, Mattle H, eds. *Neurology.* 4th ed (revised and enlarged). Stuttgart, Germany and New York: Georg Thieme Verlag; 2004;728–738.
15. Haines T, Gross A, Burnie SJ, Goldsmith CH, Perry L. Patient education for neck pain with or without radiculopathy. *Cochrane Database Syst Rev.* 2009;1:CD005106.
16. Graham N, Gross A, Goldsmith CH, et al. Mechanical traction for neck pain with or without radiculopathy. *Cochrane Database Syst Rev.* 2008;3:CD006408.
17. Persson LC, Lilja A. Pain, coping, emotional state and physical function in patients with chronic radicular neck pain. A comparison between patients treated with surgery, physiotherapy or neck collar—a blinded, prospective randomized study. *Disabil Rehabil.* 2001;23:325–335.
18. Abdi S, Datta S, Trescot AM, et al. Epidural steroids in the management of chronic spinal pain: a systematic review. *Pain Physician.* 2007;10:185–212.
19. Stav A, Ovadia L, Sternberg A, Kaadan M, Weksler N. Cervical epidural steroid injection for cervicobrachialgia. *Acta Anaesthesiol Scand.* 1993;37:562–566.
20. Castagnera L, Maurette P, Pointillart V, Vital JM, Erny P, Senegas J. Long-term results of cervical epidural steroid injection with and without morphine in chronic cervical radicular pain. *Pain.* 1994;58:239–243.
21. Peloso P, Gross A, Haines T, Trinh K, Goldsmith CH, Burnie S. Medicinal and injection therapies for mechanical neck disorders. *Cochrane Database Syst Rev.* 2007;3:CD000319.
22. Benyamin RM, Singh V, Parr AT, Conn A, Diwan S, Abdi S. Systematic review of the effectiveness of cervical epidurals in the management of chronic neck pain. *Pain Physician.* 2009;12:137–157.
23. Pasqualucci A, Varrassi G, Braschi A, et al. Epidural local anesthetic plus corticosteroid for the treatment of cervical brachial radicular pain: single injection versus continuous infusion. *Clin J Pain.* 2007;23:551–557.
24. Rowlingson JC, Kirschenbaum LP. Epidural analgesic techniques in the management of cervical pain. *Anesth Analg.* 1986;65: 938–942.
25. Ferrante FM, Wilson SP, Iacobo C, Orav EJ, Rocco AG, Lipson S. Clinical classification as a predictor of therapeutic outcome after cervical epidural steroid injection. *Spine.* 1993;18:730–736.
26. Grenier B, Castagnera L, Maurette P, Erny P, Senegas J. [Chronic cervico-brachial neuralgia treated by cervical epidural injection of corticosteroids. Long-term results]. *Ann Fr Anesth Reanim.* 1995;14:484–488.
27. Cicala RS, Westbrook L, Angel JJ. Side effects and complications of cervical epidural steroid injections. *J Pain Symptom Manage.* 1989;4:64–66.
28. Abbasi A, Malhotra G, Malanga G, Elovic EP, Kahn S. Complications of interlaminar cervical epidural steroid injections: a review of the literature. *Spine.* 2007;32:2144–2151.
29. Anderberg L, Annertz M, Persson L, Brandt L, Saveland H. Transforaminal steroid injections for the treatment of cervical radiculopathy: a prospective and randomised study. *Eur Spine J.* 2007;16:321–328.
30. Scanlon GC, Moeller-Bertram T, Romanowsky SM, Wallace MS. Cervical transforaminal epidural steroid injections: more dangerous than we think? *Spine.* 2007;32:1249–1256.
31. Malhotra G, Abbasi A, Rhee M. Complications of transforaminal cervical epidural steroid injections. *Spine.* 2009;34:731–739.
32. Lee JH, Lee JK, Seo BR, Moon SJ, Kim JH, Kim SH. Spinal cord injury produced by direct damage during cervical transforaminal epidural injection. *Reg Anesth Pain Med.* 2008;33:377–379.
33. Lee JY, Nassr A, Ponnappan RK. Epidural hematoma causing paraplegia after a fluoroscopically guided cervical nerve-root injection. A case report. *J Bone Joint Surg Am.* 2007;89:2037–2039.
34. Brouwers PJ, Kottink EJ, Simon MA, Prevo RL. A cervical anterior spinal artery syndrome after diagnostic blockade of the right C6-nerve root. *Pain.* 2001;91:397–399.

35. Rosenkranz M, Grzyska U, Niesen W, et al. Anterior spinal artery syndrome following periradicular cervical nerve root therapy. *J Neurol.* 2004;251:229–231.
36. Ludwig MA, Burns SP. Spinal cord infarction following cervical transforaminal epidural injection: a case report. *Spine.* 2005;30:E266–E268.
37. McMillan MR, Crumpton C. Cortical blindness and neurologic injury complicating cervical transforaminal injection for cervical radiculopathy. *Anesthesiology.* 2003;99:509–511.
38. Rozin L, Rozin R, Koehler SA, et al. Death during transforaminal epidural steroid nerve root block (C7) due to perforation of the left vertebral artery. *Am J Forensic Med Pathol.* 2003;24:351–355.
39. Tiso RL, Cutler T, Catania JA, Whalen K. Adverse central nervous system sequelae after selective transforaminal block: the role of corticosteroids. *Spine J.* 2004;4:468–474.
40. Beckman WA, Mendez RJ, Paine GF, Mazzilli MA. Cerebellar herniation after cervical transforaminal epidural injection. *Reg Anesth Pain Med.* 2006;31:282–285.
41. Ziai WC, Ardelt AA, Llinas RH. Brainstem stroke following uncomplicated cervical epidural steroid injection. *Arch Neurol.* 2006;63:1643–1646.
42. Suresh S, Berman J, Connell DA. Cerebellar and brainstem infarction as a complication of CT-guided transforaminal cervical nerve root block. *Skeletal Radiol.* 2007; 36:449–452.
43. Ruppen W, Hugli R, Reuss S, Aeschbach A, Urwyler A. Neurological symptoms after cervical transforaminal injection with steroids in a patient with hypoplasia of the vertebral artery. *Acta Anaesthesiol Scand.* 2008;52:165–166.
44. Muro K, O'Shaughnessy B, Ganju A. Infarction of the cervical spinal cord following multilevel transforaminal epidural steroid injection: case report and review of the literature. *J Spinal Cord Med.* 2007;30:385–388.
45. Gillilan LA. The arterial blood supply of the human spinal cord. *J Comp Neurol.* 1958;110:75–103.
46. Bruneau M, Cornelius JF, Marneffe V, Triffaux M, George B. Anatomical variations of the V2 segment of the vertebral artery. *Neurosurgery.* 2006;59:ONS20–ONS24; discussion ONS-24.
47. Huntoon MA. Anatomy of the cervical intervertebral foramina: vulnerable arteries and ischemic neurologic injuries after transforaminal epidural injections. *Pain.* 2005;117:104–111.
48. Narouze S. Ultrasonography in pain medicine: a sneak peak at the future. *Pain Pract.* 2008;8:223–225.
49. Karasek M, Bogduk N. Temporary neurologic deficit after cervical transforaminal injection of local anesthetic. *Pain Med.* 2004;5:202–205.
50. Benzon HT, Chew TL, McCarthy RJ, Benzon HA, Walega DR. Comparison of the particle sizes of different steroids and the effect of dilution: a review of the relative neurotoxicities of the steroids. *Anesthesiology.* 2007;106:331–338.
51. Okubadejo GO, Talcott MR, Schmidt RE, et al. Perils of intravascular methylprednisolone injection into the vertebral artery. An animal study. *J Bone Joint Surg Am.* 2008;90:1932–1938.
52. Dreyfuss P, Baker R, Bogduk N. Comparative effectiveness of cervical transforaminal injections with particulate and nonparticulate corticosteroid preparations for cervical radicular pain. *Pain Med.* 2006;7:237–242.
53. de Leon-Casasola OA. Transforaminal cervical epidural injections. *Reg Anesth Pain Med.* 2008;33:190–191.
54. Van Zundert J, Huntoon M, van Kleef M. Transforaminal cervical epidural steroid injections: time to stop? *Spine.* Phila Pa 1976) 2009; 34(22):2477.
55. Owlia MB, Salimzadeh A, Alishiri G, Haghighi A. Comparison of two doses of corticosteroid in epidural steroid injection for lumbar radicular pain. *Singapore Med J.* 2007;48:241–245.
56. Van Zundert J, le Polain de Waroux B. Safety of epidural steroids in daily practice: evaluation of more than 4000 administrations. In: The International Monitor, ed. *XX Annual ESRA Meeting.* Rome, Italy: ESRA; 2000;122.
57. van Kleef M, Liem L, Lousberg R, Barendse G, Kessels F, Sluijter M. Radiofrequency lesion adjacent to the dorsal root ganglion for cervicobrachial pain: a prospective double blind randomized study. *Neurosurgery.* 1996;38:1127–1131; discussion 1131–1132.
58. Slappendel R, Crul BJ, Braak GJ, et al. The efficacy of radiofrequency lesioning of the cervical spinal dorsal root ganglion in a double blinded randomized study: no difference between 40 degrees C and 67 degrees C treatments. *Pain.* 1997;73:159–163.
59. Van Zundert J, Patijn J, Kessels A, Lame I, van Suijlekom H, van Kleef M. Pulsed radiofrequency adjacent to the cervical dorsal root ganglion in chronic cervical radicular pain: a double blind sham controlled randomized clinical trial. *Pain.* 2007;127:173–182.
60. Cahana A, Van Zundert J, Macrea L, van Kleef M, Sluijter M. Pulsed radiofrequency: current clinical and biological literature available. *Pain Med.* 2006;7:411–423.
61. Persson LC, Carlsson CA, Carlsson JY. Long-lasting cervical radicular pain managed with surgery, physiotherapy, or a cervical collar. A prospective, randomized study. *Spine.* 1997;22:751–758.
62. Kadanka Z, Bednarik J, Vohanka S, et al. Conservative treatment versus surgery in spondylotic cervical myelopathy: a prospective randomised study. *Eur Spine J.* 2000;9:538–544.
63. Melzack R, Wall PD. Pain mechanisms: a new theory. *Science.* 1965;150:971–979.
64. Huntoon MA. Cervical spine: case presentation, complications, and their prevention. *Pain Med.* 2008;9:S35–S40.
65. Waldman SD. *Interventional Pain Management.* Philadelphia, PA: Saunders, W.B.; 2001.
66. Larkin TM, Carragee E, Cohen S. A novel technique for delivery of epidural steroids and diagnosing the level of nerve root pathology. *J Spinal Disord Tech.* 2003;16:186–192.
67. Racz GB, Heavner JE. Cervical spinal canal loculation and secondary ischemic cord injury—PVCS—perivenous counter spread—danger sign! *Pain Pract.* 2008;8:399–403.

5 Cervical Facet Pain

Maarten van Eerd, Jacob Patijn, Arno Lataster, Richard W. Rosenquist, Maarten van Kleef, Nagy Mekhail and Jan Van Zundert

Introduction

Neck pain is defined as pain in the area between the base of the skull and the first thoracic vertebra. Pain extending into adjacent regions is defined as radiating neck pain. Pain may radiate into the head (cervicogenic headache), shoulder, or upper arm (radicular or nonradicular pain).[1]

Neck pain is common in the general population with a 12-month prevalence that varies between 30% and 50%. Neck pain results in incapacity to perform daily activities in 2% to 11% of the cases. It occurs more often in women, with peak prevalence in middle age.

Risk factors include genetic disposition and smoking.[2] Although a correlation between type of work and neck pain has not been demonstrated, high quantitative job demands (e.g., sedentary jobs at a computer or repetitive precision work with a high level of muscular tension) and lack of social support in the work environment appear to have an effect.[3,4] Psychological factors such as avoidance behavior and catastrophizing are not related to neck symptoms, in contrast to patients with low back problems.[3] Although trauma-related neck pain (whiplash-associated disorders; WADs) and degenerative neck problems both may be caused by chronic degeneration of the facet joints, the distinction is made on etiologic basis, because WADs may involve other painful structures, certainly in the subacute phase.[3] The causes of neck pain often are unclear, but the following innervated structures in the neck may be sources of pain: vertebrae, disci intervertebrales, uncovertebral (Luschka) joints, ligaments, muscles, and facet (zygapophyseal) joints.[3] Osseous and fibrocartilaginous degenerative disorders, identified by plain radiography, are frequently seen. The relationship between degenerative signs and pain, however, is unclear. There is a great deal of research into degenerative signs of the cervical vertebral column. In the discus intervertebralis, (1) annular tears, (2) disk prolapse, (3) endplate damage and internal disk disruption have been identified as potential structural disk pathologies.[5] Other structures in the neck, such as facet joints and uncovertebral joints, also show degenerative signs. The hypothesis that disk degeneration and disk narrowing increase facet joint loading and consequently facet osteoarthritis, seems plausible, but has yet to be proven. Some researchers claim that the disk and the facet joints can be seen as independent pain generators.[6] Confirmation of degenerative disease is mainly based on radiological findings. Spondolysis (disorders of the nonsynovial joints) and osteoarthritis (facet osteoarthritis) are frequent in advanced age. Degenerative disorders are usually seen at the low and midcervical levels (C4 to C5, C5 to C6, and C6 to C7). Knowledge of the innervation of various structures in the neck is important to interpret diagnostic blocks and to direct local treatments[7] (Figure 5.1).

Patients presenting to a pain clinic usually suffer from chronic pain (pain lasting longer than 3 months). Prognostic factors for chronicity include age (older than 40 years of age), previous episodes of neck pain, trauma, and simultaneous low back pain symptoms.[8]

It is important to determine if the pain symptoms produce functional limitations (e.g., in dressing, lifting, automobile operation, reading, sleeping, and working).

Recently, the following classification for neck pain and associated symptoms has been proposed:[9]

- Grade I neck pain: no symptoms indicating serious pathology and minimal influence on daily activities.
- Grade II neck pain: no symptoms indicating serious pathology, but having influence on daily activities.
- Grade III neck pain: no symptoms indicating serious pathology, presence of neurological disorders such as decreased reflexes, muscle weakness, or decreased sensory function.

Evidence-Based Interventional Pain Medicine: According to Clinical Diagnoses, First Edition. Edited by Jan Van Zundert, Jacob Patijn, Craig T. Hartrick, Arno Lataster, Frank J.P.M Huygen, Nagy Mekhail, Maarten van Kleef.

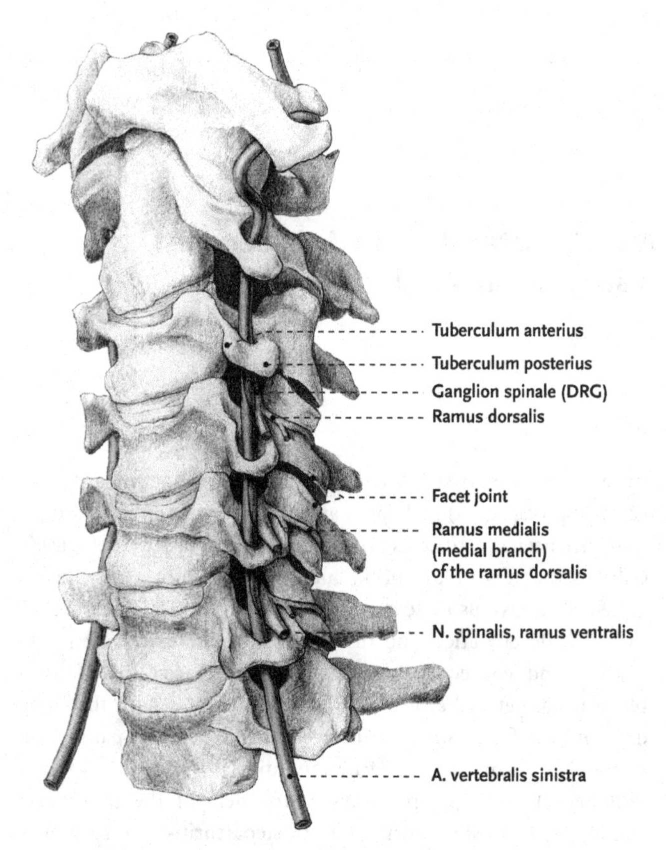

Figure 5.1. Innervation of the cervical vertebral column and the facet joints (illustration: Rogier Trompert Medical Art. www.medical-art.nl).

• Grade IV neck pain: indications of serious underlying pathology such as fracture, myelopathy, or neoplasm.

Pain originating from the cervical facet joints (facet joint syndrome)

Neck pain can be caused by the facet joints. Compared with research on lumbar facet pain, research on cervical facet dysfunction started much later. In 1988, Bogduk and Marsland[10] described the positive effect of injection of local anesthetics close to the facet joints in patients with neck pain.

While a diagnosis is defined as a clinical picture with known etiology and prognosis, a syndrome is a combination of symptoms occurring at a higher frequency in a certain population.

The cervical facet syndrome is defined as a combination of symptoms:

• axial neck pain (either not or rarely radiating past the shoulders)
• pain with pressure on the dorsal side of the spinal column at the level of the facet joints
• pain and limitation of extension and rotation
• absence of neurological symptoms

It is unclear how often neck pain originates from the facet joints. The prevalence of pain emanating from facet joints, within a population suffering from neck pain, has been reported to be 25% to 65%, depending on patient group and selection method. In the group of patients attending a pain clinic for neck pain, it is likely to be more than 50%.[11,12] This is a markedly higher percentage than facet pain in the lumbar region.

Anatomy of the facet joints

The facet joint is a diarthrotic joint with joint surfaces, synovial membrane, and a joint capsule. It forms an angle of approximately 45° with the longitudinal axis throughout the cervical spinal column. Compared with the lumbar facet joints, the cervical facet joints have a higher density of mechanoreceptors. The facet joints from C3 to C7 are innervated by the ramus medialis (medial branch) of the ramus dorsalis of the segmental nerve. Each facet joint is innervated by nerve branches from the upper and lower segment[7] (Figure 5.1).

Diagnosis

History

During the history, attention should be paid to signs and symptoms potentially indicating a serious underlying pathology ("red flags"). It is important to question the patient about previous trauma and previous or ongoing oncological treatments. Signs of potential spinal metastases are (1) history of malignancy, (2) pain starting after the age of 50, (3) continuous pain, independent of posture or movement, and (4) pain at night. When symptoms such as weight loss, fever, nausea, vomiting, dysphagia, coughing, or frequent infections are reported, extensive history and further examination is mandatory.

The most common symptom associated with pain arising from the cervical facet joints is unilateral pain, not radiating past the shoulder. The pain often has a static component, since it does not always occur in relation to movement. Rotation and retroflexion are usually reported as painful or limited. Dwyer et al. showed that injection of irritating substances into the facet joints results in a specific radiation pattern[13] (Figure 5.2). The same radiation pattern is seen with mechanical and electrical stimulation. The radiation pattern is not distinctive for facet problems but can indicate the segmental localization.

Physical examination

Neurological tests (reflexes, sensibility, and motor function) are necessary in order to exclude radiculopathy. In order to examine the function of the neck the following tests are important:

• flexion and extension—passive and active
• lateral flexion—passive and active
• rotation—passive and active
• rotation in maximal flexion—passive and active
• rotation in extension—passive and active

Rotation in a neutral position involves the rotation movement of the entire cervical spinal column. Rotation in flexion assesses the movement in the higher-cervical segments. Rotation in extension assesses the movement in the lower-cervical segments. Local pressure pain over the facet joints can indicate problems arising

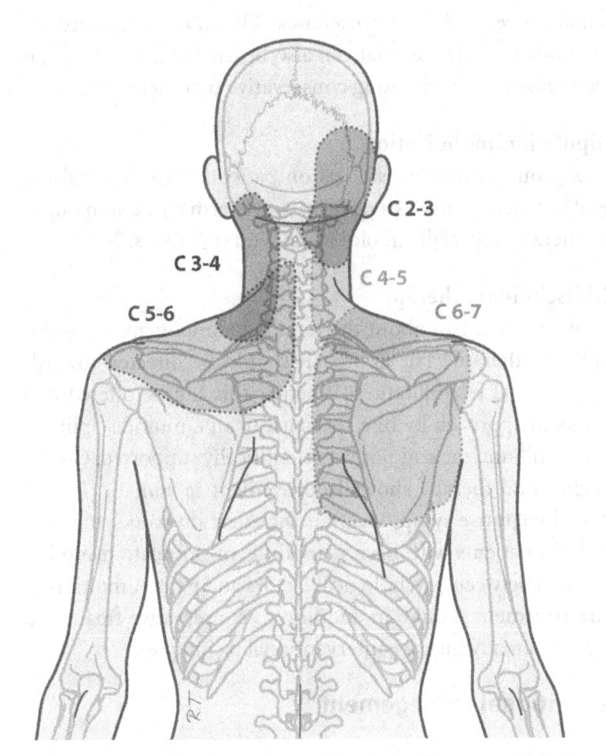

Figure 5.2. Radiation pattern of cervical facet pain (illustration: Rogier Trompert Medical Art. www.medical-art.nl).

from the facet joints. Recent research demonstrated that local pressure pain, defined as pain reported after applying pressure of at least 4 kg, is a predictor of success for consequent radiofrequency (RF) treatment (see Treatment Options).[14]

When the neck pain is accompanied by radiation to the shoulder region, shoulder pathology should be excluded.

There is no evidence to support the relationship between the results of clinical examination and the anamnesis with pain originating from the cervical facet joints.[15] In daily clinical practice, history and physical examination are useful to exclude serious pathology and to obtain a working diagnosis. An indication as to the segmental level (high-mid-low-cervical) involved can be obtained.

Additional tests

In specific cases, plain radiography of the cervical spinal column may be indicated to exclude tumor or fracture. Plain radiography does not provide information in establishing the diagnosis of facet problems, but may help in evaluating the degree of degeneration. The anterior spinal column is inspected for narrowing of the disk, anterior and posterior osteophyte formation. The posterior spinal column is inspected for facet osteoarthritis (facet sclerosis and osteophyte formation). In 1963, Kellgren et al.[16] stated that once degenerative changes are seen on plain radiography, degeneration has already reached an advanced stage.

With advancing age, degenerative changes are more frequently seen: 25% at the age of 50, up to 75% at the age of 70.[17] An age-related prevalence study concerning the facet joint involvement in chronic neck pain indicates a comparable prevalence among all age groups.[18]

Degenerative changes of the cervical spinal column are present in asymptomatic patients, indicating that degenerative changes do not always cause pain. However, the conclusion that there is no relation between degeneration and pain cannot be drawn. There are studies indicating a relation between degenerative changes and pain symptoms.[17,19]

In summary, a relation between radiologic identification of degenerative changes and pain symptoms has not been proven. If a neurological etiology of the pain symptoms is suspected, a magnetic resonance imaging (MRI) or computer tomography (CT) scan is indicated. Depending on the clinical setting, consultation of or referral to a neurologist should be considered. The use of cervical discography may help in identifying the source of pain, but its value concerning the subsequent therapeutic treatments is not established.

Diagnostic blocks

The working diagnosis of facet pain, based on history and clinical examination, may be confirmed by performing a diagnostic block. Local anesthetic can be injected intra-articularly or adjacent to the ramus medialis (medial branch) of the ramus dorsalis of the segmental nerve.[3,20] These procedures are performed under fluoroscopy. There is no consensus about the definition of a successful diagnostic block. Some authors claim that 100% pain relief should be achieved.[21] But Cohen et al. showed that there is no difference in outcome of the RF treatment of patients reporting 80% and those reporting more than 50% pain reduction after a diagnostic block.[14] In daily clinical practice, we consider a diagnostic block successful if more than 50% pain reduction is reported.

It has been demonstrated that innervation of the facet joint occurs via the ramus medialis (medial branch) of the ramus dorsalis. We prefer a block of the ramus medialis (medial branch) instead of an intra-articular block, because it is not always technically possible to position a needle into the facet joint. According to Bogduk and McGuirk,[3] the facet joints from C3 to C7 are innervated by the medial branches of the nerves above and below the joint. For a block or RF treatment, for example, of the C4 to C5 facet joint to be effective, the medial branches of the rami dorsales of C4 and C5 are to be treated.

A prognostic block can be used before RF treatment is performed. A prognostic block assumes that if an anatomical structure is injected with a local anesthetic resulting in a decrease in pain, this structure is the source of pain. This appears to be a useful concept. Research and clinical experience indicate however, that after a single block, only a small percentage (2/47; ~4%) of patients have no pain reduction.[22] This means that after a single diagnostic block, there are very few false negative results. In order to minimize the number of false positives, a number of researchers have suggested that a second block should be carried out using a local anesthetic with different duration of effect, e.g., lidocaine vs. bupivacaine (comparative double blocks). Only if the patient responds concordantly (longer or shorter pain reduction depending on the duration of action of the local anesthetic) is this indicative of facet joint pain. This is a pharmacological criterion. These researchers suggest that double blocks are the gold standard for the diagnosis of facet pain. A gold standard, however, should be generally accepted and used.

The concept of double blocks has theoretical and practical shortcomings. A decrease in the number of false positives can occur at the cost of the number of false negative reactions: patients respond positive to the local anesthetic, but not according to the previously standardized pharmacological criterion. Furthermore, a cervical injection represents a burden for the patient. Finally, it is questionable if double blocks are cost-effective.[23] A best evidence synthesis on the assessment of neck pain concluded that diagnostic facet injections have not been validated to identify facet joint pain.[24] As long as the relationship with the etiology of facet pain is not clearly established, the extra burden of performing double blocks cannot be justified. Contrary to lumbar facet blocks, only a small percentage of patients have a negative response to a single cervical facet block.

In summary, on the basis of history and physical examination, a working diagnosis of cervical facet pain is defined. Confirmation of the working diagnosis can be recommended with the diagnostic block at minimum 3 levels of the ramus medialis (medial branch) of the cervical ramus dorsalis in one session. A diagnostic block is considered positive when the patient experiences a 50% pain reduction.[14]

Differential diagnosis

Serious causes of neck pain such as tumors, infections, fractures, and systemic diseases are rare. A clinically relevant prolapsed disk or cervical spondylotic myelopathy can both cause neurological symptoms. Every patient with motor function loss and/or reflex changes and/or sensory loss must be thoroughly assessed. Metastases, cervical herniated nucleus pulposus with radiculopathy, discitis, and vertebral fractures should be excluded through history and (additional) tests. Diagnoses such as segmental dysfunction, instability, and muscle strain as diagnoses of chronic pain are not sufficiently documented to be included in the differential diagnosis.[3]

Treatment options

Conservative management

Physiotherapy/exercise therapy

In a study comparing physiotherapy with a short intervention consisting of a self-management program that encourages patients to resume normal activity patterns, physiotherapy resulted in a better outcome.[25] The improvements with both interventions are, however, small (on all outcome scales). Physical exercises have a pain reducing effect, especially if the patient received adequate information relative to the exercises. Physiotherapy, based on instructions for exercises that can also be carried out at home, is the best choice when choosing conservative treatment.

Manipulation/mobilization

In a subgroup analysis of studies on patients with neck pain in general practice, there was a positive short-term effect of manipulation therapy, especially in older (>50 years) patients.[26]

Multidisciplinary therapy

There is no consensus about the required components of multidisciplinary therapy. The approach should be directed towards biopsychosocial rehabilitation. Whether this can be offered as a multimodal approach by one specialist or in a multidisciplinary setting is still unclear and not yet scientifically supported. Cognitive behavioral therapy shows improvement in somatic, behavioral, and cognitive symptoms, but the effect on pain symptoms is small. In patients with neck pain, little, or no relationship has been found between psychological factors and pain. A multidisciplinary treatment should, in addition to conservative treatment, include minimally invasive interventional techniques.

Interventional management

Intra-articular steroid injections

No reports from quality studies regarding the effect of intra-articular steroid injections are currently known.[27] There are no comparative studies between intra-articular steroid injections and RF therapy.

Local infiltration of the ramus medialis (medial branch) of the ramus dorsalis

Medial branch block of the ramus dorsalis of the segmental nerve is primarily considered as a diagnostic aid; however, (repetitive) infiltration of local anesthetic was shown to provide therapeutic effect.[22,28] In a randomized controlled trial (RCT) comparing the effect of medial branch blocks with bupivacaine alone to blocks with the same local anesthetic plus steroid, a comparable pain reduction was observed in both groups for mean duration of 14 and 16 weeks, respectively. During the follow-up period of 1 year, the mean number of procedures was similar (3.5 and 3.4, respectively). Patients were selected for participation in this study by controlled blocks providing ≥80% pain relief.[28] These findings suggest that the addition of corticosteroid to local anesthetic does not provide better outcome. Moreover, as described above, the diagnostic procedure used in the RCT is burdensome for the patient, requiring repeat infiltrations every 14 to 16 weeks. Therefore, this cannot be recommended as first-line therapy.

RF treatment of the ramus medialis (medial branch) of the ramus dorsalis

Percutaneous RF treatment of cervical pain has been intensively studied. The data from original articles were summarized in seven systematic reviews.[20,27–29–32] There is only one RCT evaluating RF treatment of the ramus medialis (medial branch) of the ramus dorsalis, but this was in patients with WADs.[21] Consequently, this RCT cannot be rated in the evidence scoring for degenerative cervical facet joint pain. The effectiveness of RF treatment for degenerative neck pathology was shown in observational studies.[14,33,34] A retrospective chart analysis on the effect of repeat RF facet denervations illustrated that the mean duration of effect of the first intervention was 12.5 months. Patients who responded positively to the first intervention received from one to six additional interventions. After each intervention (multiple level treatment of the ramus medialis of the ramus dorsalis), more than 90% of the patients had satisfactory pain relief, and duration of effect was between 8 and 12 months.[35]

Lord et al.[21] described a technique for approaching the ramus medialis (medial branch) of the ramus dorsalis laterally as well as posteriorly. This can only be carried out in the prone position.

Good results have also been reported using an alternative technique as described by Sluijter, van Kleef and van Suijlekom.[36,37] Theoretically, a block of the ramus medialis (medial branch), close to the ramus dorsalis, based on sensory and motor stimulation parameters, could generate a similar effect as an extensive denervation over the entire length of the nerve. Even though there are no studies comparing both techniques, we consider the former to be the least invasive approach. Percutaneous cervical facet denervation is an acceptable treatment option for a clinical diagnosis of chronic degenerative cervical facet pain, given the many observational descriptions of a positive effect.

Complications of interventional management

Complications are rare. Nevertheless, one should be aware that the arteria vertebralis may be punctured if the needle is pushed too far anteriorly into the foramen intervertebrale. Verification of the needle position should be made under antero-posterior fluoroscopy to prevent intrathecal injection or injection of the local anesthetic into the spinal cord. In an observational study, the incidence of inadvertent intravascular penetration for medial branch blocks at spinal level was reported to be 3.9%, comparable with the incidence at lumbar level (3.7%). Some patients experienced short-term vasovagal reactions. The intravascular uptake of local anesthetic and contrast solution (due to direct injection into a vessel) was thought to be responsible for false negative diagnostic blocks. No systemic effects were reported.[38] A report on transient tetraplegia after cervical facet joint injection, done without imaging, illustrates the vulnerability of the cervical arteries.[39]Appropriate monitoring of the vital signs and availability of resuscitation equipment are essential.

Infections have been described, but the incidence is unknown and probably very low.[40]

A recent report on septic arthritis of the facet joints included two cases of cervical facet joints. In these cases, the port of entry could not be identified, but in one lumbar case report, percutaneous injection was directly linked to this severe complication.[41] Other potential complications of facet joint interventions are related to needle placement and drug administration; they include dural puncture, spinal cord trauma, spinal anesthesia, chemical meningitis, neural trauma, pneumothorax, radiation exposure, facet capsule rupture, hematoma formation, and side effects of corticosteroids.[42]

After RF treatment, postoperative burning pain is regularly reported. This pain disappears after 1 to 3 weeks.[43] Smith et al.[44] found contrast enhancement on MRI typical for paraspinal abscess, even without apparent infection, which was attributed to a noninfectious postinflammatory process. There are no incidence data on side effects and complications following cervical RF facet denervation. At the lumbar level, the incidence of complications was lower than 1%.[45]

Surgical treatments

Anterior cervical fusion is described as a possible technique for nonradicular neck pain. One study showed a clear effect on pain and function, but the long-term effect of this invasive treatment is unknown.[46]

Evidence for interventional management.

A summary of the available evidence is given in Table 5.1

Table 5.1. Summary of evidence for interventional management of cervical facet pain.

Technique	Score
Intra-articular injections	0
Therapeutic (repetitive) ramus medialis (medial branch) of the cervical ramus dorsalis block (local anesthetic with or without corticosteroid)	2 B+
Radiofrequency treatment of the ramus medialis (medial branch) of the cervical ramus dorsalis	2 C+

Recommendations

For patients suffering chronic neck pain caused by cervical arthrosis, not responding to conservative treatment, RF treatment of the ramus medialis (medial branch) of the ramus dorsalis of the segmental nerves from C3 to C6 can be considered.

The use of repetitive blocks with local anesthetic with or without corticosteroid places a serious burden on the patient and is therefore not recommended as first line treatment.

Clinical practice algorithm

A practice algorithm for the management of facet pain is illustrated in Figure 5.3.

Technique(s)

Percutaneous facet denervation

The (postero-) lateral approach in the supine position is described below (Figure 5.4). The advantage of this technique is that it is possible to maintain eye contact with the patient. Sedation is rarely required.

The patient is placed in the supine position with the head slightly extended on a small cushion. The C-arm is placed in an

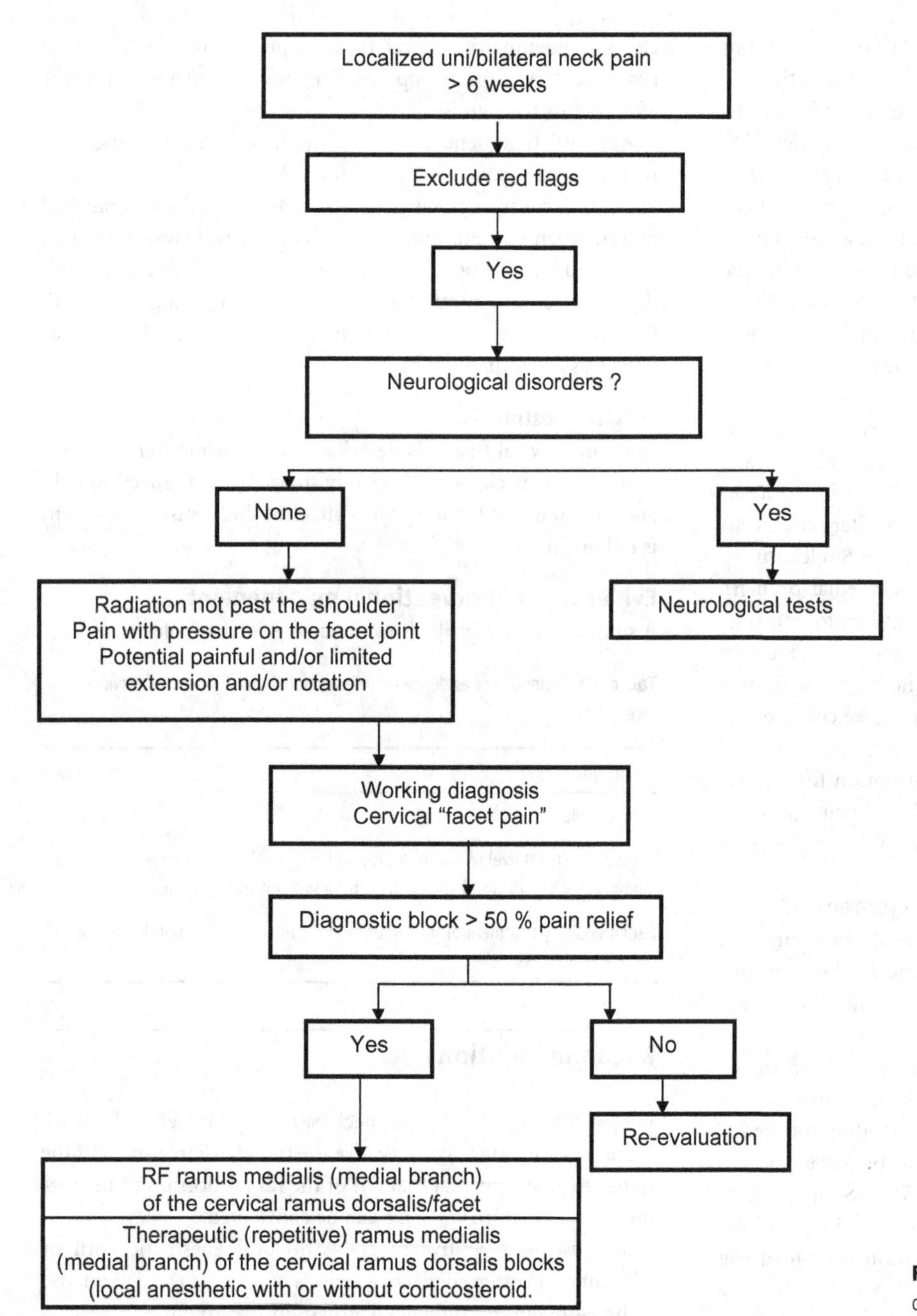

Figure 5.3. Clinical practice algorithm for treatment of cervical facet pain. RF, radiofrequency treatment.

oblique position (20 to 30° laterally). In this position, the beam runs parallel with the exiting nerve root that runs somewhat caudofrontal. In this position, the pedicles from the contralateral side are projected onto the anterior half of the corpus vertebrae Figure 5.5. In the AP projection, the C-arm is positioned 10 to 20° caudally. In this position, the discus intervertebralis space and the foramen intervertebrale are visible (Figure 5.6). The ramus medialis (medial branch) of the ramus dorsalis runs over the base of the processus articularis superior. The injection point is marked on the skin, slightly posterior and caudal to the end point of the needle that is dorsal to the posterior boundary of the facet column. The first needle is introduced in a horizontal plane, slightly cranially so that the tip of the needle points in the direction of the end point. It is important to understand that this is not a "tunnel-view" technique. The needle is slowly advanced anteriorly and cranially until bony contact with the facet column occurs. The further the needle is advanced, the more difficult it becomes to change the direction. Therefore, the position of the needle needs to be checked frequently. If the needle points too much in the direction of the foramen intervertebrale, without contacting bone, the direction needs to be corrected to be more posterior. If there is no bone contact in the posterior direction,

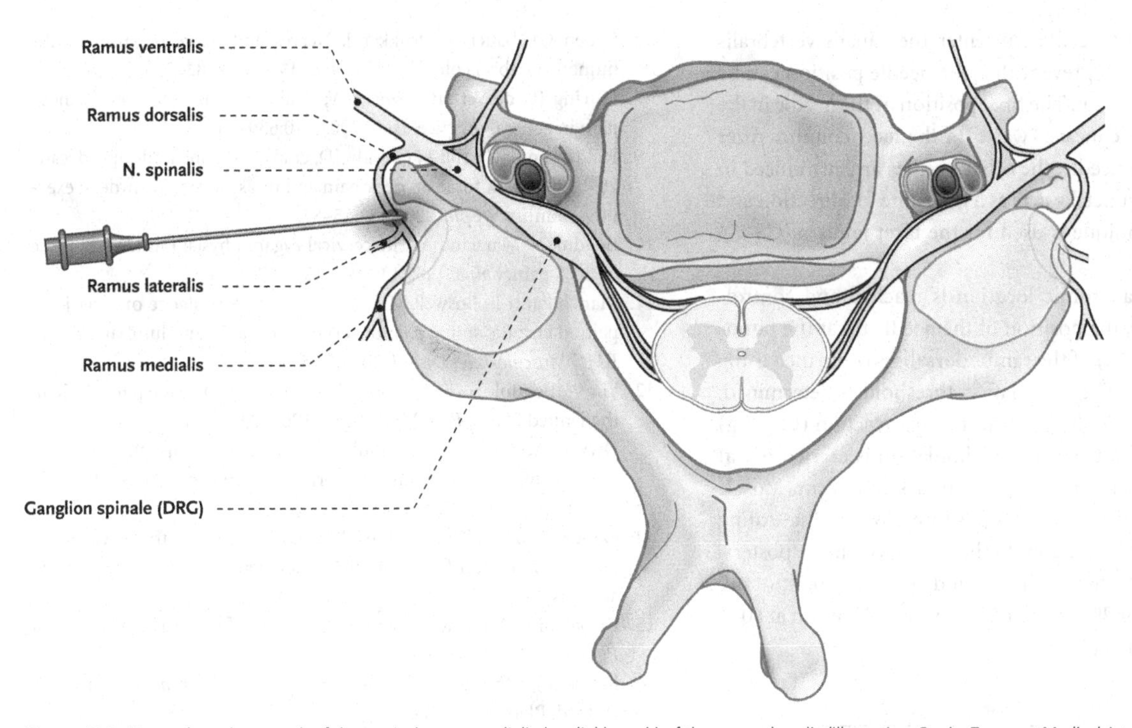

Figure 5.4. Posterolateral approach of the cervical ramus medialis (medial branch) of the ramus dorsalis (illustration: Rogier Trompert Medical Art. www.medical-art.nl).

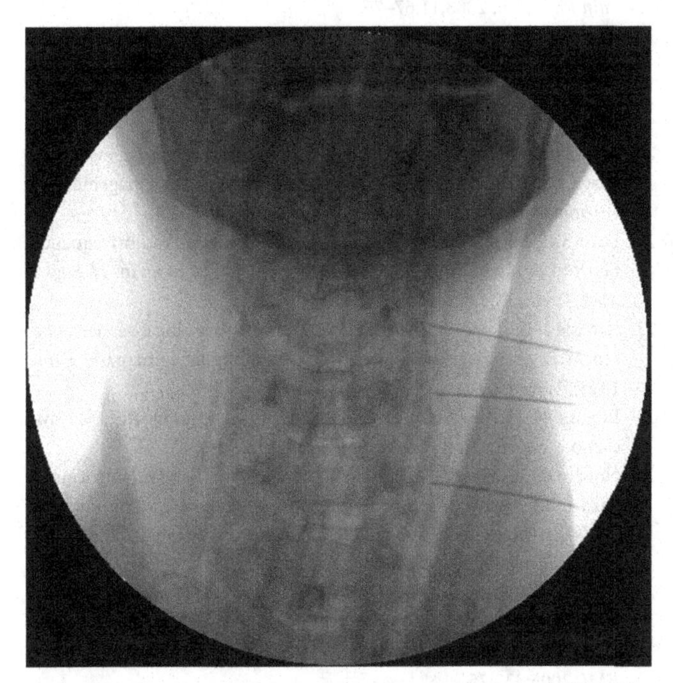

Figure 5.5. Radiofrequency treatment cervical ramus medialis (medial branch) of the ramus dorsalis /facet C4, C5, C6 left: antero posterior projection.

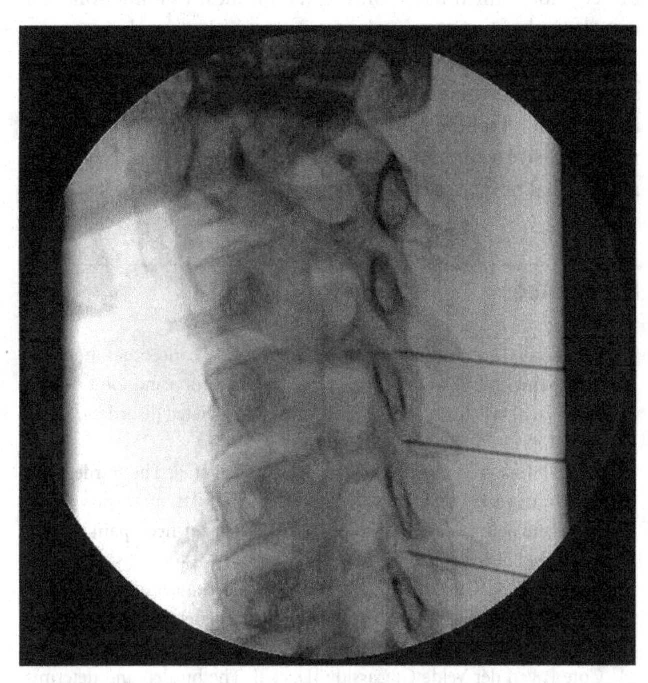

Figure 5.6. Radiofrequency treatment cervical ramus medialis (medial branch) of the ramus dorsalis/facet C4, C5, C6 left: ¾ projection.

there is a risk that the needle will enter the canalis vertebralis between the laminae. To prevent this, the needle position can be checked in the AP direction. The final position of the needle in the AP direction is in the concave "waist" of the facet column. After placement of the first needle, the other needles are introduced in the same way. The first needle acts as a guideline for direction and depth. The same technique is used for the facet joints of C3–C4 to C6–C7.

Once an optimal anatomic location is reached and controlled using fluoroscopy, the position of the needle tip at the ramus medialis (medial branch) of the ramus dorsalis is confirmed using electrical stimulation. The stimulation threshold is determined: an electrical stimulation of 50 Hz must give a reaction (tingling) in the neck at less than 0.5 V. Then stimulation is carried out at 2 Hz. Contractions of the paraspinal muscles can occur. Muscle contractions in the arm indicate a position close to the exiting segmental nerve. The needle should then be placed more posteriorly. Once the correct position has been determined, 0.5 to 1 mL local anesthetic (1% or 2% lidocaine) is given. A RF lesion at 80°C for 60 seconds is carried out.

Summary

Neck pain is common in the general population. The etiology is difficult to confirm based on history, physical examination, and radiological tests. Conservative treatment is the first choice.

At the cervical level, the facet joint appears to be an important source of pain with degenerative neck symptoms. Where there is an indication that the pain is arising from the facet joints, a minimally invasive technique such as RF treatment of the ramus medialis (medial branch) of the ramus dorsalis may be considered.

References

1. Guzman J, Hurwitz EL, Carroll LJ, et al. A new conceptual model of neck pain: linking onset, course, and care: the bone and joint decade 2000–2010 task force on neck pain and its associated disorders. *Spine.* 2008;33:S14–S23.
2. Hogg-Johnson S, van der Velde G, Carroll LJ, et al. The burden and determinants of neck pain in the general population: results of the bone and joint decade 2000–2010 task force on neck pain and its associated disorders. *Spine.* 2008;33:S39–S51.
3. Bogduk N, McGuirk B. *Management of Acute and Chronic Neck Pain. Pain Research and Clinical Management.* Philadelphia, PA: Elsevier; 2006.
4. Cote P, van der Velde G, Cassidy JD, et al. The burden and determinants of neck pain in workers: results of the bone and joint decade 2000–2010 task force on neck pain and its associated disorders. *Spine (Phila Pa 1976).* 2008;33:S60–S74.
5. Adams MA, Roughley PJ. What is intervertebral disc degeneration, and what causes it? *Spine.* 2006;31:2151–2161.
6. Bogduk N, Aprill C. On the nature of neck pain, discography and cervical zygapophysial joint blocks. *Pain.* 1993;54:213–217.
7. Groen GJ, Baljet B, Drukker J. Nerves and nerve plexuses of the human vertebral column. *Am J Anat.* 1990;188:282–296.
8. Hoving JL, de Vet HC, Twisk JW, et al. Prognostic factors for neck pain in general practice. *Pain.* 2004;110:639–645.
9. Haldeman S, Carroll L, Cassidy JD, et al. The bone and joint decade 2000–2010 task force on neck pain and its associated disorders: executive summary. *Spine.* 2008;33:S5–S7.
10. Bogduk N, Marsland A. The cervical zygapophysial joints as a source of neck pain. *Spine.* 1988;13:610–617.
11. Manchikanti L, Boswell MV, Singh V, et al. Prevalence of facet joint pain in chronic spinal pain of cervical, thoracic, and lumbar regions. *BMC Musculoskelet Disord.* 2004;5:15.
12. Yin W, Bogduk N. The nature of neck pain in a private pain clinic in the United States. *Pain Med.* 2008;9:196–203.
13. Dwyer A, Aprill C, Bogduk N. Cervical zygapophyseal joint pain patterns. I: a study in normal volunteers. *Spine.* 1990;15: 453–457.
14. Cohen SP, Bajwa ZH, Kraemer JJ, et al. Factors predicting success and failure for cervical facet radiofrequency denervation: a multi-center analysis. *Reg Anesth Pain Med.* 2007;32:495–503.
15. Kirpalani D, Mitra R. Cervical facet joint dysfunction: a review. *Arch Phys Med Rehabil.* 2008;89:770–774.
16. Kellgren J, Jeffrey M, Ball J. *The Epidemiology of Chronic Rheumatism.* Oxford: Blackwell; 1963.
17. Friedenberg ZB, Miller WT. Degenerative disc disease of the cervical spine. *J Bone Joint Surg Am.* 1963;45:1171–1178.
18. Manchikanti L, Manchikanti KN, Cash KA, et al. Age-related prevalence of facet-joint involvement in chronic neck and low back pain. *Pain Physician.* 2008;11:67–75.
19. van der Donk J, Schouten JS, Passchier J, et al. The associations of neck pain with radiological abnormalities of the cervical spine and personality traits in a general population. *J Rheumatol.* 1991;18:1884–1889.
20. Manchikanti L, Boswell MV, Singh V, et al. Comprehensive evidence-based guidelines for interventional techniques in the management of chronic spinal pain. *Pain Physician.* 2009;12:699–802.
21. Lord SM, Barnsley L, Wallis BJ, et al. Percutaneous radio-frequency neurotomy for chronic cervical zygapophyseal-joint pain. *N Engl J Med.* 1996;335:1721–1726.
22. Barnsley L, Lord S, Bogduk N. Comparative local anaesthetic blocks in the diagnosis of cervical zygapophysial joint pain. *Pain.* 1993;55:99–106.
23. Bogduk N, Holmes S. Controlled zygapophysial joint blocks: the travesty of cost-effectiveness. *Pain Med.* 2000;1:24–34.
24. Nordin M, Carragee EJ, Hogg-Johnson S, et al. Assessment of neck pain and its associated disorders: results of the bone and joint decade 2000–2010 task force on neck pain and its associated disorders. *J Manipulative Physiol Ther.* 2009;32:S117–S140.
25. Klaber Moffett JA, Jackson DA, Richmond S, et al. Randomised trial of a brief physiotherapy intervention compared with usual physiotherapy for neck pain patients: outcomes and patients' preference. *BMJ.* 2005;330:75.
26. Schellingerhout JM, Verhagen AP, Heymans MW, et al. Which subgroups of patients with non-specific neck pain are more likely to benefit from spinal manipulation therapy, physiotherapy, or usual care? *Pain.* 2008;139:670–680.
27. Falco FJ, Erhart S, Wargo BW, et al. Systematic review of diagnostic utility and therapeutic effectiveness of cervical facet joint interventions. *Pain Physician.* 2009;12:323–344.

28. Manchikanti L, Singh V, Falco FJ, et al. Cervical medial branch blocks for chronic cervical facet joint pain: a randomized, double-blind, controlled trial with one-year follow-up. *Spine.* 2008;33: 1813–1820.
29. Geurts JW, van Wijk RM, Stolker RJ, et al. Efficacy of radiofrequency procedures for the treatment of spinal pain: a systematic review of randomized clinical trials. *Reg Anesth Pain Med.* 2001;26:394–400.
30. Niemisto L, Kalso E, Malmivaara A, et al. Radiofrequency denervation for neck and back pain: a systematic review within the framework of the cochrane collaboration back review group. *Spine.* 2003;28:1877–1888.
31. Manchikanti L, Singh V, Vilims BD, et al. Medial branch neurotomy in management of chronic spinal pain: systematic review of the evidence. *Pain Physician.* 2002;5:405–418.
32. Boswell MV, Trescot AM, Datta S, et al. Interventional techniques: Evidence-based practice guidelines in the management of chronic spinal pain. *Pain Physician.* 2007;10:7–111.
33. McDonald GJ, Lord SM, Bogduk N. Long-term follow-up of patients treated with cervical radiofrequency neurotomy for chronic neck pain. *Neurosurgery.* 1999;45:61–67; discussion 67–68.
34. Barnsley L. Percutaneous radiofrequency neurotomy for chronic neck pain: outcomes in a series of consecutive patients. *Pain Med.* 2005;6:282–286.
35. Husted DS, Orton D, Schofferman J, et al. Effectiveness of repeated radiofrequency neurotomy for cervical facet joint pain. *J Spinal Disord Tech.* 2008;21:406–408.
36. Sluijter ME. *Radiofrequency Part 2.* Meggen (LU), Switzerland: Flivopress, SA; 2003.
37. van Kleef M, van Suijlekom JA. Treatment of chronic cervical pain, brachialgia, and cervicogenic headache by means of radiofrequency procedures. *Pain Pract.* 2002;2:214–223.
38. Verrills P, Mitchell B, Vivian D, et al. The incidence of intravascular penetration in medial branch blocks: cervical, thoracic, and lumbar spines. *Spine.* 2008;33:E174–E177.
39. Heckmann JG, Maihofner C, Lanz S, et al. Transient tetraplegia after cervical facet joint injection for chronic neck pain administered without imaging guidance. *Clin Neurol Neurosurg.* 2006;108: 709–711.
40. Rathmell JP, Lake T, Ramundo MB. Infectious risks of chronic pain treatments: injection therapy, surgical implants, and intradiscal techniques. *Reg Anesth Pain Med.* 2006;31:346–352.
41. Michel-Batot C, Dintinger H, Blum A, et al. A particular form of septic arthritis: septic arthritis of facet joint. *Joint Bone Spine.* 2008;75:78–83.
42. Boswell MV, Colson JD, Sehgal N, et al. A systematic review of therapeutic facet joint interventions in chronic spinal pain. *Pain Physician.* 2007;10:229–253.
43. Haspeslagh SR, Van Suijlekom HA, Lame IE, et al. Randomised controlled trial of cervical radiofrequency lesions as a treatment for cervicogenic headache [isrctn07444684]. *BMC Anesthesiol.* 2006; 16:1.
44. Smith M, Ferretti G, Mortazavi S. Radiographic changes induced after cervical facet radiofrequency denervation. *Spine J.* 2005;5: 668–671.
45. Kornick C, Kramarich SS, Lamer TJ, et al. Complications of lumbar facet radiofrequency denervation. *Spine.* 2004;29:1352–1354.
46. Garvey TA, Transfeldt EE, Malcolm JR, et al. Outcome of anterior cervical discectomy and fusion as perceived by patients treated for dominant axial-mechanical cervical spine pain. *Spine.* 2002;27:1887–1895; discussion 1895.

6 Cervicogenic Headache

Hans van Suijlekom, Jan Van Zundert, Samer Narouze, Maarten van Kleef and Nagy Mekhail

Introduction

The prevalence of Cervicogenic headache (CEH), according to the criteria of Sjaastad et al.[1] is 1%.[2] Depending upon the population studied (population-based vs. hospital-based) and the criteria used, the prevalence has been reported between 2.5% and 13.8%.[3,4]

Besides the criteria for CEH from the Cervicogenic Headache International Study Group[1] (CHISG) (Table 6.1), the International Headache Society also published diagnostic criteria for CEH (Table 6.2).[5] Both definitions are used in clinical practice.

CEH is a clinically defined headache syndrome arising from cervical nociceptive structures. Bogduk stated that all structures (e.g., facet joints, disci intervertebrales, muscles and ligaments) that can be innervated by the segmental nerves from C1–C3 are possible sources for CEH.[6] The Quebec Headache Study group in 1993 stated that cervical facet dysfunction is probably the most important clinical source.[7]

The nucleus trigeminocervicalis is central to the postulated mechanism of CEH. This nucleus is formed by the pars caudalis of the spinal nucleus nervi trigemini and the grey matter from the upper 3 cervical spinal cord segments.[8] Nociceptive afferents of the nervus trigeminus and the first 3 cervical nerves interact here and form multiple collateral nerve endings.[9] In the nucleus trigeminocervicalis nerve endings appear to overlap and converge on second-order neurons.[10] This convergence forms the basis of the referred pain. Convergence between the nervus trigeminus and cervical afferents can result in cervical pain which is felt in the sensory receptive fields of the nervus trigeminus.[11]

Diagnosis

History

The patient usually seeks help for the headache symptoms arising from the neck. For the case history, a number of general questions should be posed such as: duration of the symptoms, frequency, localization, provocative factors, signs of migraine, trauma, medications, treatments already applied, family history, and so forth. By posing specific questions, a clear working diagnosis can be obtained (Table 6.1). CEH is principally a unilateral headache but can also occur bilaterally. The pain usually begins in the neck and radiates outward to the fronto-temporal and possibly to the supra-orbital area. The headache is usually nagging and non-pulsating in character. The pain can occur in attacks; the duration of an attack is unpredictable (hours to days). The pattern of the attacks can also change into a chronic fluctuating headache. Symptoms which suggest the involvement of the cervical spinal column are essential, such as limited movement of the neck, provocation of the neck/headache symptoms with mechanical stimuli, etc. (Table 6.1). Migraine-like symptoms such as nausea, vomiting, and photophobia are, if present, usually mild in character. Positive response to a diagnostic/prognostic block with a local anesthetic confirms the diagnosis of CEH.

Physical examination

Physical examination of the neck encompasses several elements:

1 Movement tests of the cervical spinal column: passive flexion, retroflexion, lateroflexion, and rotation should be assessed on limitation of movement.
2 Segmental palpation of the cervical facet joints.
3 Assessment of the following "pressure points":
   - Nervus occipitalis major (occipital-temporal part of the skull);
   - Nervus occipitalis minor (attachment of the musculus sternocleidomastoideus to the skull);
   - Third cervical nerve root (facet joint C2–C3);
   - Pressure pain anterior, posterior, and on the ventral musculus trapezius border;[12]
   - The assessment of the "pressure points" aims at getting an indication of the segmental level, where the nociceptive stimulus possibly occurs. It should be noted that there is

Evidence-Based Interventional Pain Medicine: According to Clinical Diagnoses, First Edition. Edited by Jan Van Zundert, Jacob Patijn, Craig T. Hartrick, Arno Lataster, Frank J.P.M Huygen, Nagy Mekhail, Maarten van Kleef.

Table 6.1. Diagnostic criteria for CEH according to Sjaastad.[1]

1. Symptoms that indicate pain arises from the neck:
   a. Provocation of the headache radiating from the neck by:
      Neck movement and/or continuous backward tilting of the head; and/or
      External pressure on the occipital or higher cervical region on the symptomatic side.
   b. Limited movement of the neck.
   c. Ipsilateral neck, shoulder- or arm-pain of a mostly nonradicular nature.
2. Positive response to diagnostic/prognostic block with a local anesthetic.
3. Unilateral headache.

The diagnosis of CEH can be made if the patient fulfills **1a** and **2**. If the patient does not exhibit the symptoms **1a**, the combination of **1b**, **1c**, **2**, and **3** is, however, very suggestive of CEH. A bilateral form of CEH is also possible.
CEH, Cervicogenic headache.

Table 6.2. Diagnostic criteria for CEH according to IHS.[5]

A. Pain, referred from a source in the neck and perceived in one or more regions of the head and/or face, fulfilling criteria C and D.

B. Clinical, laboratory, and/or imaging evidence of a disorder or lesion within the cervical spine or soft tissues of the neck known to be, or generally accepted as, a valid cause of headache.

C. Evidence that the pain can be attributed to the neck disorder or lesion based on at least one of the following:

Demonstration of clinical signs that implicate a source of pain in the neck;

Abolition of headache following diagnostic block of a cervical structure or its nerve supply using placebo- or other adequate controls.

D. Pain resolves within 3 months after successful treatment of the causative disorder or lesion.

IHS, International Headache Society.

no scientific evidence for the assessment of pressure points. Assessment is empirical and subjective. Further research is required to assess the value of such tests.

Additional tests

The relationship between radiographic changes and pain is certainly not unequivocal.[13,14] Conventional radiologic tests are therefore unsuitable in order to either include or exclude involvement of the cervical spinal column. If there are indications of "red flags," one should always carry out further diagnostic tests, such as magnetic resonance imaging and computed tomography scans.

Differential diagnosis

In the differential diagnosis of CEH, just as with other headaches, organic disorders such as a space-occupying lesion in the posterior fossa cerebellaris and other tumors, sinus thrombosis, arthritis of the cervical spinal column, etc. should be excluded. Differential diagnoses which should be noted include:

1 Migraine without aura;
2 Tension headache;
3 Cluster headache;
4 Hemicrania continua;
5 Chronic paroxysmal hemicrania (CPH).

A main diagnostic problem is to distinguish CEH from migraine without aura. Similarities include:

1 Unilaterality of the headache;
2 Occurrence predominantly in women;
3 Possible occurrence of nausea and vomiting.

However, there are also fundamental differences between migraine and CEH:

1 Unilaterality without "side shift" in CEH, while in migraine without aura there can be a shift of the headache during the same headache attack as well as between the individual headache attacks.
2 CEH usually begins in the neck while migraine usually begins in the fronto-temporal region.
3 CEH can be provoked by mechanical pressure in the upper lateral area of the cervical spinal column, on the symptomatic side, and/or with continuous backward tilting of the head; whereas, this usually does not occur with migraine.
4 In CEH, there is often a limitation of movement in the neck, which is not characteristic of migraine.
5 A nonradicular, ipsilateral diffuse shoulder/arm pain sometimes occurs in CEH but not in migraine.

Unilateral CEH is easy to differentiate from muscle tension headache, although in the bilateral form this is more difficult. However, with help from the following characteristics of CEH, it is usually possible to differentiate between CEH and muscle tension headache: provocation of the headache symptoms by mechanical pressure and/or continuous backward tilting of the head, limitation in movement of the neck, and a non-radicular, ipsilateral diffuse shoulder/arm pain.

CEH is easy to differentiate from cluster headache. Cluster headache is an excruciating unilateral headache that usually has a circadian rhythm. It can last from 20 minutes up to 3 hours. During the attack, it is often difficult for the patient to stay still secondary to the severity of the pain. Also, cluster headache is characterized by associated autonomic symptoms.

Hemicrania continua is a unilateral chronic daily headache, which can fluctuate in intensity during the day. Pathognomically, however, the headache responds well to indomethacin.

Chronic Paroxismal Hemicrania (CPH) is characterized by a high frequency of severe unilateral headache attacks of a short duration (10 to 30 minutes). CPH also responds well to indomethacin.

It is possible that a patient can experience more than one type of headache simultaneously. With a very careful case history and physical examination, it is often possible to analyze these headache types and, where possible, to treat them individually.

Treatment options

Conservative treatment

Generally, a conservative treatment should be the first option before interventional treatment is started. Conservative pain treatments include among others: medication, physiotherapy, manual therapy, and transcutaneous electrical nerve stimulation (TENS). There is no one preferred method. Usually patients with CEH, seen in a pain management centre, have already been extensively treated with conservative therapies.

TENS

TENS is an example of a noninvasive regularly used nerve stimulation technique. Farina et al.[15] demonstrated in their nonrandomized study that TENS is an effective treatment method for CEH. A randomized study in patients with CEH patients, showed a significant improvement in headache symptoms after 3 months of TENS therapy compared with the placebo group.[16]

Interventional management

Various interventional procedures for CEH have been published. A generally acceptable treatment method for CEH is not yet available. This is mainly because of the fact that the cause of CEH in general is unknown, so that many of the treatments are of a symptomatic nature.

A number of invasive procedures for patients with CEH are described below. The selection of the type of invasive treatment is guided by the case history and physical examination.

Local injections

Injections of the nervus occipitalis major with a local anesthetic with or without corticosteroids give a temporary positive effect for CEH.[17–19] A randomized study by Naja et al.[20] showed significant pain reduction after a follow-up of 2 weeks. This study was continued in the form of a prospective study whereby significant pain reduction was still achieved after a follow-up of 6 months. In this last study, 87% of the patients required an extra injection. In addition to an injection of the nervus occipitalis major, an injection of the nervus occipitalis minor was performed.[21]

Injection into the atlanto-axial joint with a local anesthetic and corticosteroid, in patients with CEH, was carried out when the clinical picture suggested atlantoaxial joint pain. There was no statistically significant difference after 6 months in this retrospective study.[22]

Radiofrequency (RF) treatment

If during a physical examination of a patient with CEH a diagnosis of segmental paravertebral pressure pain in the cervical spinal column is made, this can indicate the involvement of the cervical facet joints. In this case, a block of the ramus medialis of the cervical ramus dorsalis (cervical medial branch block) followed by percutaneous RF treatment can be performed.

In 1986, Hildebrandt et al.,[23] in an open study, reported a good result for 37%, an acceptable result for 28%, and no improvement for 35% of the patients with head and neck pain. It is not known whether these patients had CEH. The average follow-up was 12 months (range 3 to 30).

In a prospective study in patients with CEH according to the criteria of Sjaastad, receiving RF treatment of the ramus medialis (medial branch) of the cervical ramus dorsalis, the results were outstanding to good in 65%, average in 14%, and no improvement was seen in 21% of the patients, with an average follow-up of 16.8 months (range 12 to 22).[24]

Later, 2 randomized controlled trials studying the effect of RF treatment of the ramus medialis (medial branch) of the cervical ramus dorsalis in patients with CEH were published. Stovner et al.[25] included 12 patients with CEH according to the criteria of Sjaastad, and treated 6 patients with cervical facet denervation of C2 to C6 and 6 patients with a sham intervention. Follow-up after 3, 12 and 24 months showed no difference between the 2 groups. Physical examination of the cervical facet joints was not carried out in this study.

Haspeslagh et al.[26] included 30 patients with unilateral CEH according to the criteria of Sjaastad. Fifteen of these patients were treated with cervical facet denervation which was by failure of this intervention followed by an RF treatment of the ganglion spinale C2 and/or C3 (dorsal root ganglion, DRG) in 3 patients. The other 15 patients were treated with a series of injections of the nervus occipitalis major and ultimately followed with TENS therapy if necessary. Even though no significant difference between the 2 groups was found, there were patients in both groups with a significant visual analog scale reduction and/or a positive effect on the global perceived effect scale. After a follow-up of 1 year there were 8 (53%) patients in the RF group and 7 (46%) in the injection/TENS group with a significant pain reduction. Physical examination for painful facet joints was an inclusion criterion of this study.

Govind and colleagues reported, in their retrospective study, 88% success rate (43/49 patients) with a median duration of headache relief of 297 days in patients with headache stemming from the C2–C3 joint.[27] They performed a RF treatment of the nervus occipitalis tertius. The most common side effect is incomplete lesioning of the nervus occipitalis tertius because of its variable anatomy.[28]

Surgical treatments

Neurolysis of the nervus occipitalis major in patients with CEH, according to the criteria of Sjaastad, gave significant pain reduction after 1 week. Follow-up after a year showed that in 92% of the patients, the symptoms had completely returned.[29]

Microsurgical decompression of the C2 ganglion spinale (DRG) in 35 patients with CEH, according to the criteria of Sjaastad, showed that 37% of the patients were pain free, and in 51% a clear improvement was seen.[30] The average follow-up was 21 (3 to 70) months. During microsurgical decompression of the ganglion spinale (DRG), ligament structures and veins around the ganglion were "removed" by means of electrocoagulation. Stechinson claims that the results from Pikus et al. can also be attributed to the effects of electrocoagulation nearby the ganglion spinale (DRG), a sort of "radiofrequency lesion".[31]

Evidence for interventional management

A summary of the available evidence is given in Table 6.3.

Table 6.3. Summary of evidence for interventional management of cervicogenic headache.

Technique	Score
Injection of nervus occipitalis major with corticosteroid + local anesthetic.	1 B+
Injection of atlanto–axial joint with corticosteroid + local anesthetic.	2 C−
Radiofrequency treatment of the ramus medialis (medial branch) of the cervical ramus dorsalis.	2 B±
Pulsed radiofrequency treatment of the cervical ganglion spinale (DRG) (C2–C3).	0

DRG, dorsal root ganglion.

Recommendations

In patients with CEH, that is resistant to conservative treatment options, injection of the nervus occipitalis major with corticosteroids and local anesthetic is recommended.

If the results are unsatisfactory, RF treatment of the ramus medialis (medial branch) of the cervical ramus dorsalis can be considered, preferably in relation to a study.

RF and pulsed radiofrequency (PRF) treatment of the cervical ganglion spinale (DRG) level C2–C3 can be considered in the context of a study.

Based upon the available literature, the algorithm for techniques can be recommended (Figure 6.1). Neurosurgical treatments will not be discussed further in this chapter.

Clinical practice algorithm

A practice algorithm for the management of CEH is provided in Figure 6.1.

Technique(s)

Nervus occipital injection

For a description of the technique, we refer to chapter 8: "Occipital neuralgia."[32]

Percutaneous facet denervation

For a description of this technique, we refer to chapter 5: "Cervical facet pain."[33]

Summary

CEH is mainly characterized by unilateral headache symptoms which arise from the neck and radiates to the fronto-temporal and possibly to the supra-orbital region.

Physical examination encompasses movement tests of the cervical spinal column and segmental palpation of the cervical facet joints.

Injection of the nervus occipitalis major is recommended after unsatisfactory results with conservative treatments.

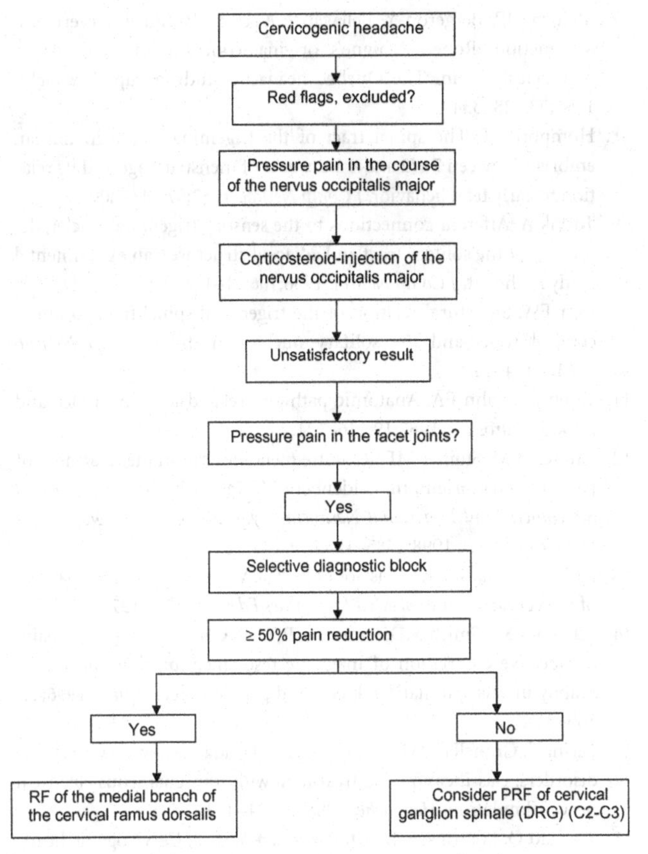

Figure 6.1. Clinical practice algorithm for the treatment of cervicogenic headache. RF, radiofrequency.

In the case of an unsatisfactory outcome after injection of the nervus occipitalis major, RF treatment of the ramus medialis (medial branch) of the cervical ramus dorsalis can be considered. If the result is unsatisfactory, PRF treatment of the ganglion spinale (DRG) of C2 and/or C3 can be considered in the context of a study.

References

1. Sjaastad O, Fredriksen TA, Pfaffenrath V. Cervicogenic headache: diagnostic criteria. The cervicogenic headache international study group. *Headache.* 1998;38:442–445.
2. Monteiro J. *Cefaleias: Estudo Epidemiologico e Clinico de Uma Populacao Urbana.* Porto: University Hospital Porto; 1995.
3. Nilsson N. The prevalence of cervicogenic headache in a random population sample of 20–59 years olds. *Spine.* 1995;20:1884–1888.
4. Sjaastad O, Bakketeig LS. Prevalence of cervicogenic headache: Vågå study of headache epidemiology. *Acta Neurol Scand.* 2008;117: 173–180.
5. IHC IHSCS. International classification of headache disorders. 2nd ed. *Cephalalgia.* 2004;24:1–160.
6. Bogduk N. The anatomical basis for cervicogenic headache. *J Manipulative Physiol Ther.* 1992;15:67–70.

7. Meloche JP, Bergeron Y, Bellavance A, et al. Painful intervertebral dysfunction: Robert Maigne's original contribution to headache of cervical origin. The Quebec headache study group. *Headache.* 1993;33:328–334.
8. Humphrey T. The spinal tract of the trigeminal nerve in human embryos between 7 1/2 and 8 1/2 weeks of menstrual age and its relation to early fetal behavior. *J Comp Neurol.* 1952;97:143–209.
9. Torvik A. Afferent connections to the sensory trigeminal nuclei, the nucleus of the solitary tract and adjacent structures; an experimental study in the rat. *J Comp Neurol.* 1956;106:51–141.
10. Kerr FW. Structural relation of the trigeminal spinal tract to upper cervical roots and the solitary nucleus in the cat. *Exp Neurol.* 1961;4:134–148.
11. Taren JA, Kahn EA. Anatomic pathways related to pain in face and neck. *J Neurosurg.* 1962;19:116–121.
12. Van Kleef M, Sluijter ME. Radiofrequency lesions in the treatment of pain of spinal origin. In: Gildenberg PL, Tasker RR, eds. *Textbook of Stereotactic and Functional Neurosurgery.* New York: The Mc Graw-Hill Companies; 1998:1585–1599.
13. Heller CA, Stanley P, Lewis-Jones B, et al. Value of x ray examinations of the cervical spine. *Br Med J (Clin Res Ed).* 1983;287:1276–1278.
14. Schellhas KP, Smith MD, Gundry CR, et al. Cervical discogenic pain. Prospective correlation of magnetic resonance imaging and discography in asymptomatic subjects and pain sufferers. *Spine.* 1996;21: 300–311.
15. Farina S, Granella F, Malferrari G, et al. Headache and cervical spine disorders: classification and treatment with transcutaneous electrical nerve stimulation. *Headache.* 1986;26:431–433.
16. Sjaastad O, Fredriksen TA, Stolt-Nielsen A, et al. Cervicogenic headache: A clinical review with special emphasis on therapy. *Funct Neurol.* 1997;12:305–317.
17. Anthony M. Headache and the greater occipital nerve. *Clin Neurol Neurosurg.* 1992;94:297–301.
18. Gawell M, Rothbart P. Occipital nerve block in the management of headache and cervical pain. *Cephalalgia.* 1991;12:9–13.
19. Vincent M. Greater occipital nerve blockades in cervicogenic headache. *Funct Neurol.* 1998;13:78–79.
20. Naja ZM, El-Rajab M, Al-Tannir MA, et al. Occipital nerve blockade for cervicogenic headache: a double-blind randomized controlled clinical trial. *Pain Pract.* 2006;6:89–95.
21. Naja ZM, El-Rajab M, Al-Tannir MA, et al. Repetitive occipital nerve blockade for cervicogenic headache: expanded case report of 47 adults. *Pain Pract.* 2006;6:278–284.
22. Narouze SN, Casanova J, Mekhail N. The longitudinal effectiveness of lateral atlantoaxial intra-articular steroid injection in the treatment of cervicogenic headache. *Pain Med.* 2007;8:184–188.
23. Hildebrandt J. Percutaneaus nerve block of the cervical facets—a relatively new method in the treatment of chronic headache and neck pain. *Man Med.* 1986;2:48–52.
24. Van Suijlekom JA, van Kleef M, Barendse G, et al. Radiofrequency cervical zygapophyeal joint neurotomy for cervicogenic headache. A prospective study in 15 patients. *Funct Neurol.* 1998;13:297–303.
25. Stovner LJ, Kolstad F, Helde G. Radiofrequency denervation of facet joints C2–C6 in cervicogenic headache: a randomized, double-blind, sham-controlled study. *Cephalalgia.* 2004;24:821–830.
26. Haspeslagh SR, Van Suijlekom HA, Lame IE, et al. Randomised controlled trial of cervical radiofrequency lesions as a treatment for cervicogenic headache [isrctn07444684]. *BMC Anesthesiol.* 2006; 16:1.
27. Govind J, King W, Bailey B, et al. Radiofrequency neurotomy for the treatment of third occipital headache. *J Neurol Neurosurg Psychiatry.* 2003;74:88–93.
28. Lord SM, Barnsley L, Bogduk N. Percutaneous radiofrequency neurotomy in the treatment of cervical zygapophysial joint pain: a caution. *Neurosurgery.* 1995;36:732–739.
29. Bovim G, Fredriksen TA, Stolt-Nielsen A, et al. Neurolysis of the greater occipital nerve in cervicogenic headache. A follow up study. *Headache.* 1992;32:175–179.
30. Pikus HJ, Phillips JM. Outcome of surgical decompression of the second cervical root for cervicogenic headache. *Neurosurgery.* 1996;39:63–70.
31. Stechison MT. Outcome of surgical decompression of the second cervical root for cervicogenic headache. *Neurosurgery.* 1997;40:1105–1106.
32. Vanelderen P, Lataster A, Levy R, et al. Evidence-based interventional pain medicine according to clinical diagnoses: 8. occipital neuralgia. *Pain Pract.* 2010;10: DOI:10.1111/j.1533-2500.2009.00355.x.
33. Van Eerd M, Patijn J, Lataster A, et al. Evidence-based interventional pain medicine according to clinical diagnoses: 5. cervical facet pain. *Pain Pract.* 2010;10: DOI:10.1111/j.1533-2500.2009.00346.x.

7 Whiplash-Associated Disorders

Hans van Suijlekom, Nagy Mekhail, Nileshkumar Patel, Jan Van Zundert, Maarten van Kleef and Jacob Patijn

Introduction

Whiplash-associated disorder (WAD) is the official name for the constellation of symptoms affecting the neck that are triggered by an accident with an acceleration–deceleration mechanism. The occurrence of WAD is typical in motor vehicle accidents specifically with an impact from behind or from the flanks, but WAD can also result from other injuries including diving.

Research in Europe shows that the prevalence of neck pain caused by car accidents has risen from 3.4 per 100,000 in 1970 to 1974, to 40.2 per 100,000 in 1990 to 1994.[1] In 1995, the Quebec Task Force made a theoretical classification of WADs,[2] which was recently updated.[3] This makes it easier to compare international research.

- Grade 0: no complaints in the neck. No physical signs.
- Grade I neck pain: no symptoms indicating serious pathology and minimal influence on daily activities.
- Grade II neck pain: no symptoms indicating serious pathology, but having influence on daily activities.
- Grade III neck pain: no symptoms indicating serious pathology, presence of neurological disorders such as decreased reflexes, muscle weakness, or decreased sensory function.
- Grade IV neck pain: indications of serious underlying pathology such as fracture, myelopathy, or neoplasm.

This article will primarily cover the current understanding of the pathophysiology and pain intervention approach for patients with WAD I and II. Spitzer et al.[2] indicates that the natural course of whiplash is fairly favorable. Approximately 85% of the patients resumed their activities within 6 months after an accident. It is generally assumed that the symptoms become chronic in 15% to 30% of the WAD patients.[4]

Diagnosis

History

Typical symptoms of acute whiplash injury include: (1) pain in the neck, shoulders, and, potentially, in the arms; (2) headache, particularly in the occipital area, sometimes radiating to the forehead above both eyes; and (3) restricted mobility of the neck as a result of neck stiffness immediately after the accident. Concomitant symptoms include dizziness, visual impairments, nausea, tinnitus, deafness, paresthesias in the hands, localized spasm and tenderness, unilateral brachialgia due to shoulder complaints, lower back pain, posttraumatic stress disorder (depression), and cognitive function disorders.

The importance of history taking is to be able to rule out grades III and IV neurological symptoms that can indicate damage to the nervous system and skeletal structures. The term acute whiplash syndrome applies to the first 3 weeks after the accident. Thereafter, a sub-acute stage starts during which most of the symptoms disappear while administering conservative therapy. If the symptoms persist after 3 months, it is considered chronic whiplash syndrome.[4]

Physical examination

The physical examination aims to either exclude or demonstrate nervous system damage. At the same time, fractures should be ruled out. A thorough neurological examination of the neck should be carried out, focusing on the sensibility and motor function of the arms and hands, and radicular provocation tests (Spurling). Clinical signs of WAD typically include localized spasm and tenderness as well as limitation in the active range of motion, including lateroflexion and extension. Patients with

Evidence-Based Interventional Pain Medicine: According to Clinical Diagnoses, First Edition. Edited by Jan Van Zundert, Jacob Patijn, Craig T. Hartrick, Arno Lataster, Frank J.P.M Huygen, Nagy Mekhail, Maarten van Kleef.

neck pain have tenderness and spasms that are not evident in the asymptomatic individuals.[5] Even so, palpation may reveal localized tenderness, and range of motion may be restricted, but neither of these features yield a definitive diagnosis in the WAD I and II patients. They merely point to some abnormality that warrants further interventions.

Additional tests

The objective of physical examination is to pinpoint the source of pain, and hopefully, the information obtained from the assessments will direct to effective treatments.

Additional tests should be carried out when indicated. A magnetic resonance imaging scan (MRI) of the neck is not useful with WAD I and II, but can still be considered in case of suspected neurological problems.[4] Research has demonstrated that an MRI scan during the chronic stage of a whiplash injury rarely shows a traumatic defect.[6] Choosing an MRI is guided by clinical evaluation in case of unexplained neurologic abnormalities and in preparation of surgical intervention. MRI is perhaps the best screening tool for missed and occult fractures, infections, and tumors. Apart from these criteria, utility of MRI is limited.

Electrophysiologic examination by electromyography (EMG) and nerve conduction velocity (NCV) tests are not justified in WAD I and II given the absence of radicular pain. Even for the assessment of radiculopathy, electrophysiologic tests are not more valuable than a careful neurologic evaluation.

Hence, forced by the overwhelming lack of evidence for the conventional investigational approach (use of X-rays, MRI, EMG/NCVs), one has to resort to *physiologic* tests. Pain is a sensory experience. As such, in dealing with WAD I and II patients, imaging and electrophysiologic investigations cannot reliably diagnose the source of pain. Rather, these latter tests are useful corollaries to physiologic tests, to confirm the findings of the physiologic tests and clinical evaluation.

In the chronic whiplash patients, where conservative treatment has failed and physical examination reveals possible dysfunction of the cervical facet joints, a diagnostic blockade of these joints is appropriate.[7]

Differential diagnosis

The relation with the acceleration–deceleration trauma is found in the medical history. Differential diagnosis that specifically must not be overlooked includes: (1) infections; (2) tumors; and (3) neurologic disorders. The "red flags" that will alert the clinician are unexplained fevers, night sweats, unexplained weight loss, decrease in appetite, general malaise, history of cancers, weakness, neurologic symptoms, immunosupression, illicit drug use, as well as other alerts in the evaluation of systems.

Treatment options

Conservative management

A review article by Verhagen et al. within the Cochrane Collaboration describes the effect of conservative treatments for acute whiplash patients with WAD grades I and II.[8] The treatments in these studies varied from immobilization by means of a cervical collar to early active mobilization and multimodal treatment. These studies concluded that active treatment strategies are slightly more effective than passive treatment strategies and any treatment (whether passive or active) is more effective than no treatment at all. There is no clear evidence which treatment is better. The Dutch Institute for Healthcare Improvement working group recommends that patients with WAD (grades I to II) should be given a clear explanation about why they are experiencing the symptoms and precisely what they should expect, providing the natural course of the condition.[4]

Two studies on the medical treatment of chronic WAD exemplify the lack of effectiveness of pharmaceutical interventions. In a randomized study, Schreiber et al. investigated the effect of fluoxetine vs. amitriptyline on pain in 40 patients with back pain or neck pain as a result of a whiplash accident.[9] There were no significant differences. Another study showed no significant effect of melatonin compared with placebo for sleep disorders.[10]

Interventional management

Interventional treatments are only considered after a minimum of 6 months because in that time period, the clinical signs have sufficiently stabilized. Interventional treatments for WAD historically include injection of steroids into the epidural space, into trigger points, or facet joints, injection of botulinum toxins in muscles with increased tenderness, and percutaneous radiofrequency (RF) treatment.

While cervical epidural steroids appear to have short-term benefit for the radicular symptoms, no study has demonstrated the effectiveness in an axial, nonradicular whiplash population in WAD I and II categories.

A randomized study by Barnsley et al. in 1994 investigated the effect of intra-articular depot corticosteroid versus local anesthetic injections in the cervical facet joints of chronic whiplash patients.[7] There were no significant differences noted.

Trigger point injections are as effective as simple ultrasound, but not more effective than physical therapy.[11]

Freund and Schwartz[12] published a randomized, placebo-controlled pilot study in 2000 with 26 chronic whiplash patients (WAD grade II) on the effect of botulinum toxin on neck pain and neck function. The treatment group (group I) received 5 injections of 0.2-mL (20 U) botulinum toxin type A and the control group (group II) received 5 injections of 0.2-mL saline solution. The follow-up parameters were visual analog scale for neck pain and function measurements using the Vernon–Mior index. After a 4-week follow-up, there was no significant difference in the effect parameters between the two groups. Likewise, others have failed to demonstrate the effectiveness of botulinum toxins in treatment of chronic neck pain even when the pain is primarily associated with myofascial spasms.[13]

In a randomized, double-blind, placebo-controlled clinical trial of Padberg et al. in 2007, botulinum toxin was not proven to be effective in treatment of neck pain in chronic WAD.[14]

The effect of RF treatment of the cervical facet joints is well documented. In 1996, Lord et al. published a randomized, double-blind study with 24 chronic whiplash patients on the effect of percutaneous RF treatment of the ramus medialis (medial branch) of the ramus dorsalis of the cervical facet joints.[15] Patients ($n = 54$) were selected double-blindly for this study. Each patient underwent 3 blocks of the rami mediales (medial branches) of the 2 rami dorsales supplying the putatively symptomatic facet joint. The blocks were performed with lidocaine 2%, bupivacaine 0.5%, or a saline solution, and were randomly administered (double blind, placebo controlled). Patients with complete relief of pain for the duration of the local anesthetic and those who reported no relief with normal saline were deemed to have true facetogenic pain. Twenty-four such patients were included in the study. Patients were randomized in two groups of 12 patients: Group I underwent RF treatment at multiple levels of the cervical ramus medialis (medial branch) of the ramus dorsalis. Group II received a sham treatment. After 27 weeks, 7 (58%) of the patients from group I and 1 (8%) from group II were pain free. The mean time of pain symptom recurrence to at least 50% of the preoperative level was 263 days in 12 patients in group I and 8 days in 12 patients in group II. Others have also demonstrated the utility of cervical RF treatment, in litigant and nonlitigant populations.[16,17] Prushansky et al.[18] conducted a prospective study of 40 patients with chronic whiplash injury-associated disorders who underwent RF treatment. The authors found an improvement in 70% of patients based on a number of parameters including the Neck Disability Index and cervical range of motion. In 1999, McDonald et al.[19] published a prospective long-term follow-up study of the long-term effect of RF treatment of the ramus medialis (medial branch) of the ramus dorsalis of the cervical facet joints in 28 chronic whiplash patients with neck pain. Twenty patients (71%) reported complete pain reduction. The mean time of pain symptom recurrence to at least 50% of the preoperative level was 219 days (0 to 1,095 days) in all 28 patients and 422 days if only the positive results were evaluated. In 11 patients (55%), the procedure was repeated for the recurrence of the pain symptoms, resulting in complete pain reduction. Several procedures were carried out in 4 patients (20%) who reported complete pain reduction lasting a minimum of 90 days in each case. As the treated nerves regenerate, the complete relief can be reinstated by repeating the procedure.[20]

Psychological disorders are a characteristic of many chronic pain syndromes. Wallis et al. showed that in the above-mentioned patient group, the psychological stress factors, measured using the McGill Pain Questionnaire and the SCL-90-R (Symptom Checklist-90 Revised), entirely normalized in the patients in which the pain after the RF treatment had completely disappeared.[17]

Complications of interventional management

Complications of RF treatment of the ramus medialis (medial branch) of the cervical ramus dorsalis are described in chapter 5 on cervical facet pain.[21]

Evidence for interventional management

A summary of the available evidence is given in Table 7.1.

Recommendations

RF lesions of the ramus medialis (medial branch) of the ramus dorsalis of the cervical segmental nerves are recommended for therapy-resistant neck complaints when there is an indication for involvement of the cervical facet joints in this pain syndrome.

Clinical practice algorithm

The practice algorithm for the treatment of WAD is given in Figure 7.1.

Table 7.1. Summary of evidence for interventional management of whiplash-associated disorders.

Technique	Evaluation
Botulinum toxin type A	2 B–
Intra-articular injection	2 C–
Radiofrequency treatment of the ramus medialis (medial branch) of the cervical ramus dorsalis	2 B+

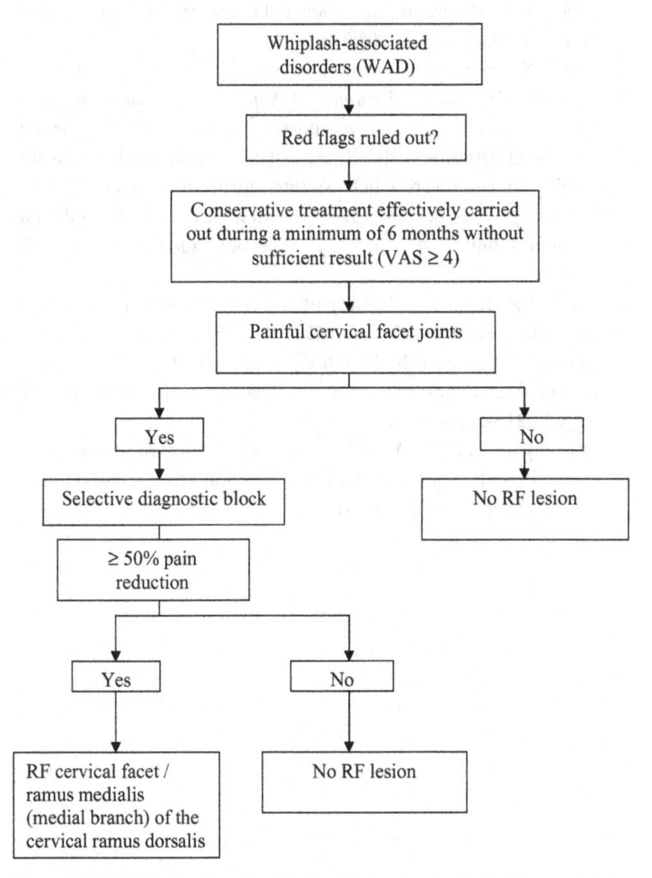

Figure 7.1. Clinical Practice algorithm for the treatment of whiplash-associated disorders (WAD). RF, radiofrequency; VAS, visual analog scale.

Technique(s)

RF facet denervation is described in the chapter on cervical facet pain.[21]

Summary

WADs are comprised of a range of symptoms of which the neck complaints and headaches are the most significant spine-related symptoms.

Six months of conservative treatment are recommended.

The prevalence of cervical facetogenic pain is high in the whiplash population. If the facet joints are painful, a RF treatment of the ramus medialis (medial branch) of the ramus dorsalis at the cervical facets joints can be recommended.

References

1. Versteege G. Sprain of the neck and whiplash associated disorders: anesthesiology and pain management. PhD Thesis, Groningen University, Groningen, 2001.
2. Spitzer WO, Skovron ML, Salmi LR, et al. Scientific monograph of the Quebec Task Force on whiplash-associated disorders: redefining "whiplash" and its management. *Spine.* 1995;20:1S–73S.
3. Haldeman S, Carroll L, Cassidy JD, et al. The bone and joint decade 2000–2010 task force on neck pain and its associated disorders: executive summary. *Spine.* 2008;33:S5–S7.
4. Dutch Neurology Association. [Nederlandse Vereniging voor Neurologie]. *Diagnosis and Treatment of People with Whiplash Associated Disorder I/II* [Diagnose en Behandeling van mensen met Whiplash Associated Disorder I/II]. Utrecht, the Netherlands: Institute for Quality in Healthcare CBO [Kwaliteitsinstituut Voor de Gezondheidszorg CBO]. http://www.neurologie.nl/uploads/136/1149/richtlijn_Whiplash.versie.maart.2008.def.pdf (accessed May 30, 2008).
5. Sandmark H, Nisell R. Validity of five common manual neck pain provoking tests. *Scand J Rehabil Med.* 1995;27:131–136.
6. Bonuccelli U, Pavese N, Lucetti C, et al. Late whiplash syndrome: a clinical and magnetic resonance imaging study. *Funct Neurol.* 1999;14:219–225.
7. Barnsley L, Lord SM, Wallis BJ, et al. Lack of effect of intraarticular corticosteroids for chronic pain in the cervical zygapophyseal joints. *N Engl J Med.* 1994;330:1047–1050.
8. Verhagen AP, Scholten-Peeters GG, de Bie RA, et al. Conservative treatments for whiplash. *Cochrane Database Syst Rev.* 2004;1: CD003338.
9. Schreiber S, Vinokur S, Shavelzon V, et al. A randomized trial of fluoxetine versus amitriptyline in musculo-skeletal pain. *Isr J Psychiatry Relat Sci.* 2001;38:88–94.
10. Wieringen S, Jansen T, Smits M, et al. Melatonin for chronic whiplash syndrome with delayed melatonin onset. *Clin Drug Investig.* 2001;21:813–820.
11. Esenyel M, Caglar N, Aldemir T. Treatment of myofascial pain. *Am J Phys Med Rehabil.* 2000;79:48–52.
12. Freund BJ, Schwartz M. Treatment of whiplash associated neck pain [corrected] with botulinum toxin-a: a pilot study. *J Rheumatol.* 2000;27:481–484.
13. Wheeler AH, Goolkasian P, Gretz SS. Botulinum toxin A for the treatment of chronic neck pain. *Pain.* 2001;94:255–260.
14. Padberg M, de Bruijn SF, Tavy DL. Neck pain in chronic whiplash syndrome treated with botulinum toxin. A double-blind, placebo-controlled clinical trial. *J Neurology.* 2007;254:290–295.
15. Lord SM, Barnsley L, Wallis BJ. Percutaneous radiofrequency neurotomy in the treatment of cervical zygapophy-seal joint pain. *N Engl J Med.* 1996;335:1721–1726.
16. Sapir DA, Gorup JM. Radiofrequency medial branch neurotomy in litigant and nonlitigant patients with cervical whiplash: a prospective study. *Spine (Phila Pa 1976).* 2001;26:26.
17. Wallis BJ, Lord SM, Bogduk N. Resolution of psychological distress of whiplash patients following treatment by radiofrequency neurotomy: a randomised, double-blind, placebo controlled trial. *Pain.* 1997;73:15–22.
18. Prushansky T, Pevzner E, Gordon C, et al. Cervical radiofrequency neurotomy in patients with chronic whiplash: a study of multiple outcome measures. *J Neurosurgery.* 2006;4:365–373.
19. McDonald GJ, Lord SM, Bogduk N. Long-term follow-up of patients treated with cervical radiofrequency neurotomy for chronic neck pain. *Neurosurgery.* 1999;45:61–67.
20. Husted DS, Orton D, Schofferman J, et al. Effectiveness of repeated radiofrequency neurotomy for cervical facet joint pain. *J Spinal Disord Tech.* 2008;21:406–408.
21. Van Eerd M, Patijn J, Lataster A, et al. Evidence-based interventional pain medicine according to clinical diagnoses: 5. Cervical facet pain. *Pain Pract.* 2010;10: DOI:10.1111/j.1533-2500.2009.00346.x.

8 Occipital Neuralgia

Pascal Vanelderen, Arno Lataster, Robert Levy, Nagy Mekhail, Maarten van Kleef and Jan Van Zundert

Introduction

The International Headache Society (IHS) defines occipital neuralgia as paroxysmal shooting or stabbing pain in the dermatomes of the nervus occipitalis major or nervus occipitalis minor.[1] The pain originates in the suboccipital region and radiates over the vertex. Hypo- or dysesthesia in the affected area can accompany the pain. Pressure over the nervus occipitalis major or minor usually elicits the pain.

No data are available about the prevalence or incidence of occipital neuralgia. The nervus occipitalis major is more frequently involved (90%) as compared with the nervus occipitalis minor (10%). In 8.7%, both nervi occipitales are responsible for the neuralgia.[2]

Often, damage or irritation of the nervus occipitalis major or minor is the cause of the neuralgia. Vital et al.[3] described 2 bends that divide the course of the nervus occipitalis major into 3 parts. The nervus occipitalis major is formed by the ramus dorsalis of the C2 nerve root. The first part runs between the origin of the nerve and the musculus obliquus capitis inferior underneath of which the nerve makes its first bend in a medial direction. The second part of the nerve runs cranially between the musculus semispinalis capitis on the one side and the musculus obliquus capitis inferior, musculus rectus capitis posterior, and the musculus rectus capitis anterior on the other side. When perforating the musculus semispinalis capitis toward the surface, the nerve makes its second bend in a lateral direction. The third part of the nerve runs further laterally where the aponeurosis of the musculus trapezius is perforated and the nerve begins its subcutaneous course. The nervus occipitalis major usually branches after perforating the aponeurosis.

There are various potential causes of irritation: vascular, neurogenic, muscular, and osteogenic.

1 Vascular
   - Irritation of the nerve roots C1/C2 by an aberrant branch of the arteria inferior posterior cerebelli (posterior inferior cerebellar artery)[4]
   - Dural arteriovenous fistula at the cervical level[5]
   - Bleeding from a bulbocervical cavernoma[6]
   - Cervical intramedullar cavernous hemangioma[7]
   - Giant cell arteritis[8–10]
   - Fenestrated arteria vertebralis pressing on C1/C2 nerve roots[11]
   - Aberrant course of the arteria vertebralis[12]

2 Neurogenic
   - Schwannoma in the area of the craniocervical junction: schwannoma of the nervus occipitalis[13,14]
   - C2 myelitis[15]
   - Multiple sclerosis[16]

3 Muscular/tendinous[17]

4 Osteogenic
   - C1/C2 arthrosis, atlantodental sclerosis[18]
   - Hypermobile arcus posterior of the atlas[19]
   - Cervical osteochondroma[20]
   - Osteolytic lesion of the cranium[21]
   - Exuberant callus formation after fracture C1/C2[22]

5 After vitrectomy surgery[23]

Diagnosis

History

Patients complain of a shooting or stabbing pain in the neck radiating over the cranium. Constant pain can persist between the

Evidence-Based Interventional Pain Medicine: According to Clinical Diagnoses, First Edition. Edited by Jan Van Zundert, Jacob Patijn, Craig T. Hartrick, Arno Lataster, Frank J.P.M Huygen, Nagy Mekhail, Maarten van Kleef.

paroxysms. The pain can be perceived in the retro-orbital area caused by overlap of the C2 dorsal root and the nucleus trigeminus pars caudalis.[23] Vision impairment/ocular pain (67%), tinnitus (33%), dizziness (50%), nausea (50%), and congested nose (17%) can be present because of connections with cranial nerves VIII, IX, and X, and the cervical sympathicus.[24]

Physical examination

Upon clinical examination, hypo- or dysesthesia in the area of the nervus occipitalis major or minor as well as tenderness to pressure over the course of the nervus occipitalis major or minor can be observed. A positive Tinel's sign (pain upon percussion over the nerve) can be present.

Clinical presentation and a temporary improvement with a local anesthetic diagnostic block of the nervus occipitalis major and/or minor confirm the diagnosis.[1] False-positive results occur with migraine and cluster headaches.[25]

Additional tests

Radiography is recommended to rule out underlying pathologies. Open-mouth X-ray of the cervical spine shows possible arthritis of the C2 facet joints. A computer tomography scan of the craniocervical junction is indicated in case of suspected neoplastic or degenerative osseous pathology. It is important to note that degenerative changes of the cervical spinal column do not necessarily correspond with the symptoms the patient is presenting. Magnetic resonance imaging is ideal for visualizing disorders of the cervical and occipital soft tissues.

Differential diagnosis

Tumors, infection, and congenital anomalies (Arnold-Chiari malformation) should be ruled out. Occipital neuralgia can be mistaken for migraine, cluster headache, tension headache, and hemicrania continua. Other structures may cause similar pain, such as the upper cervical facet joints (C2-C3), osteoarthritis of the atlantooccipital or atlantoaxial joint, giant cell arteritis, and tumors of the cervical spinal column.[26]

Treatment options

Conservative management

Conservative treatment focuses on reducing secondary muscle tension and on improving posture. Pharmacological treatment may include tricyclic antidepressants and antiepileptics (carbamazepine, gabapentin, and pregabalin).

Interventional management

Infiltration of the nervi occipitales with local anesthetic and corticosteroids

The most common site to infiltrate the nervus occipitalis major is along its course, where the nerve penetrates the aponeurosis of the musculus trapezius. Here, the nerve is most often constricted.[27] Vital et al. found that this site is located on a line that connects the middle of the 2 ears, 3.18 cm from the midline.[3] Becser et al. found that the subcutaneous pathway of the nerve starts at the level of the intermastoid line at 13 mm from the midline.[28] Loukas et al. investigated the best site to infiltrate the nervus occipitalis major based on external landmarks.[29] On average, the nervus occipitalis major is situated 3.8 cm lateral from the midline and one quarter of the distance along a line connecting the protuberantia occipitalis externa to the processus mastoideus (or 2 cm lateral and 2 cm inferior to the protuberantia occipitalis externa). This is in accordance with the findings of Vital et al.[3] Natsis et al. defined the optimal site for infiltration of the nervus occipitalis major 1.5 cm lateral and 2 to 2.5 cm inferior to the protuberantia occipitalis externa.[30] Great variability in the course of the nervus occipitalis major is described.[31]

In a small ($n = 10$) retrospective study by Kuhn et al., the nervus occipitalis major was infiltrated with corticosteroids after a positive test block with bupivacaine.[24] The authors found pain relief for less than 1 week in 10% of patients, 1 week in 30%, 2 weeks in 30%, 1 month in 10%, and more than 2.5 months in 20% of patients. Hammond and Danta found a short-term effect (less than 1 week) in 64% of the patients after 1 infiltration with local anesthetics; 36% of the patients had an effect lasting longer than 1 month.[2]

Botulinum toxin a infiltrations

Injections with botulinum toxin type A in 6 patients relieved the sharp, shooting pain associated with occipital neuralgia, yet had no effect on the dull, aching pain.[32] Quality-of-life measures exhibited some improvement. No significant reduction in pain medication was demonstrated. However, in a retrospective case series of 6 patients with occipital neuralgia, Kapural et al. were able to demonstrate a pain reduction after injection of botulinum toxin A (visual analog scale [VAS]) declined from 8 ± 1.8 to 2 ± 2.7) as well as an improvement in the pain disability index.[33] The mean duration of pain relief averaged 16.3 ± 3.2 weeks.

Pulsed radiofrequency treatment of the nervi occipitales

To date, 1 case report and 1 prospective trial have been published concerning pulsed radio-frequency (PRF) treatment in occipital neuralgia.[34,35] Both used 20-millisecond bursts with a frequency of 2 Hz and a maximum temperature of 42°C for 4 minutes to the nervi occipitales. In the case report, the patient showed 70% pain relief lasting 4 months. After recurrence of pain, the treatment was repeated with again 70% pain relief lasting 5 months. Of the 19 patients included in the prospective trial, 68.4%, 57.9%, and 52.6% reported an improvement of 50% or more 1, 2, and 6 months after PRF treatment, respectively. The mean VAS score before treatment was 7.5 (standard error of the mean [SEM] ± 0.4) and declined to 3.5 (SEM ± 0.8), 3.5 (SEM ± 0.7), and 3.9 (SEM ± 0.8) at 1, 2, and 6 months, respectively ($P < 0.001$, $P < 0.001$, $P = 0.006$). There was a statistically significant improvement in the use of medication and in quality-of-life parameters.

PRF treatment of the C2 ganglion spinale (dorsal root ganglion (DRG))

A prospective audit looked into the effects of PRF treatment adjacent to the cervical ganglion spinale (DRG). In 4 of the 18 patients, the procedure was carried out at C2 level as a treatment for headache. Two of these 4 patients had a long-term effect (18 and >24 months), whereas no improvement was observed in the other 2 patients.[36]

Subcutaneous neurostimulation of the nervi occipitales

Weiner and Reed first reported 13 patients who underwent 17 implant procedures for medically refractory occipital neuralgia. With follow-up ranging from 18 months to 6 years, good to excellent results were seen in 12 of 13 patients as defined by greater than 50% pain relief and requiring little or no pain medications. The thirteenth patient was explanted following resolution of the symptoms.[37]

Slavin et al.[38] carried out a trial stimulation in 14 patients with therapy-resistant occipital neuralgia. A definitive neurostimulator was implanted subcutaneously in 10 patients who had a reduction in pain of greater than 50%. After a mean follow-up of 22 months, 70% of the patients still had good results. This confirms the results of an earlier study by Slavin et al.[39] where 13 of 18 patients experienced >50% pain reduction as a result of test stimulation with a favorable follow-up effect, of mean 28 months, in 85% of the patients implanted. Other studies also report comparable results.[40,41]

Complications of interventional management

Although infection and bleeding are possible complications of any percutaneous technique, these have only been reported with subcutaneous lead implantation for neurostimulation together with lead migration, hardware erosions, electrode fractures, disconnections, and sepsis.[42] One case report describes sudden unconsciousness because of an inadvertent subarachnoidal injection through an os occipitale defect after craniotomy.[43] Other possible side-effects of occipital nerve infiltrations include temporary dizziness and gait uncertainty, injection site soreness, bradycardia, and focal alopecia.[44–47]

Evidence for interventional management

A summary of the available evidence is given in Table 8.1.

Table 8.1. Summary of evidence for interventional management of occipital neuralgia.

Technique	Evaluation
Single infiltration of the nervi occipitales with local anesthetic and corticosteroids	2 C+
Pulsed radiofrequency treatment of the nervi occipitales	2 C+
Pulsed radiofrequency treatment of the cervical ganglion spinale (dorsal root ganglion)	0
Subcutaneous stimulation of the nervi occipitales	2 C+
Botulinum toxin A injection	2 C±

Recommendations

A single infiltration of the nervus occipitalis major with local anesthetic and corticosteroids can be considered for the treatment of occipital neuralgia. The effects of botulinum toxin A infiltrations are contradictory. PRF treatment of the nervus occipitalis can be considered if infiltration with local anesthetic and corticosteroids fails to provide sufficient pain relief. PRF treatment of the ganglion spinale (dorsal root ganglion) C2 or C3 is only recommended in a clinical trial setting. Subcutaneous nerve stimulation can be considered in severe disabling pain unresponsive to other treatments. Considering its relatively high cost and the invasive nature of the treatment, occipital nerve stimulation should be considered later in the treatment algorithm and should be performed in experienced centers.

Clinical practice algorithm

The treatment algorithm of occipital neuralgia is given in Figure 8.1.

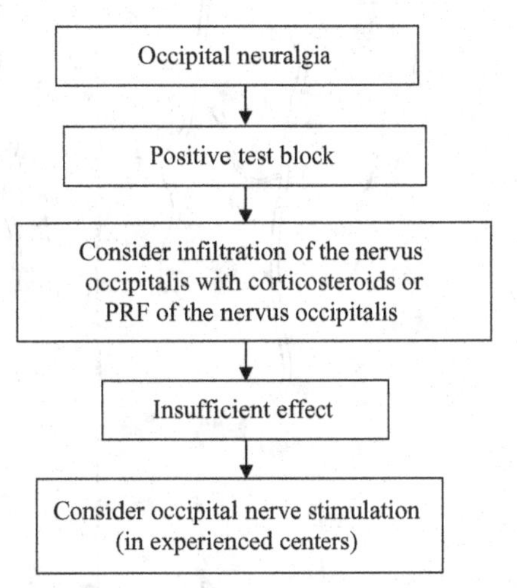

Figure 8.1. Clinical practice algorithm for the treatment of occipital neuralgia. PRF, pulsed radio-frequency.

Technique(s)

Infiltration of the nervus occipitalis major and minor

The infiltration sites of the nervus occipitalis major and minor are determined by external landmarks as described by Vital and Becser (see Figure 8.2).[3] The needle (22G) is introduced until there is bone contact or paresthesia is elicited. Subsequently, the needle is slightly withdrawn, and the local anesthetic and corticosteroids are injected.

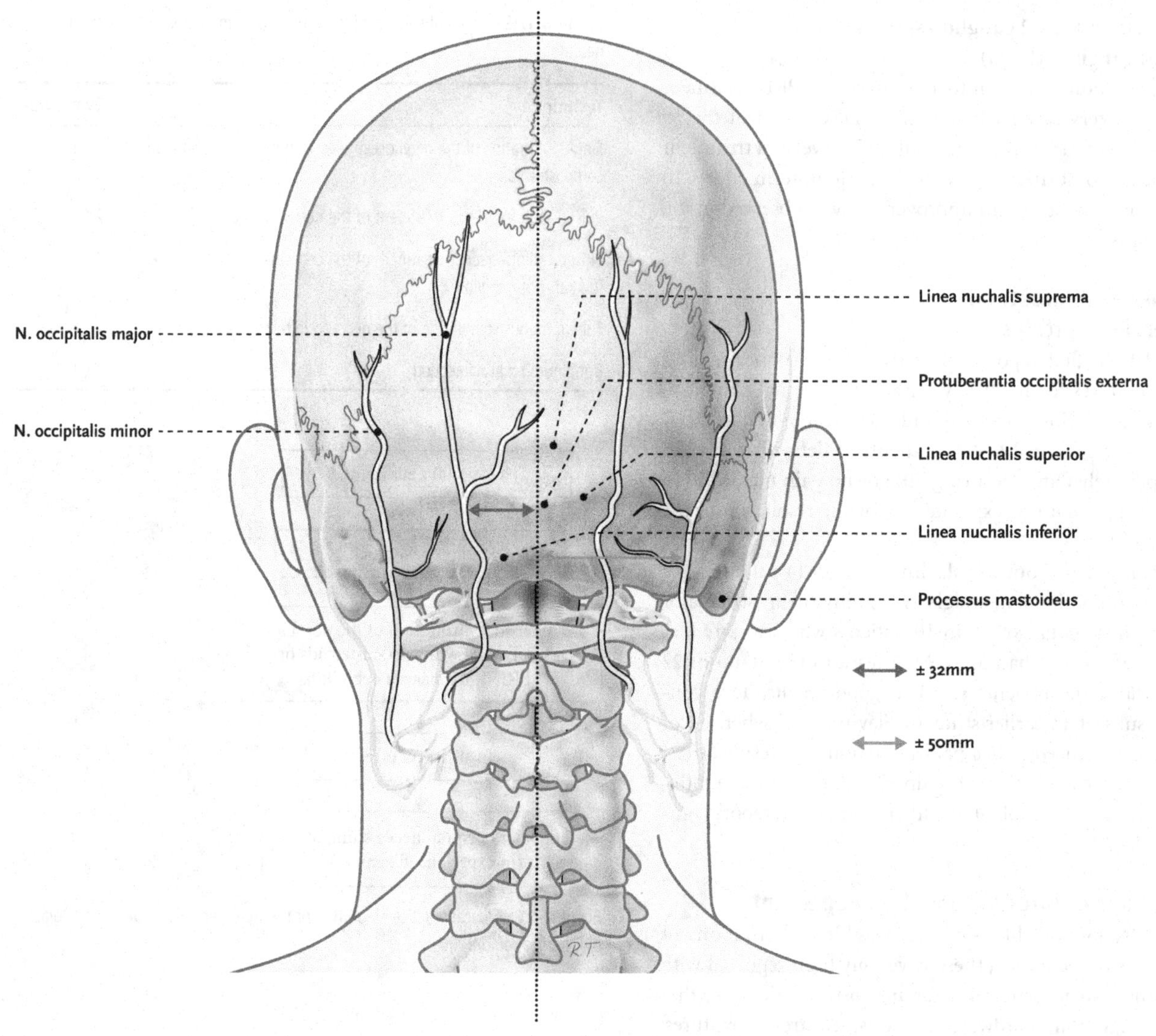

Figure 8.2. Landmarks for injection of the nervus occipitalis. Illustration: Rogier Trompert Medical Art (www.medical-art.nl).

PRF treatment of the nervus occipitalis major and minor

The puncture site (22G needle, 5 cm, 1 cm active tip) is located according to the external landmarks described by Vital and Becser.[3] The thermocouple is introduced after perforation of the skin. The nervus occipitalis major and minor are located with a 50-Hz, 0.5-V current until the patient reports paresthesia in the dermatomes of the nervus occipitalis major and minor. Subsequently, a PRF treatment (45 V, 20 milliseconds, 2 Hz) lasting 120 seconds with a maximum temperature of 42°C is performed twice.

Occipital neurostimulation

The first stage of the procedure (the trial) is performed under mild sedation and local anesthesia to monitor the patient's feedback and ensure the most optimal coverage of the painful areas by the stimulation. The patient is placed in a prone position. After disinfection and sterile draping, a curved needle is inserted at the upper lateral end of the neck and advanced toward the midline of the craniovertebral junction along the contour of the C1 arcus vertebralis under fluoroscopic guidance, crossing over the anatomic course of the nervus occipitalis major or minor. When positioning of the needle is considered satisfactory, standard 4-contact electrodes are advanced through the needle, and the tip of the electrode containing 4 discrete contacts is placed in close proximity of the nervus occipitalis major or minor. Correct position of the electrode is verified by intraoperative test stimulation of the awake patient, and fluoroscopically, once adequate coverage has been achieved, the electrode is sutured in place with nonabsorbable sutures using 2 plastic anchors provided by the manufacturer to minimize the possibility of movement. In case of a successful trial, defined as more than 50% of pain reduction, the patient undergoes the second part of the surgical procedure under general anesthesia. The first incision is made along the retroauricular area in a vertical direction. The soft tissues are dissected down to the fascia, and a small pocket is created above the fascia. The temporary electrode is removed, and the standard 4-contact electrode is then positioned into the same anatomic location. Once the electrode is positioned in the right place, the needle is removed, and the electrode is anchored to the occipital fascia with nonabsorbable sutures using a plastic anchor. Next, a subcutaneous pocket is created below the clavicula on the same side to accommodate the neurostimulator. Extension cables are advanced through a subcutaneous tunnel, establishing connection between the electrode and the neurostimulator. At the end, all incisions are closed, cleaned, and covered with sterile dressings.[38]

Summary

Occipital neuralgia is responsible for neck pain and headache. No absolute data are available about its prevalence and incidence.

History, clinical examination, and a positive test block with local anesthetic can provide an indication for the diagnosis.

A single infiltration of the nervus occipitalis major with corticosteroids and local anesthetic is advised.

If the symptoms are resistant to infiltration with local anesthetic and corticosteroids, PRF of the nervus occipitalis can be considered. If pain persists, PRF of the ganglion spinale (DRG) C2 or C3 can be considered in a clinical trial setting.

Because of the cost and invasiveness, subcutaneous nerve stimulation is placed last in the treatment algorithm and should only be performed in experienced centers.

References

1. IHC IHSCS. International Classification of Headache Disorders. The international classification of headache disorders: 2nd edition. *Cephalalgia.* 2004;24:1–160.
2. Hammond SR, Danta G. Occipital neuralgia. *Clin Exp Neurol.* 1978;15:258–270.
3. Vital JM, Grenier F, Dautheribes M, et al. An anatomic and dynamic study of the greater occipital nerve (n. of Arnold). Applications to the treatment of Arnold's neuralgia. *Surg Radiol Anat.* 1989;11: 205–210.
4. White JB, Atkinson PP, Cloft HJ, et al. Vascular compression as a potential cause of occipital neuralgia: a case report. *Cephalalgia.* 2008;28:78–82.
5. Hashiguchi A, Mimata C, Ichimura H, et al. Occipital neuralgia as a presenting symptom of cervicomedullary dural arteriovenous fistula. *Headache.* 2007;47:1095–1097.
6. Bruti G, Mostardini C, Pierallini A, et al. Neurovascular headache and occipital neuralgia secondary to bleeding of bulbocervical cavernoma. *Cephalalgia.* 2007;27:1074–1079.
7. Cerrato P, Bergui M, Imperiale D, et al. Occipital neuralgia as isolated symptom of an upper cervical cavernous angioma. *J Neurol.* 2002;249:1464–1465.
8. Pfadenhauer K, Weber H. Giant cell arteritis of the occipital arteries—a prospective color coded duplex sonography study in 78 patients. *J Neurol.* 2003;250:844–849.
9. Gonzalez-Gay MA, Garcia-Porrua C, Branas F, et al. Giant cell arteritis presenting as occipital neuralgia. *Clin Exp Rheumatol.* 2001;19:479.
10. Jundt JW, Mock D. Temporal arteritis with normal erythrocyte sedimentation rates presenting as occipital neuralgia. *Arthritis Rheum.* 1991;34:217–219.
11. Kim K, Mizunari T, Kobayashi S, et al. [Occipital neuralgia caused by the compression of the fenestrated vertebral artery: a case report]. *No Shinkei Geka.* 1999;27:645–650.
12. Sharma RR, Parekh HC, Prabhu S, et al. Compression of the C-2 root by a rare anomalous ectatic vertebral artery. Case report. *J Neurosurg.* 1993;78:669–672.
13. Garza I. Craniocervical junction schwannoma mimicking occipital neuralgia. *Headache.* 2007;47:1204–1205.
14. Ballesteros-Del Rio B, Ares-Luque A, Tejada-Garcia J, et al. Occipital (Arnold) neuralgia secondary to greater occipital nerve schwannoma. *Headache.* 2003;43:804–807.
15. Boes CJ. C2 myelitis presenting with neuralgiform occipital pain. *Neurology.* 2005;64:1093–1094.
16. De Santi L, Monti L, Menci E, et al. Clinicalradiologic heterogeneity of occipital neuralgiform pain as multiple sclerosis relapse. *Headache.* 2009;49:304–307.
17. Cox CL Jr, Cocks GR. Occipital neuralgia. *J Med Assoc State Ala.* 1979;48:23–27, 32.
18. Tancredi A, Caputi F. Greater occipital neuralgia and arthrosis of C1-2 lateral joint. *Eur J Neurol.* 2004;11:573–574.
19. Postacchini F, Giannicola G, Cinotti G. Recovery of motor deficits after microdiscectomy for lumbar disc herniation. *J Bone Joint Surg Bri.* 2002;84:1040–1045.
20. Baer-Henney S, Tatagiba M, Samii M. Osteochondroma of the cervical spine causing occipital nerve neuralgia. Case report. *Neurol Res.* 2001;23:777–779.
21. Piovesan EJ, Werneck LC, Kowacs PA, et al. [Greater occipital neuralgia associated with occipital osteolytic lesion. Case report]. *Arq Neuropsiquiatr.* 1999;57:114–119.
22. Clavel M, Clavel P. Occipital neuralgia secondary to exuberant callus formation. Case report. *J Neurosurg.* 1996;85:1170–1171.
23. Mason JO 3rd, Katz B, Greene HH. Severe ocular pain secondary to occipital neuralgia following vitrectomy surgery. *Retina.* 2004;24:458–459.
24. Kuhn WF, Kuhn SC, Gilberstadt H. Occipital neuralgias: clinical recognition of a complicated headache. A case series and literature review. *J Orofac Pain.* 1997;11:158–165.
25. Ashkenazi A, Levin M. Greater occipital nerve block for migraine and other headaches: is it useful? *Curr Pain Headache Rep.* 2007;11: 231–235.
26. Handel T, Kaplan R. Occipital neuralgia. In: Frontera WR, ed. *Essentials of Physical Medicine and Rehabilitation.* Philadelphia, PA: Hanley and Belfus; 2002.
27. Ashkenazi A, Levin M. Three common neuralgias. How to manage trigeminal, occipital, and postherpetic pain. *Postgrad Med.* 2004;116: 16–18 21–14, 31–12 passim.
28. Becser N, Bovim G, Sjaastad O. Extracranial nerves in the posterior part of the head. Anatomic variations and their possible clinical significance. *Spine.* 1998;23:1435–1441.

29. Loukas M, El-Sedfy A, Tubbs RS, et al. Identification of greater occipital nerve landmarks for the treatment of occipital neuralgia. *Folia Morphol (Warsz).* 2006;65:337–342.
30. Natsis K, Baraliakos X, Appell HJ, et al. The course of the greater occipital nerve in the suboccipital region: a proposal for setting landmarks for local anesthesia in patients with occipital neuralgia. *Clin Anat.* 2006;19:332–336.
31. Tubbs RS, Salter EG, Wellons JC, et al. Landmarks for the identification of the cutaneous nerves of the occiput and nuchal regions. *Clin Anat.* 2007;20:235–238.
32. Taylor M, Silva S, Cottrell C. Botulinum toxin type-a (botox) in the treatment of occipital neuralgia: a pilot study. *Headache.* 2008;48:1476–1481.
33. Kapural L, Stillman M, Kapural M, et al. Botulinum toxin occipital nerve block for the treatment of severe occipital neuralgia: a case series. *Pain Pract.* 2007;7:337–340.
34. Navani A, Mahajan G, Kreis P, et al. A case of pulsed radiofrequency lesioning for occipital neuralgia. *Pain Med.* 2006;7:453–456.
35. Vanelderen P, Rouwette T, Devooght P, et al. Pulsed radiofrequency for the treatment of occipital neuralgia: a prospective study with 6 month follow-up. *Reg Anesth Pain Med.* 2010;35(2):148–151.
36. Van Zundert J, Lamé IE, de Louw A, et al. Percutaneous pulsed radiofrequency treatment of the cervical dorsal root ganglion in the treatment of chronic cervical pain syndromes: a clinical audit. *Neuromodulation.* 2003;6:6–14.
37. Weiner R, Reed K. Peripheral neurostimulation for control of intractable occipital neuralgia. *Neuromodulation.* 1999;2: 217–222.
38. Slavin KV, Nersesyan H, Wess C. Peripheral neurostimulation for treatment of intractable occipital neuralgia. *Neurosurgery.* 2006;58:112–119. discussion 112–119.
39. Slavin KV, Colpan ME, Munawar N, et al. Trigeminal and occipital peripheral nerve stimulation for craniofacial pain: a single-institution experience and review of the literature. *Neurosurg Focus.* 2006; 21:E5.
40. Norenberg E, Winkelmuller W. [The epifacial electric stimulation of the occipital nerve in cases of therapy-resistant neuralgia of the occipital nerve]. *Schmerz.* 2001;15:197–199.
41. Kapural L, Mekhail N, Hayek SM, et al. Occipital nerve electrical stimulation via the midline approach and subcutaneous surgical leads for treatment of severe occipital neuralgia: a pilot study. *Anesth Analg.* 2005;101:171–174.
42. Slavin KV. Peripheral nerve stimulation for neuropathic pain. *Neurotherapeutics.* 2008;5:100–106.
43. Okuda Y, Matsumoto T, Shinohara M, et al. Sudden unconsciousness during a lesser occipital nerve block in a patient with the occipital bone defect. *Eur J Anaesthesiol.* 2001;18:829–832.
44. Naja ZM, El-Rajab M, Al-Tannir MA, et al. Repetitive occipital nerve blockade for cervicogenic headache: expanded case report of 47 adults. *Pain Pract.* 2006;6:278–284.
45. Saadah HA, Taylor FB. Sustained headache syndrome associated with tender occipital nerve zones. *Headache.* 1987;27:201–205.
46. Leinisch-Dahlke E, Jurgens T, Bogdahn U, et al. Greater occipital nerve block is ineffective in chronic tension type headache. *Cephalalgia.* 2005;25:704–708.
47. Afridi SK, Shields KG, Bhola R, et al. Greater occipital nerve injection in primary headache syndromes—prolonged effects from a single injection. *Pain.* 2006;122:126–129.

9 Painful Shoulder Complaints

Frank Huygen, Jacob Patijn, Olav Rohof, Arno Lataster, Nagy Mekhail, Maarten van Kleef and Jan Van Zundert

Introduction

The incidence of shoulder complaints in daily general practice is high. An estimate of 24 episodes for every 1,000 patients in general practice has been calculated with a prevalence of 35 for every 1,000 patients per year, 60% of whom are women.[1] Although 60% of the patients with shoulder complaints recover after one year, shoulder pain has a tendency to recur from time to time.[1]

It is not always clear why a patient develops shoulder complaints except when it is due to trauma. Pathologies such as an aseptic inflammation of the synovial membranes of the glenohumeral joint, the acromioclavicular and sternoclavicular joints, and inflammation of the outer soft tissue surrounding these joints can cause shoulder complaints. A systematic review establishes that there is a relationship between artherosclerosis and shoulder pain.[2] In addition, function disorders of the cervical spinal column and the cervicothoracic transition play a role in the etiology of shoulder complaints. It is therefore also of great importance to involve the cervical spinal column and cervicothoracic transition in the examination of the shoulder function. Shoulder complaints may be due to many causes and/or be part of an already existing ailment.

Diagnosis

History

In general, the symptom pattern is characterized by pain that prevents the patient from sleeping on the affected side. The localization and radiation pattern of the pain can provide an indication as to whether one is dealing with a primary disease of the shoulder joint or with a cause external to the shoulder joint. Other serious conditions such as pain in other joints, fever, malaise, weight loss, dyspnea, and angina pectoris should be ruled out: specifically for nontraumatic shoulder pain that has an abnormal natural course. Above all, a Pancoast tumor must be ruled out. The findings from the shoulder examination are therefore of great importance.

Physical examination and categorization of shoulder pain

Three shoulder tests are important for the examination of shoulder complaints: shoulder abduction, shoulder external rotation, and horizontal shoulder adduction. With these three tests it is possible to establish the most important shoulder pathologies, which are usually expressed as a brachialgia.

Normal active and passive shoulder abduction

During the active and passive shoulder abduction, the examiner stands behind the patient, who is sitting. When the right shoulder is being examined, the examiner fixates the patient's body by placing his left (fixating) hand on the patient's left shoulder keeping his left thumb at the C7 level. This is to prevent the patient from lateral flexion toward the left during the abduction of the right shoulder. With the examining (open) right hand placed on the patient's elbow, the active abduction of the arm is guided to the point where the patient stops because of pain, and if possible, passive shoulder abduction is further executed. The abduction is executed in the frontal plane as much as possible by keeping the examiner's (open) right hand somewhat to the ventral side of the patient's elbow (Figure 9.1) to prevent ventral translation of the arm during the abduction. Under normal circumstances, a spontaneous external rotation of the humerus will occur between 145° and 180° abduction of the arm. This is due

Evidence-Based Interventional Pain Medicine: According to Clinical Diagnoses, First Edition. Edited by Jan Van Zundert, Jacob Patijn, Craig T. Hartrick, Arno Lataster, Frank J.P.M Huygen, Nagy Mekhail, Maarten van Kleef.

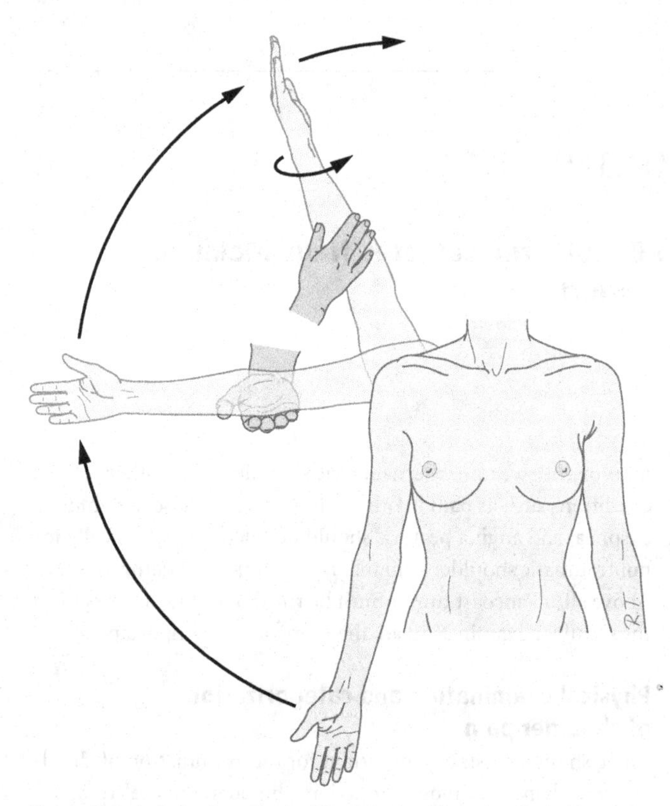

Figure 9.1. Active and passive shoulder abduction. Illustration: Rogier Trompert. Medical Art. (www.medical-art.nl)

to the fact that, to perform this abduction trajectory, the tuberculum majus of the humerus must rotate posteriorly under the acromion. It is very important that the abduction is executed in the frontal plane as much as possible because a normal abduction can usually be executed in other movement planes independent from a disturbed shoulder function and potential shoulder pathology can subsequently be missed.

Normal active and passive shoulder external rotation

During active and passive shoulder external rotation, the examiner stands behind the patient, who is sitting. When the right shoulder is being examined, the examiner fixates the patient's right elbow against the patient's body with his left hand (Figure 9.2). This is to prevent the right shoulder from abduction during the external rotation. With the examining right hand placed on the wrist, active external rotation of the shoulder is guided to the point where the patient stops because of pain, and if possible, the passive shoulder external rotation is further executed.

Normal active and passive horizontal shoulder adduction

The examiner stands on the patient's side that is being examined during the active and passive horizontal shoulder adduction. When the right shoulder is being examined, the examiner places his left (fixating) hand on the patient's left shoulder keeping his left thumb at the C7 level. This is to prevent the patient from lateral flexion to the left during the horizontal shoulder adduction of the right shoulder (Figure 9.3). With the examining right

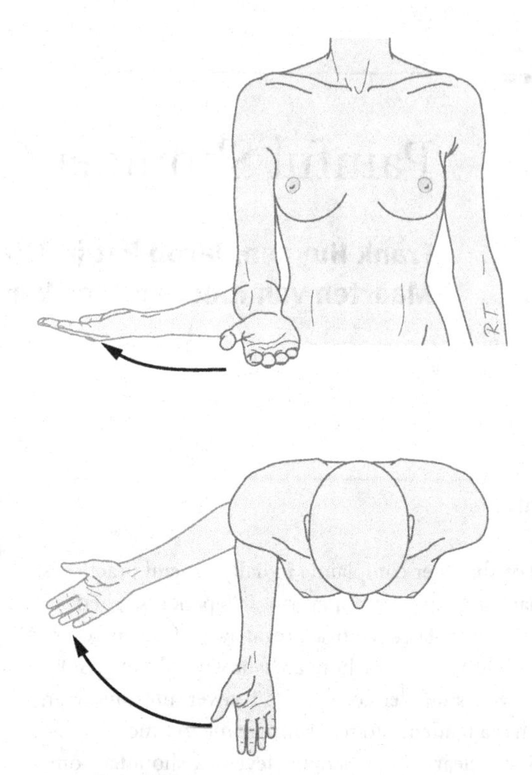

Figure 9.2. Shoulder external rotation. Illustration Rogier Trompert. Medical Art. (www.medical-art.nl)

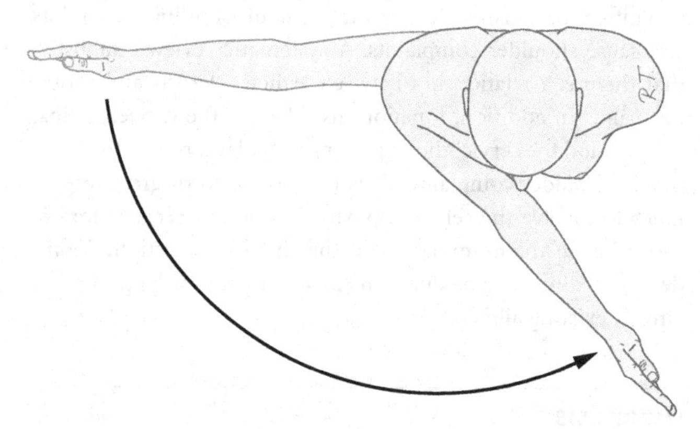

Figure 9.3. Shoulder adduction. Illustration Rogier Trompert. Medical Art. (www.medical-art.nl)

hand placed on the patient's right elbow, the active horizontal shoulder adduction is guided to the point where the patient stops because of pain and, if possible, the passive horizontal shoulder adduction is further executed.

Because the etiology of the shoulder complaints is usually unclear or even unknown, the findings from the active and passive range of motion examination are used to classify the shoulder complaints.[3] On the basis of the active and passive abduction, external rotation and horizontal adduction of the shoulder, one can detect the underlying cause of the shoulder complaints and categorize it in the following three groups:[4]

Table 9.1. Shoulder complaints with limited range of motion.

Affections	Passive external rotation	Active abduction in neutral pos. arm	Passive abduction in external rotation arm	Passive horizontal abduction
Osteoarthritis/Arthritis of the glenohumeral joint	+++	+++	+++	+
Capsulitis of the glenohumeral joint	+++	+++	+++	+
Rotator cuff syndrome	++	+++	+++	+
Osteoarthritis/Arthritis of the acromioclavicular joint	–	+++	+++	+++
Degenerative disorders of the subacromial space (e.g. calcium deposits)	–	+++	–	–

+, degree limited; –, normal; Pos., position.

- Shoulder complaints with limited range of passive motion
- Shoulder complaints without limited range of passive motion but with pain on shoulder abduction or retro-abduction
- Shoulder complaints without limited range of passive motion and no painful abduction trajectory

Shoulder complaints with a limited range of passive motion
Table 9.1 shows the shoulder complaints with a limited range of motion. It does not include shoulder affections that are considered to be the result of a systemic condition such as rheumatoid arthritis, for example.

Shoulder complaints without limited range of passive motion but with a painful abduction course
Table 9.2 represents the shoulder complaints without limited range of motion but with a painful arc in the active as well as the passive shoulder abduction. In addition, one or more structures in the subacromial space can be affected. This is also called the *impingement syndrome* in orthopedics. Subacromial bursitis is a common clinical affection.

Shoulder complaints without limited range of passive motion and without a painful abduction course
If the active and passive motion examination of the shoulder reveals no disorder, the pain is usually caused by structures external to the shoulder or the shoulder pain can be part of a radiating pattern such as brachialgia resulting from cervical radicular syndrome or a brachial plexus lesion. This also includes neurological conditions such as Parsonage–Turner syndrome (amyotrophic shoulder neuralgia)[5] and the referred pain syndromes of the shoulder; the latter can have a visceral genesis. An exception is the unstable shoulder as in habitual shoulder dislocation. Table 9.3 provides an overview of the most common shoulder complaints without limited range of passive motion.

Additional tests

Diagnostics and laboratory tests are not indicated during the initial phase of uncomplicated shoulder complaints. Additional blood tests (C-reactive protein, hemoglobin, erythrocyte sedimentation rates, rheumatoid factor) must be carried out in case of persisting shoulder complaints if a systemic condition or other serious affection is suspected.[6] Radiographs, ultrasound, and a magnetic resonance imaging examination are indicated with prolonged persistence of shoulder complaints. A bone scan is indicated when metastasis or primary tumor is suspected.

Table 9.2. Shoulder complaints without limited range of motion but with a painful course.

Affections	Passive external rotation	Active abduction in neutral pos. arm	Passive abduction in external rotation arm	Passive horizontal abduction
Impingement	–	+++	–	–
Subacromial bursitis	–	+++	–	–

+, degree limited; –, normal; Pos., position.

Treatment options

In general, shoulder complaints are initially treated conservatively. When indicated, interventional treatments usually involve local injections with corticosteroids and a local anesthetic. Interventional treatments are usually limited to shoulder complaints based on capsulitis of the shoulder joint, either arising spontaneously or in the context of a postoperative capsulitis. In addition, interventional treatments can be considered for impingement syndrome or a subacromial bursitis, diseases of the acromioclavicular joint, and diseases of the glenohumeral joint such as frozen shoulder.

Conservative management

The initial conservative treatment consists of nonsteroidal anti-inflammatory drugs,[1] possibly in combination with manual medicine[7] and/or exercise therapy, particularly when there is a functional disorder of the cervical spinal column and cervicothoracic passage. The local application of heat and cold has been insufficiently studied.[1]

Interventional management

Depending on the conditions, a local injection with an anesthetic and corticosteroid is given to treat subacromial bursitis,

Table 9.3. Shoulder complaints without limited range of passive motion.

Affections	Passive external rotation	Active abduction in neutral pos. arm	Passive abduction in external rotation arm	Passive horizontal abduction
Shoulder instability (habitual dislocation)	–	+++	–	–
Amyotrophic shoulder neuralgia (Parsonage–Turner syndrome)	–	–	–	–
Cervical radicular syndrome	–	–	–	–
Brachial plexus lesion	–	–	–	–
Cervical spondylarthrosis	–	–	–	–
Referred pain syndromes				
Gallbladder conditions	–	–	–	–
Pneumothorax	–	–	–	–
Cardiovascular conditions	–	–	–	–
Subdiaphragm pathology	–	–	–	–
Intrathoracic tumors	–	–	–	–
Metastases	–	–	–	–

+, degree limited; –, normal; Pos., position.

diseases of the acromioclavicular joint, adhesive capsulitis (frozen shoulder) and a rotator cuff disease.[1] On the basis of a Cochrane review,[8] there is little evidence to either support or reject the efficacy of corticosteroid injections.

• With impingement syndrome or subacromial bursitis, usually 40 mg of depot corticosteroids with a local anesthetic are administered.[8] Active abduction should be pain free immediately after the injection when carried out properly. There is limited evidence for its efficacy in the short term.[1]

• In case of acromioclavicular joint diseases, an intra-articular injection is indicated for persistent pain.[9] Passive abduction should be pain-free and normalized in terms of limited range of motion immediately after the injection if it is carried out properly.

• In case of glenohumeral joint diseases, such as frozen shoulder, an intra-articular injection with an anesthetic and corticosteroids can be considered when there is severe pain.[1] There is limited evidence for this treatment, but after 3 to 6 months the injections are no longer more beneficial than other conservative treatments.[1]

The natural course of an uncomplicated frozen shoulder is that of a self-limiting disease from which most of the patients completely recover.[10] In the first phase (2 to 9 months) the pain is prominent, in the second phase (4 to 12 months) the limited range of motion is more prominent than the pain, and in the last phase (5 to 24 months) recovery gradually occurs.

A continuous cervical epidural infusion of local anesthetic and small doses of opioids has been used to provide continuous analgesia in patients with adhesive capsulitis of the shoulder (frozen shoulder).[11] The tunneled epidural catheter was maintained for an average of 6 weeks to facilitate rehabilitation. As yet, only this observational retrospective study is available.

A pulsed radiofrequency (PRF) treatment of the nervus suprascapularis can be considered for a frozen shoulder or a capsulitis of the shoulder joint. As yet, only retrospective studies are available that investigated the effect of PRF treatment of the nervus suprascapularis for shoulder pain.[12–17]

Table 9.4. Summary of evidence for interventional management of painful shoulder complaints.

Technique	Evaluation
Corticosteroid injections	2 B±
Continuous cervical epidural infusion (frozen shoulder)	2 C+
PRF nervus suprascapularis	2 C+

PRF, pulsed radiofrequency.

Evidence for interventional management

A summary of the available evidence is given in Table 9.4.

Recommendations

Primarily, shoulder complaints should be treated conservatively with pharmaceuticals and manual and/or exercise therapy. Interventions with a local injection of anesthetics and corticosteroids and PRF treatment of the nervus suprascapularis can only be considered for specific affections that are therapy resistant. Continuous cervical epidural infusion of local anesthetic and a small dose of opioids can be considered for frozen shoulder and capsulitis, to facilitate the rehabilitation preferably as part of a study.

Technique(s)

Subacromial bursitis

The patient should be in a supine position. After sterile preparation of the area, 4 mL bupivacaine 0.25% with 40 mg depot corticosteroid is injected. The lateral corner of the acromion is identified. The bursa subacromialis is injected exactly in the center. In case of serious calcification in the bursa subacromialis, calcification should be surgically removed. The most important complication of injection is an infection. Small subcutaneous bleedings may result in a temporary increase in pain after the injection.

Acromioclavicular joint disorders

Intra-articular injection of the acromioclavicular joint is applied with the patient in a supine position. After sterile prep, 1 mL bupivacaine 0.25% with 40 mg depot corticosteroid is injected. The top (most cephalad portion) of the acromion is identified. The intra-articular space is identified 2.5 cm medial from this point. There should be some resistance when injecting because it involves a relatively small intra-articular space. The tip of the needle is probably situated inside the connective tissue layers of the joint capsule if there is substantial resistance. With too little resistance, the intra-articular space is possibly no longer intact and an MRI should be made. The most important complication is infection.

Glenohumeral joint

Intra-articular injection of the shoulder is performed with the patient in a supine position. After sterile covering, 2 mL bupivacaine 0.25% with 40 mg depot corticosteroid is injected. The midpoint of the acromion is identified. The intra-articular space is identified 2.5 cm underneath this point. There should be little resistance during injection. If the resistance is high, the tip of the needle is probably situated inside the connective tissue layers of the capsule. The most important complication is infection. Twenty-five per cent of the patients complain of temporary worsening of the pain after the injection.

Nervus suprascapularis

A PRF treatment of the nervus suprascapularis is carried out as described below. The patient is sitting on the edge of the bed with the neck in slight lateral flexion. It is not necessary to use imaging techniques for this procedure. The localization and treatment using anatomical landmarks is more efficient, less expensive, with less radiation hazard and better results.

The anatomy and innervation of the shoulder, with particular attention given to the nervus suprascapularis and the landmarks for the PRF treatment are represented in Figure 9.4.

The spina scapulae is palpated and demarcated from the cranial side. Across the middle of a line running from the acromion to the margo medialis scapulae (medial scapular border), a line is drawn parallel to the cervical spinal column; the lateral angle is then divided into two equal parts with a line and an X (the

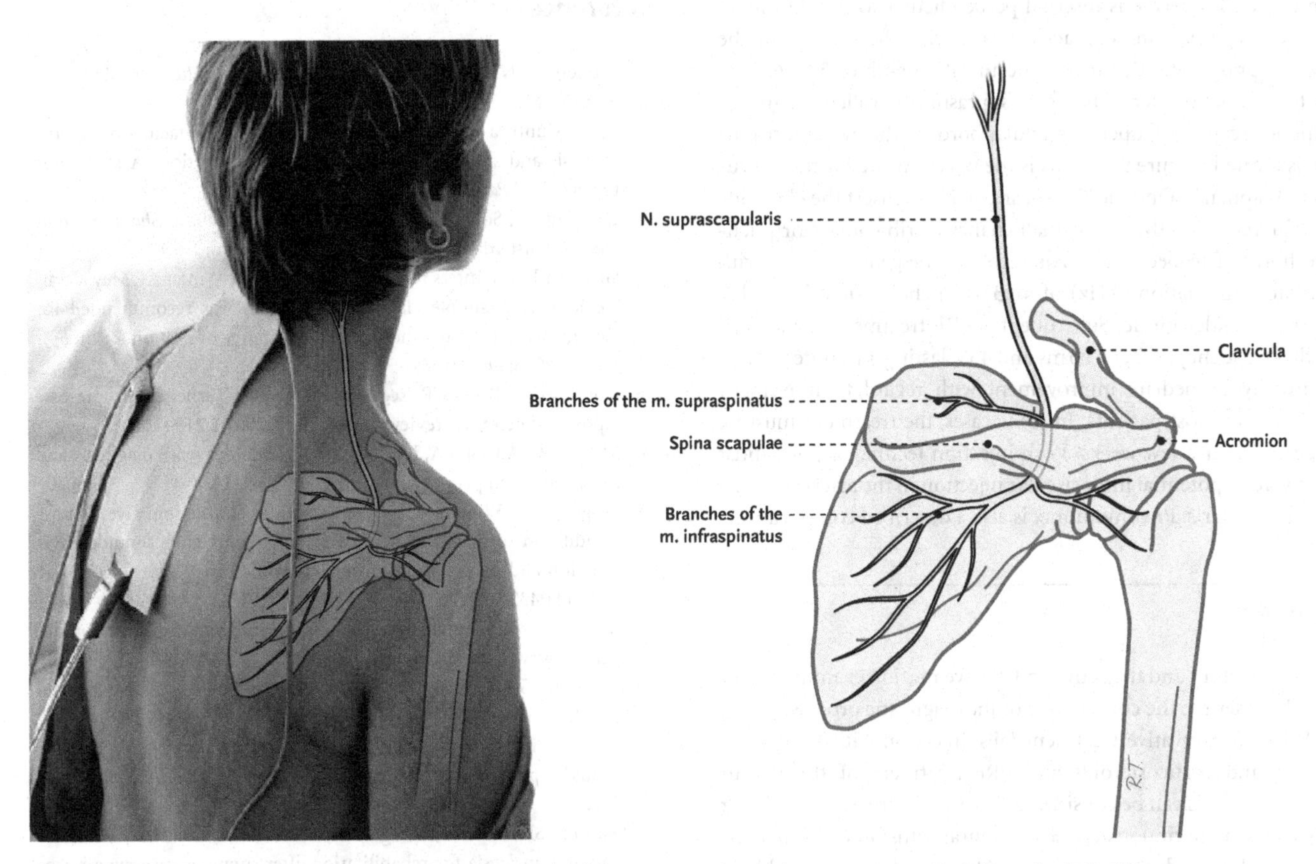

Figure 9.4. Anatomy of the shoulder joint, landmarks for the pulsed radiofrequency treatment of the nervus suprascapularis. Illustration Rogier Trompert, Medical Art. www.medical-art.nl

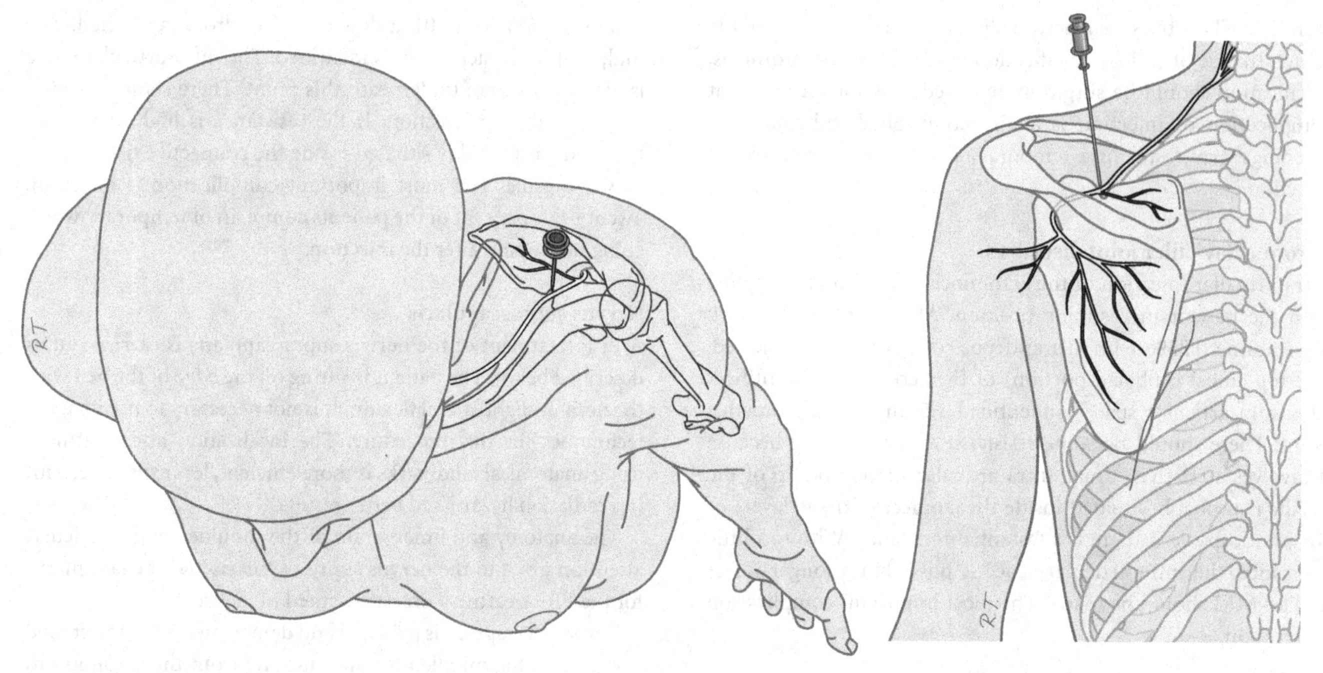

Figure 9.5. Injection site for the treatment of the nervus suprascapularis. Illustration Rogier Trompert Medical Art. (www.medical-art.nl)

injection site) is drawn on this line 2.5 cm from the angular point. An SMK 10/5 needle is inserted perpendicular to the skin in all directions until bone contact is made with the scapula in the fossa supraspinata; this usually occurs at a depth of 5 to 6.5 cm. At the cranial border of the fossa supraspinata, called the margo superior scapulae (superior scapular border), the incisura scapulae is located (Figure 9.5). This is the injection site for the nervus suprascapularis. One should be careful not to insert the electrode too far ventrally; there is a small chance of rib contact or pneumothorax. The electrode is connected to the generator and with a motor stimulation (2 Hz) of <0.3 V twitches should be visible in the shoulder girdle. Subsequently, PRF treatment is executed with a frequency of 2 Hz, 20 ms and 45 V lasting 4 minutes. There is usually immediate improvement with regard to movement and pain in most patients. In some cases, the treatment must be repeated after a few weeks. With injection techniques, one must be aware of potential intravascular injection in the arteria or vena suprascapularis. Pneumothorax is also a described complication.

Summary

Clinical history and the active and passive motion examination of the shoulder are the cornerstone of the diagnostic process.

When conservative treatment fails, injection with local anesthetics and corticosteroids and PRF treatment of the nervus suprascapularis can be considered. In case of a frozen shoulder or capsulitis, a continuous cervical epidural infusion of local anesthetic and small doses of opioids can be considered, preferably in the context of a study.

References

1. Winters D. NHG-standaard schouderklachten. *Huisarts Wet.* 2008; 51:555–565.
2. Viikari-Juntura E, Shiri R, Solovieva S, et al. Risk factors of atherosclerosis and shoulder pain—is there an association? A systematic review. *Eur J Pain.* 2008;12:412–426.
3. De Winter J, Sobel J. *Diagnosis and Classification of Shoulder Complaints.* Amsterdam: Free University Amsterdam; 1999.
4. Groenier KH, Winters JC, van Schuur WH, De Winter AF, Meyboom-De Jong B. A simple classification system was recommended for patients with restricted shoulder or neck range of motion. *J Clin Epidemiol.* 2006;59:599–607.
5. Hussey AJ, O'Brien CP, Regan PJ. Parsonage-Turner syndrome-case report and literature review. *Hand (N Y).* 2007;2:218–221.
6. Mitchell C, Adebajo A, Hay E, Carr A. Shoulder pain: diagnosis and management in primary care. *BMJ.* 2005;331:1124–1128.
7. Bergman GJ, Winters JC, Groenier KH, et al. Manipulative therapy in addition to usual medical care for patients with shoulder dysfunction and pain: a randomized, controlled trial. *Ann Intern Med.* 2004;141:432–439.
8. Buchbinder R, Green S, Youd J. Corticosteroid injections for shoulder pain (review). *The Cochrane Library.* 2008;3:CD004016.
9. Arroll B, Goodyear-Smith F. Corticosteroid injections for painful shoulder: a meta-analysis. *Br J Gen Pract.* 2005;55:224–228.
10. Burbank KM, Stevenson JH, Czarnecki GR, Dorfman J. Chronic shoulder pain: part II. Treatment. *Am Fam Physician.* 2008;77:493–497.
11. Narouze SN, Govil H, Guirguis M, Mekhail NA. Continuous cervical epidural analgesia for rehabilitation after shoulder surgery: a retrospective evaluation. *Pain Physician.* 2009;12:189–194.

12. Shah RV, Racz GB. Pulsed mode radiofrequency lesioning of the suprascapular nerve for the treatment of chronic shoulder pain. *Pain Physician.* 2003;6:503–506.
13. Rohof OJJM. Radiofrequency treatment of peripheral nerves. *Pain Pract.* 2002;2:257–260.
14. Rohof OJJM, Dongen VCPCv. Pulsed radiofrequency of the suprascapular nervi in the treatment of chronic intractable shoulder pain. 2nd World Congress of Pain, Pain Practice Edition. Edited by Raj PP. Istanbul, Blackwell Science, 2001, pp 114.
15. Liliang PC, Lu K, Liang CL, Tsai YD, Hsieh CH, Chen HJ. Pulsed radiofrequency lesioning of the suprascapular nerve for chronic shoulder pain: a preliminary report. *Pain Med.* 2009;10:70–75.
16. Keskinbora K, Aydinli I. [Long-term results of suprascapular pulsed radiofrequency in chronic shoulder pain]. *Agri.* 2009;21: 16–21.
17. Kane TP, Rogers P, Hazelgrove J, Wimsey S, Harper GD. Pulsed radiofrequency applied to the suprascapular nerve in painful cuff tear arthropathy. *J Shoulder Elbow Surg.* 2008;17:436–440.

10 Thoracic Pain

Maarten van Kleef, Robert Jan Stolker, Arno Lataster, José W. Geurts, Honorio T. Benzon and Nagy Mekhail

Introduction

Thoracic pain symptoms are relatively rare, comprising an estimated 5% of the patients referred to an outpatient pain clinic.[1–3] Thoracic pain symptoms are significant, but the number of publications on the etiology of thoracic pain is limited. Patients with thoracic pain should always be thoroughly examined because important underlying pathology could be the cause of the symptoms. Diagnoses such as angina pectoris, herpes zoster infection, thoracic disc herniations, pulmonary tumors or pleural tumors, and aneurysms can also give rise to prolonged thoracic pain of unknown origin.[4] Chronic thoracic pain after surgical interventions, such as thoracotomy, mastectomy, and coronary artery bypass surgery are relatively often the cause of thoracic pain.[5–7] Referred pain from internal organs often results in diffuse thoracic pain and can be caused by pulmonary embolisms, esophageal carcinoma, achalasia, or pancreatic diseases.

The diagnosis in thoracic pain is difficult and often "spine related". The cause of this pain may come from the nerve endings of the periosteum, nervi intercostales, ligaments, intervertebral discs, and facetal joints.[8] Consequently, thoracic pain syndromes of spinal origin are commonly seen in medical practice, spinal osteoporotic fractures needs to be ruled out in these patients. These types of pain are often nociceptive. Postoperative pain frequently appears after thoracotomies, sternotomies, and mastectomies; and often causes neuropathic pain.

Because there are many causes of thoracic pain, we limit our discussion to pain symptoms for which interventional pain management might be possible, ie, thoracic radicular pain and pain originating from the thoracic facet joints.

Thoracic radicular pain symptoms

Diagnosis

Thoracic radicular pain is characterized by radiating pain in the area innervated by a nervus intercostalis. The symptoms are usually unilateral and the pain is rarely felt in the area covered by two nerves. Thoracic radicular pain is not a typical clinical syndrome, as in the lumbar area. Different causes can give rise to thoracic radicular pain (Table 10.1). There are different pain patterns possible: constant pain or intermittent pain, nociceptive or neuropathic pain, or a combination of these. The cause of the pain may be malignant. In contrast to the signs and symptoms of a lumbar disc herniation, a disc herniation at the thoracic level does not cause radicular symptoms but tractus pyramidalis signs. The areas innervated by the nervus intercostalis are overlapping which often makes it difficult to find a relationship between the pain pattern and the nerve or nerve root involved. Thoracic radicular pain can be caused by an unknown neuralgia of the nervus intercostalis, compression of a segmental nerve upon its emergence from the foramen intervertebrale, or as a result of rib pathology. There is an exceptional form that appears most in middle-aged patients termed the 12th rib syndrome.[9] This syndrome refers to irritation of the nervus subcostalis caused by compression against the crista iliaca. The pain is often experienced in the segment of the 11th and 12th rib.

History

Initially, questions should be asked about the localization of the pain. It is important to determine a potential cause (Table 10.1). The specific clinical history can be brief in the event of surgery

Evidence-Based Interventional Pain Medicine: According to Clinical Diagnoses, First Edition. Edited by Jan Van Zundert, Jacob Patijn, Craig T. Hartrick, Arno Lataster, Frank J.P.M Huygen, Nagy Mekhail, Maarten van Kleef.
 This article was previously published in *Pain Practice* 2010; **10**: 327–338.

Table 10.1. Causes of thoracic radicular pain.

Neuralgia
• Intercostal neuralgia
• Neuralgia of the abdominal wall
Pain radiating from the spinal cord
• Osteoporosis
• Vertebral collapse
• Vertebral metastases
Scar pain
• Post-thoracotomy
• Postmastectomy
• Post-thoracoscopy
• Intercostobrachial neuralgia
• Postlobectomy
• Pfannenstiel incision
Rib pathology
• Fracture/pseudarthrosis
• Rib resection

and traumas. It is important to ask if the symptoms are related to respiration or if it worsens upon coughing. General symptoms such as weight loss and chronic cough should not be omitted. In the event of intercostal neuralgia, a heavy pain, which is shooting and sharp, occurs along the nervus intercostalis. This pain is not affected by position or manipulation. Pain resulting from rib pathology or compression of nervi intercostales is often position dependent, is often worse on sitting and less when lying down.[10]

Physical examination

Examination of the thoracic spinal column consists of inspection at rest and during movement, and palpation of the vertebrae and the paravertebral region. Provocation of pain specifically with different movements of the spine can be an indication of a spinal cause of the pain. The sensation of the thorax and abdomen should be examined. Hypo-/hyperalgesia, allodynia, and loss of sensation are indications that it might be neuropathic pain.

Pressure pain on the sternum and sternocostal junctions is usually associated with a local pain pattern (eg, Tietze's syndrome), but it can sometimes be accompanied by radicular pain. Pressure pain over a rib can be an indication of the level of the pain generator. Pressure pain may be noted over the course of the distal section of the 11th and/or 12th rib, particularly in older patients.

Compression on the thorax can be a sensitive examination, eliciting pain originating from the sternocostal joints and pain from the sternocostal junction. Palpation of the abdomen is necessary to rule out intra-abdominal pathology.

Additional test

Since thoracic radicular pain is not a clinical syndrome and its cause is not always unambiguously derived from the clinical history or physical examination, additional examination is indicated in most cases. In the event of a collapsed vertebra, an X-ray of the spinal column is sufficient. Along with a clinical history of a trauma, with or without a history of osteoporosis, the diagnostics can be completed.

A magnetic resonance imaging (MRI) could be necessary to rule out malignant causes of the pain and epidural metastases. This is particularly important if there is a history of malignancy, or in cases of acute development of severe pain or progressive pain symptoms, but also if recent physical examination showed the development of symptoms of neurological impairment. A thoracic X-ray can be useful in the event of thoracic wall pathology. If there are abnormalities, the patient should be referred to a pulmonary physician for further evaluation. In cases of doubt or when intra-abdominal pathology is suspected, then an ultrasound or a computed tomography (CT) scan may be indicated.

Diagnostic selective nerve blocks

It is difficult to determine which nerve is causing the pain based on clinical examination because the innervations of a nervus intercostalis overlap. Therefore, diagnostic blocks of nervi intercostales are performed. Blocks of the nervi spinales at level Th11 or Th12 can also be carried out by using the same technique commonly used at the lumbar level. Intercostal blocks can be carried out above the Th10 level to localize the level of the pain. Obviously, one must be careful not to cause pneumothorax. The advantage of intercostal blocks is that spread of the drug to the epidural space is less probable, because of its more peripheral location. Theoretically, this guarantees better selectivity of the test block.

Intercostal blocks should be performed under radiological control after the level has been established. First, the rib is identified and then the needle is carefully inserted a few millimeters deeper. The exact needle position is monitored after injection of 0.5 mL of contrast in the area of the nerve sheath. When the sulcus costae is outlined or the image of the nervus intercostalis appears, 1 mL of local anesthetics can be injected. If this does not occur, then the needle needs to be inserted slightly deeper. After the injection, there should be a >50% reduction of pain during the local anesthetic blockade. Usually, three levels are tested because there is often an overlap of segments. The level at which the largest temporary pain symptom reduction occurs is selected for treatment.

Differential diagnosis

The differential diagnosis of thoracic radicular pain may be difficult. Pain originating from sternocostal junctions and the sternum such as described above with Tietze's syndrome can be treated with an injection of local anesthetic solution, potentially with corticosteroids.[9]

Radiation of pain with a thoracic facet syndrome can present as radicular pain. In this case, the dermatomal area of innervation is often not affected entirely, but mostly the dorsal (proximal) section.

Pain from costovertebral joints usually occurs in ankylosing spondylitis (Bechterew's disease). The first, 11th, and 12th ribs (the ribs with just one facet plane), and the sixth through the eighth ribs (the longest ribs) are most frequently affected.[11]

Pain related to costovertebral joints is usually unilateral, and nagging or burning in character. The onset of pain may be acute. The pain on the skin is usually projected in the paravertebral section of the dermatome, but can also be localized in more than one segment due to the bilateral innervation. Sometimes the pain manifests itself as atypical chest pain. There is often hyperalgesia in the adjacent epidermal region. There might be pressure pain across the joints and pain induced by the manipulation of the corresponding rib. This last symptom is typical for pain originating from the costovertebral joints. Other symptoms are similar to pain originating from the thoracic facet joints. If the pain is localized in the areas innervated from Th10 through Th12, then differential diagnosis of a renal cause of the pain can be considered. In rare cases, mesothelioma can present as thoracic radicular pain, the painful region usually involves more than one or two segments. If the cause is not determined than it is usually intercostal neuralgia or, in lower thoracic segments, abdominal wall neuralgia.

Treatment options

Conservative management

Medical treatment with analgesics can be applied according to the World Health Organization pain ladder. In the event of neuropathic pain, co-analgesics such as antiepileptics and antidepressants can be administered. Transcutaneous electrical nerve stimulation (TENS) is an option for the treatment of thoracic radicular pain. Results for this specific treatment are not known. Physical therapy is usually applied in the form of manual therapy and focuses on the facet joints or costovertebral joints.

Interventional management

Interventional pain treatments consist of intercostal block, percutaneous radiofrequency (RF) treatment of the ganglion spinale (dorsal root ganglion, DRG) and pulsed radiofrequency (PRF) treatment of the ganglion spinale (DRG) or of the nervus intercostalis.

Intercostal block

There are no recent publications that evaluated the effectiveness of intercostal blocks for the abovementioned pain symptoms.

(Pulsed) radiofrequency treatment

Two publications report good results from RF treatment in thoracic radicular pain management. Stolker et al. evaluated 45 patients with thoracic radicular pain.[12] There was a significant reduction of pain in more than 70% of the patients 13 to 46 months after the treatment. A similar study was conducted by van Kleef and Spaans.[3] They found that 52% of the patients had significant pain reduction for 9 to 39 months. The effectiveness of the treatment was smaller when several segments were involved in the pain syndrome. There are no studies that compared RF treatment and treatment with PRF. There is one small retrospective study with a brief follow-up in which the treatment with PRF treatment of the nervi intercostales was compared with that of the ganglia spinalia (DRGs).[13] PRF of the DRG resulted in a higher percentage of success, and the duration of the pain relief was longer (5 months vs. 3 months). The effect of classic RF treatment is better and lasts longer, but it damages the ganglion spinale (DRG).

Complications of interventional management

The most prevalent complication of interventional treatment is postprocedural pain. Local pain occurs for a few days after almost all procedures. Twenty percent of the patients who received RF treatment reported that the postprocedural pain lasted for a few weeks. The most significant complication of thoracic blocks is pneumothorax; drainage maybe necessary in a number of cases. The patient is usually discharged from the outpatient clinic a few hours after the procedure. It should be emphasized that the presence of pneumothorax should be checked first. When in doubt, a thoracic X-ray should be made to rule it out.

Other interventional treatments

In cases of compression fractures resulting from osteoporosis, or even metastases, vertebroplasty can be considered.[14]

Evidence for interventional management

A summary of the available evidence for interventional treatment of thoracic radicular pain is given in Table 10.2.

Recommendations

In cases of chronic thoracic radicular pain, an intercostal block can be performed as part of the diagnostic blocks. In case of therapy resistant pain, RF treatment or PRF treatment of the ganglion spinale can be considered.

Clinical practice algorithm

The practice algorithm is illustrated in Figure 10.1.

Techniques

RF treatment of the thoracic ganglion spinale (DRG) above Th7

The treatment is performed in a prone patient without sedation so that the communication with the patient is optimal. Because there is frequent overlap of the one thoracic segmental segment

Table 10.2. Summary of evidence for interventional management of thoracic radicular pain.

Technique	Evaluation
Intercostal block	0
Radiofrequency treatment of thoracic ganglion spinale (DRG)	2 C+
Pulsed radiofrequency treatment of thoracic ganglion spinale (DRG)	2 C+

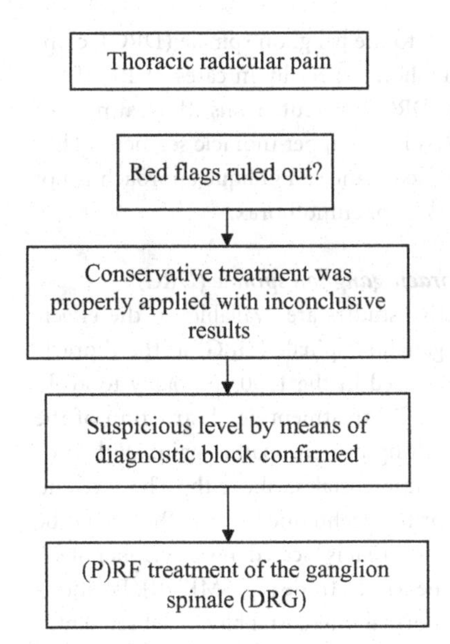

Figure 10.1. Clinical practice algorithm for the treatment of thoracic radicular pain. PRF, pulsed radiofrequency; DRG, ganglion spinale (dorsal root ganglion).

to the other, it is advisable to perform two or more diagnostic blocks in order to identify the segment involved. An intercostal block can be performed in order to confirm the involvement of a thoracic segmental nerve.[15] The RF treatment is performed at the level where the most significant pain relief can be gained. In the higher thoracic region, the classic posterolateral approach cannot be employed because the foramen intervertebrale is located more anteriorly and the proper injection site is difficult to reach due to the angle with the ribs. This is the reason why an alternative technique is applied to reach the ganglion spinale (DRG) at Th7 and higher.

Approach of the ganglion spinale above Th7

A dorsal approach is chosen with the patient in a prone position. The position of the needle tip is the craniodorsal part of the foramen intervertebrale, which is the same as in the classical dorsolateral approach. The site of insertion of the needle is the middle point (outer half) of the pediculus arcus vertebrae in the anterior posterior (AP) view. This approach is supported by data from a cadaver study which showed that the ganglion spinale (DRG) is located more laterally.[16] The injection site is confirmed with a lateral fluoroscopic view. This should focus on the median dorsal quadrant of the foramen intervertebrale where the ganglion spinale (DRG) is located. After local anesthetic injection, a small hole is drilled through the lamina arcus vertebrae under fluoroscopic monitoring and a 16G Kirschner wire is inserted. While drilling, lateral radiological monitoring should be used to ascertain that the Kirschner wire does not shoot past the target area. The RF cannula is then inserted through a 14G needle that was placed through the drilled hole until it reaches the proper position in the foramen intervertebrale. It is important that the 14G needle is kept properly in position by an assistant so that the

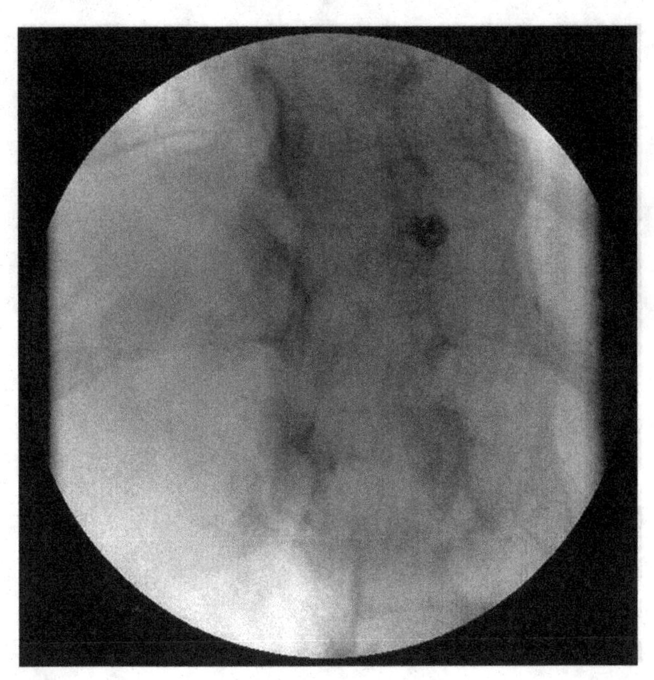

Figure 10.2. Radiofrequency treatment of the ganglion spinale (DRG) Th10: oblique view.

drilled hole is not missed. The final position of the RF cannula is monitored with a lateral fluoroscopic view. The needle should be located in the craniomedial dorsal part of the foramen intervertebrale.

The cannula stylet is replaced by the RF electrode and stimulation at 50 Hz is started. The patient should notice tingling in the selected dermatome at 0.4 to 1.0 V. Stimulation at 2 Hz should cause muscle contractions of the intercostal muscles with a stimulation threshold that is lower than 1.5 times the sensory threshold. When the electrode is placed properly, 0.4 mL iohexol contrast agent is injected to see if there is intradural or intravascular spread. Then 1 to 2 mL of lidocaine (1 or 2%) is injected and a 60-second RF treatment at 67°C is made.

RF treatment of the thoracic ganglion spinale (DRG) below Th7 (Figure 10.2, 10.3 and 10.4)

For the low thoracic levels, one can treat the ganglion spinale (DRG) with a technique used at the lumbar level. The foramen intervertebrale is noted on the X-ray image at 15° oblique position. Under AP fluoroscopic monitoring, the tip of the 10-cm-long needle is noted to be caudal to the pediculus arcus vertebrae at the lateral half. In transverse view, the tip is located in the craniodorsal part of the foramen intervertebrale. The stylet is removed and the electrode is placed. Upon stimulation at 50 Hz of current between 0.4 and 0.8 V, a tingling sensation is noted at the corresponding dermatome; motor stimulation is at 2 Hz with the threshold value at least twice as high as the sensory threshold value. The anesthetic lidocaine 2% is injected after the correct position of the needle is confirmed with a water-soluble contrast agent and an intravascular injection is ruled out. Subsequently,

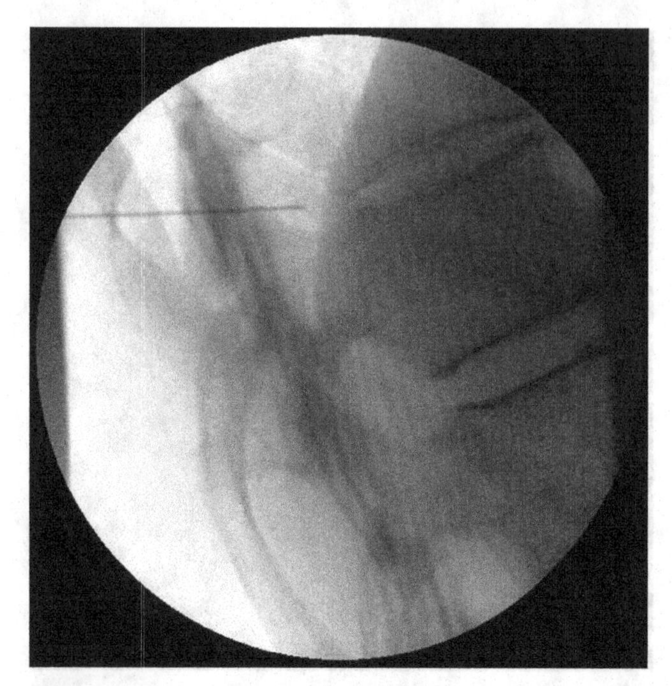

Figure 10.3. Radiofrequency treatment of the ganglion spinale (DRG) Th10: lateral view.

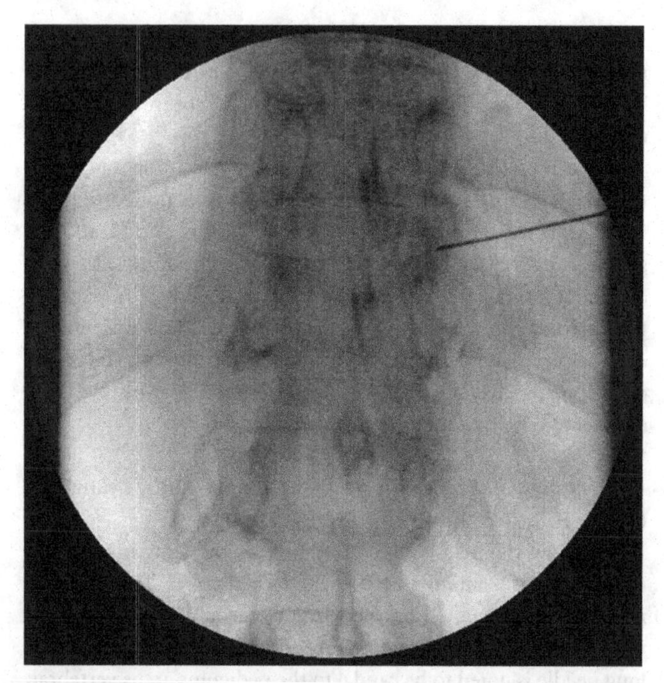

Figure 10.4. Radiofrequency treatment of the ganglion spinale (DRG) Th10: anterior posterior view. The needle is in the middle of the facet column.

a RF treatment of 67°C for 60 seconds is made. In the event that one wants to perform a PRF treatment, there is a minimum for the sensory threshold value. Although this treatment is often not painful, a local anesthetic injection is still necessary because contractions may occur that can dislocate the electrode. If a RF treatment is applied, a minimum threshold value is needed, otherwise the electrode gets too close to the ganglion spinale (DRG), completely destroying the ganglion, especially in cases of RF of the thoracic ganglia spinalia (DRGs). Percutaneous RF treatment of the ganglion spinale (DRG) in the upper thoracic segment (Th8-Th10) has always been difficult since an oblique approach is not possible because of the risk of pneumothorax.

PRF treatment of the thoracic ganglion spinale (DRG)

Presently, only retrospective studies are available on the effects of RF treatments of the ganglion spinale (DRG) at the thoracic level. The use of PRF increased in the 1990s probably to avoid the disadvantages of classic RF treatment, ie, destruction of the neural tissue possibly resulting in neuropathic pain. With PRF, it is possible to treat nervi intercostales. Above the Th7 level, no hole needs to be drilled for this technique because PRF could be applied to the segmental nerve that is located more peripherally. A cannula is used to insert the RF electrode (eg, SMK 10). Positioning is similar to that of a normal intercostal block. Subsequently, the electrode is placed in the cannula and stimulation current of 50 Hz is administered. Tingling sensation results from a stimulation of less than 0.6 mA. A tetanic contraction of the musculi intercostales sometimes occurs when the strength of the current is increased since the nervus intercostalis is a mixed nerve. The effectiveness of this treatment is not completely known. If this technique is not effective, then a classic RF treatment can be considered.

Summary

Thoracic radicular pain has an extensive differential diagnosis. Physicians should be aware of potentially malignant causes of this pain symptom and, in the event of an increase or change in symptoms, should perform adequate diagnostics tests. Usually, a CT or an MRI scan seems to be reasonable prior to starting symptomatic treatment (interventional treatment). Determination of the affected level should be carried out by a number of intercostal blocks of the suspected segments. The segment that provides the most temporary pain relief can be selected for treatment. Currently, limited results are known about PRF treatment of the ganglion spinale (DRG) at the thoracic level. However, it seems to be a reasonable choice at the present time in view of the less invasive character of this treatment. If the effect of PRF is short and the pain involves one or two segments, then RF treatment of the ganglion spinale (DRG) can be performed. Extensive skills are required to execute this procedure above the level of Th7 so this treatment should take place in specialized centers.

Thoracic facet pain

It is known that thoracic facet joints can be a source of thoracic pain. A recent study showed that, in a population with localized thoracic pain, the prevalence of thoracic facet joint pain amounts to 42%. According to this study, the facet joints in the cervical region contribute to 55% of the spinal pain.[17] In contrast, facet-mediated pain accounts for 30% in the lumbar region.

The innervation of the thoracic facet joints has not been conclusively shown, consequently, the technique of RF facet treatment has not been finalized.[18,19] The technique that we describe will probably have to be altered in the future.

Thoracic facet joints are directed more vertically than the lumbar facet joints. As all facet joints, they are innervated by the rami mediales (medial branches) of the rami dorsales of the segmental nerves. Each facet joint shows a bisegmental innervation by the ramus medialis (medial branch) of the same level and the ramus medialis (medial branch) of the vertebral level above it. There is debate about the precise pathways of the nerves.[20,21] The thoracic rami mediales (medial branches) run through the space between the processus transversi and are in contact with the superolateral portion of the processus transversi. They then continue to run medially and inferiorly across the posterior surface of the processus transversus where they innervate the musculi multifidi. While the arched course essentially remains the same, the nerves branch off at a point superior to the superolateral corner of the processus transversus (Figure 10.5).

Diagnosis

History

There are two publications on the symptoms of thoracic facet pain,[20,21] wherein the authors investigated the patterns of referral pain associated with the thoracic facet joints. Both groups claim a typical radiation pattern of the several thoracic facet joints (Figure 10.6).

Our experience is that the diagnosis of thoracic facet pain should be considered if the patient complains of paravertebral pain that worsens with prolonged standing, hyperextension, or rotation of the thoracic spinal column. The pain is often bilateral and affects several segments. Sometimes, the patient reports that the pain is felt more ventrally; hyperesthesia sometimes occurs in the adjacent dermatomes.

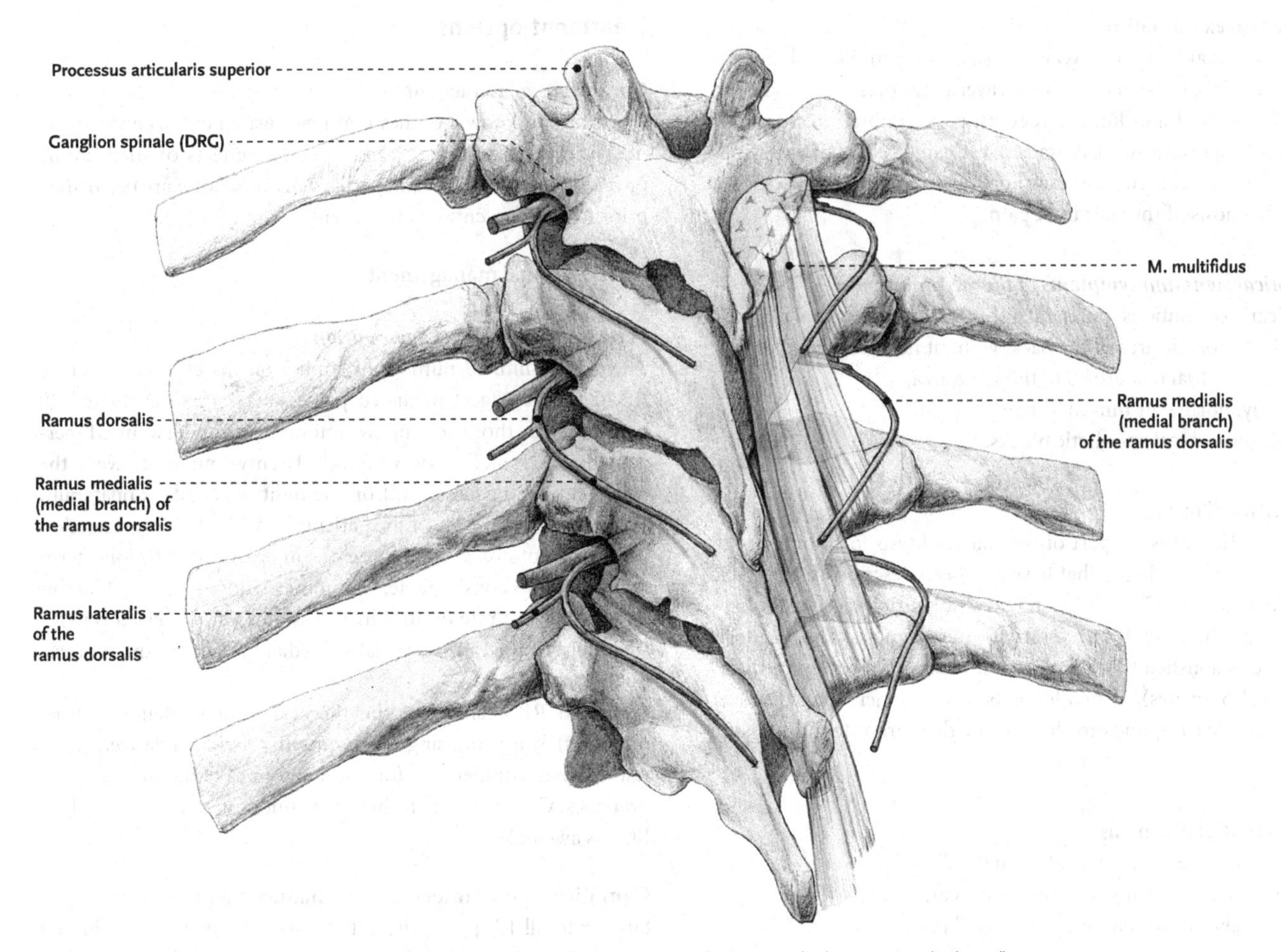

Figure 10.5. Anatomy and innervation of the thoracic spinal column. (illustration Rogier Trompert Medical Art www.medical-art.nl).

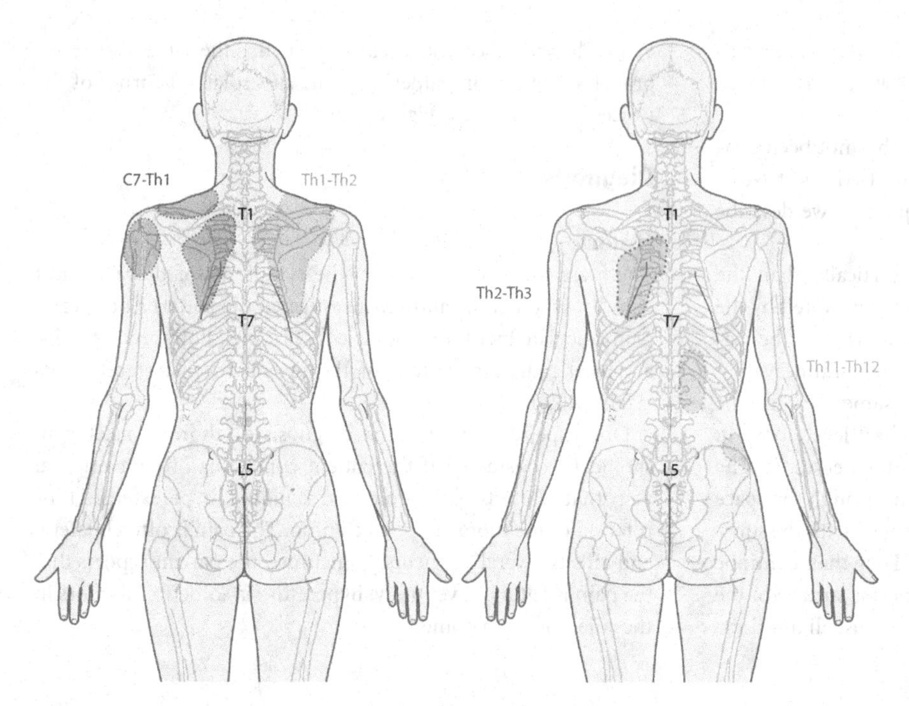

Figure 10.6. Radiation pattern of thoracic facet pain. (illustration Rogier Trompert Medical Art www.medical-art.nl).

Physical examination

Physical examination reveals no signs of neurological impairment. Pain can be elicited by paravertebral pressure. Analogous to the cervical and lumbar regions, paravertebral pressure pain could be a predictor of thoracic facet pain.[22] None of the symptoms noted on a physical examination appears to be specific for the diagnosis of thoracic facet pain.

Clinical signs and symptoms of thoracic facet pain

- Nearly continuous unilateral or bilateral paravertebral pain in a distinct thoracic area of the back, without neurological findings;
- Paravertebral tenderness in the same area;
- X-ray: normal or minimal changes;
- Diagnosis local anesthetic blocks.

Additional tests

CT or MRI scans are part of the standard tests for thoracic pain to rule out pathologies that have also been described for thoracic segmental pain. This could reveal disc and/or facet pathology, although these are not necessary for the diagnosis. The diagnosis can be established by diagnostic test blocks of the rami mediales (medial branches), at two levels per joint, innervating the facet joint that corresponds to the level of the paravertebral pressure pain.

Differential diagnosis

Thoracic pain: always exclude "red flags"

- Intrathoracic pathology (aneurysm, cancer);
- Intra-abdominal pathology (referred pain);
- Thoracic disc herniations.

Treatment options

Conservative management

There are no known studies that investigated other conservative management of thoracic joint pain. The effects of medication, physical therapy, TENS, and perhaps manipulation are performed prior to an interventional treatment.

Interventional management

Percutaneous RF facet denervation

There are a limited number of studies on the efficacy of classic RF in thoracic facet-mediated pain. Stolker et al. evaluated 40 patients with thoracic pain symptoms who underwent 51 percutaneous RF facet denervations.[19] Twenty-four underwent the procedure on the left side,21 on the right side, and six bilaterally. They showed that 82% of the patients had 50% to 75% reduction in pain symptoms 2 months after the intervention. The long-term relief was also considerable. In another study, Tzaan and Tasker noted a success rate of 40% in 15 patients who received one RF treatment of the ramus medialis (medial branch) of the thoracic rami dorsales.[23]

Cooled RF ablation of the thoracic rami mediales (medial branches) is a promising technique. It provides relatively large lesions that compensate for the anatomic variability of these branches. Currently, the technique is under investigation and no RCT is available.

Complications of interventional management

Similar to all RF procedures, it is possible that the pain briefly increases after the procedure. One must constantly be aware of pneumothorax as a complication in the thoracic region. Observation of proper techniques should minimize this risk, while constant monitoring should result in immediate diagnosis and the institution of appropriate treatments.

Evidence for interventional management

A summary of the available evidence for interventional treatment of thoracic facet pain is given in Table 10.3.

Recommendations

RF treatment of the rami dorsales of the thoracic segmental nerve can be considered for patients with thoracic facet pain who have a temporary reduction in pain symptoms after a diagnostic block of the nerves innervating the affected thoracic facet joint.

Clinical practice algorithm

The practice algorithm for management of thoracic facet pain is illustrated in Figure 10.7.

Techniques

RF treatment of thoracic facet joints

The patient lies prone on the operating table. In contrast to the intra-articular diagnostic blocks, there is controversy surrounding the RF treatment of the rami mediales (medial branches) of the rami dorsales at the thoracic level. The following technique is recommended. The C-arm is positioned in the axial plane and the proper level is identified by a steel ruler. A perfect AP fluoroscopic view shows the end plates of the vertebrae to be neatly projected over each other. The C-arm is turned obliquely and the final position of the tip of the needle is the junction between the processus articularis superior of the facet joint and the processus transversus (Figure 10.8). The site of insertion of the needle is marked on the skin and a RF needle is inserted parallel to the C-arm until contact is made with the bone at the junction between the processus articularis superior and the processus transversus. The needle is then positioned slightly more cranially and laterally, monitored from a lateral position (Figure 10.9). The tip of the needle should be posterior to the line that connects the anterior aspects of the foramen intervertebrale. Subsequently, neuro-stimulation initially takes place with 50 Hz first, then with 2 Hz. The 2 Hz stimulation causes contraction of the paravertebral muscles at intensities below 0.5 to 0.7 V. After local anesthetic is injected, a 60-second 20 V RF treatment at 80°C is made. We usually carry out this RF treatment at three adjacent levels due to the multisegmental innervation of the facet joints.

Table 10.3. Summary of evidence for interventional management of thoracic facet pain.

Technique	Evaluation
Radiofrequency treatment of the ramus medialis (medial branch) of the thoracic rami dorsales	2 C+

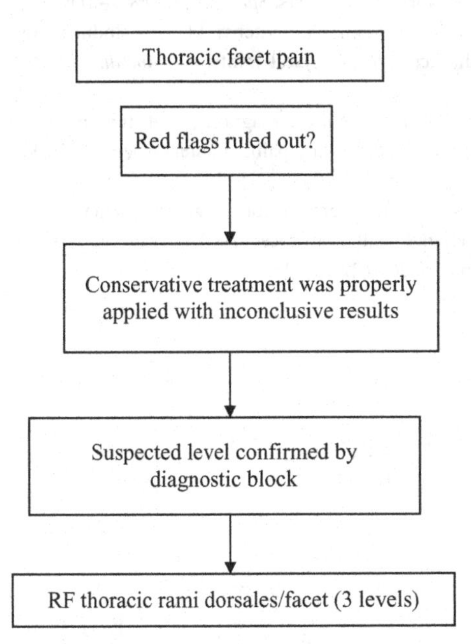

Figure 10.7. Clinical practice algorithm for the treatment of thoracic facet pain. RF, radiofrequency.

Summary

Thoracic facet pain is not a clinical entity, it is determined as a diagnosis of exclusion. The diagnosis can be confirmed after the pain is temporary relieved after a diagnostic facet block. If the pain relief is at least 50%, then RF treatment of the innervation of these facet joints can be applied. The scientific evidence for this procedure is limited.

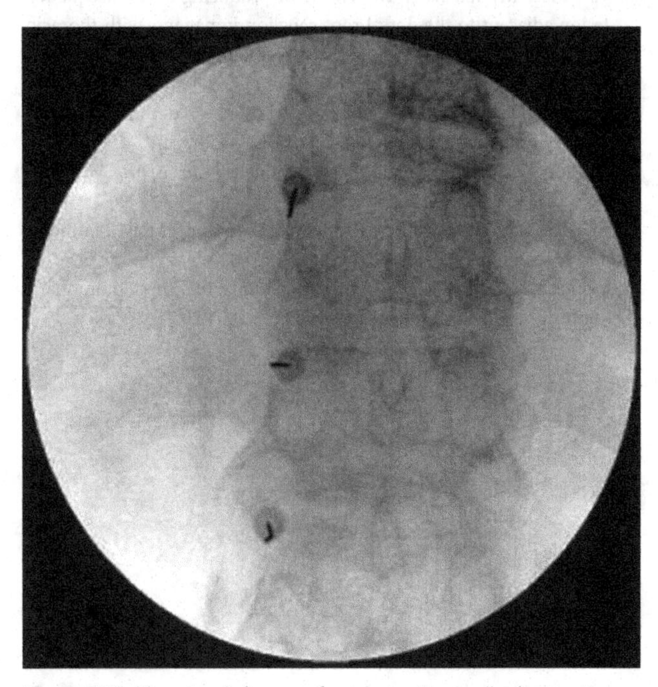

Figure 10.8. Thoracic radiofrequency facet denervation needle placement in anterior posterior view.

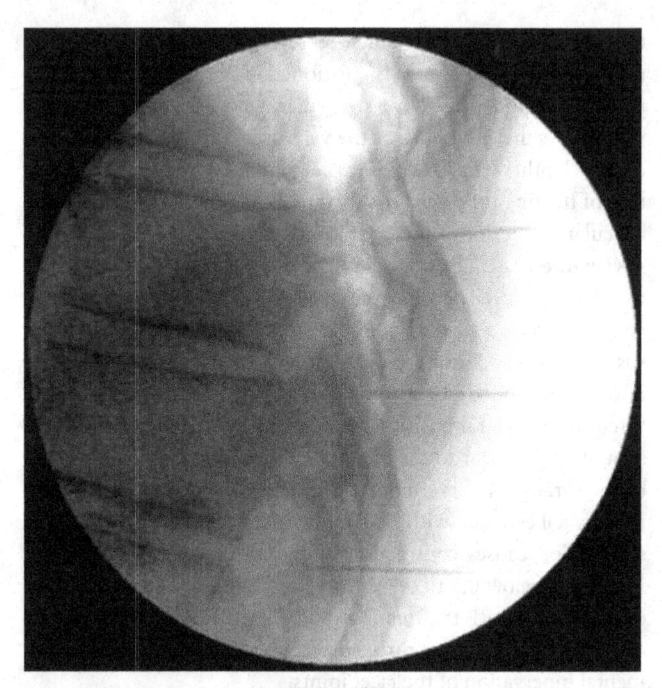

Figure 10.9. Thoracic radiofrequency facet denervation: lateral view.

References

1. Lou L, Gauci CA. Radiofrequency treatment in thoracic pain. *Pain Pract.* 2002;2:224–225.
2. Manchikanti L. Facet joint pain and the role of neural blockade in its management. *Curr Rev Pain.* 1999;3:348–358.
3. van Kleef M, Spaans F. The effects of producing a radiofrequency lesion adjacent to the dorsal root ganglion in patients with thoracic segmental pain by radiofrequency percutanious partial rhizotomy. *Clin J Pain.* 1995;11:325–332.
4. Berger A, Henry L, Goldberg M. Surgical palliation of thoracic malignancies. *Surg Oncol Clin N Am.* 2004;13:429–453, viii.
5. Karlson KA. Thoracic region pain in athletes. *Curr Sports Med Rep.* 2004;3:53–57.
6. Kost RG, Straus SE. Postherpetic neuralgia—pathogenesis, treatment, and prevention. *N Engl J Med.* 1996;335:32–42.
7. Wanek S, Mayberry JC. Blunt thoracic trauma: flail chest, pulmonary contusion, and blast injury. *Crit Care Clin.* 2004;20:71–81.
8. Bonica J, Sola A. Chest pain caused by other disorders. In: Bonica JJ, ed. *The Management of Pain.* Philadelphia, PA: Lea & Febiger; 1991:1144–1145.
9. Wright JT. Slipping-rib syndrome. *Lancet.* 1980;2:632–634.
10. McBeath AA, Keene JS. The rib-tip syndrome. *J Bone Joint Surg Am.* 1975;57:795–797.
11. Sidiropoulos PI, Hatemi G, Song IH, et al. Evidence-based recommendations for the management of ankylosing spondylitis: systematic literature search of the 3e initiative in rheumatology involving a broad panel of experts and practising rheumatologists. *Rheumatology (Oxford).* 2008;47:355–361.
12. Stolker RJ, Vervest ACM, Groen GJ. The treatment of chronic thoracic segmental pain by radiofrequency percutaneous partial rhizotomy. *J Neurosurg.* 1994;80:986–992.
13. Cohen SP, Sireci A, Wu CL, et al. Pulsed radiofrequency of the dorsal root ganglia is superior to pharmacotherapy or pulsed radiofrequency of the intercostal nerves in the treatment of chronic postsurgical thoracic pain. *Pain Physician.* 2006;9:227–235.
14. Boswell MV, Shah RV, Everett CR, et al. Interventional techniques in the management of chronic spinal pain: evidence-based practice guidelines. *Pain Physician.* 2005;8:1–47.
15. Dooley JF, McBroom RJ, Taguchi T, et al. Nerve root infiltration in the diagnosis of radicular pain. *Spine.* 1988;13:79–83.
16. Stolker RJ, Vervest AC, Ramos LM, et al. Electrode positioning in thoracic percutaneous partial rhizotomy: an anatomical study. *Pain.* 1994;57:241–251.
17. Manchikanti L, Boswell MV, Singh V, et al. Prevalence of facet joint pain in chronic spinal pain of cervical, thoracic, and lumbar regions. *BMC Musculoskelet Disord.* 2004;5:15.
18. Chua WH, Bogduk N. The surgical anatomy of thoracic facet denervation. *Acta Neurochir (Wien).* 1995;136:140–144.
19. Stolker RJ, Vervest AC, Groen GJ. Percutaneous facet denervation in chronic thoracic spinal pain. *Acta Neurochir (Wien).* 1993;122:82–90.
20. Dreyfuss P, Tibiletti C, Dreyer SJ. Thoracic zygapophyseal joint pain patterns. A study in normal volunteers. *Spine.* 1994;19:807–811.
21. Fukui S, Ohseto K, Shiotani M. Patterns of pain induced by distending the thoracic zygapophyseal joints. *Reg Anesth.* 1997;22:332–336.
22. Cohen SP, Raja SN. Pathogenesis, diagnosis, and treatment of lumbar zygapophysial (facet) joint pain. *Anesthesiology.* 2007;106:591–614.
23. Tzaan WC, Tasker RR. Percutaneous radiofrequency facet rhozotomy—experience with 118 procedures and reappraisal of its value. *Can J Neurol Sci.* 2000;27:125–130.

11 Lumbosacral Radicular Pain

Koen Van Boxem, Jianguo Cheng, Jacob Patijn, Maarten van Kleef, Arno Lataster, Nagy Mekhail and Jan Van Zundert

Introduction

A lumbosacral radicular syndrome (LRS) is characterized by a radiating pain in one or more lumbar or sacral dermatomes; it may or may not be accompanied by other radicular irritation symptoms and/or symptoms of decreased function. In the literature, this disorder can also be referred to as sciatica, ischias, or nerve root pain. A consensus approach toward standardization of back pain definitions clearly highlights huge differences in the description of low back pain, which makes comparison of epidemiological data extremely difficult.[1] The terms radicular pain and radiculopathy are also sometimes used interchangeably, although they certainly are not synonyms. In the case of radicular pain, only radiating pain is present, while in the case of radiculopathy, sensory and/or motor loss that can be objectified can be observed. Both syndromes frequently occur together and radiculopathy can be a continuum of radicular pain. In this review, lumbosacral radicular pain is considered as pain radiating into one or more dermatomes caused by nerve root irritation/ inflammation and/ or compression.

The annual prevalence in the general population, described as low back pain with leg pain traveling below the knee, varied from 9.9% to 25%. Also the point prevalence (4.6% to 13.4%) and lifetime prevalence (1.2% to 43%) are very high,[2] which means that lumbosacral radicular pain is presumably the most commonly occurring form of neuropathic pain.[3,4] The most important risk factors are: being male, obesity, smoking, history of lumbalgia, anxiety and depression, work which requires lengthy periods of standing and bending forward, heavy manual labor, lifting heavy objects, and being exposed to vibration.[5]

Pain completely or partially resolves in 60% of the patients within 12 weeks of onset.[6] However, about 30% of the patients still have pain after 3 months to 1 year. Apparently, the female population with LRS has a considerably worse outcome compared with the male population. The estimated unadjusted odds for a longterm poor outcome was 3.3 times higher for female patients than for males.[7]

In patients under 50 years of age, a herniated disk is the most frequent cause of an LSR. After the age of 50, radicular pain is often caused by degenerative changes in the spine (eg, stenosis of the foramen intervertebrale).[8]

Diagnosis

History

The patient may experience the radiating pain as sharp, dull, piercing, throbbing, or burning. Pain caused by a herniated disk classically increases by bending forward, sitting, coughing, or (excessive) stress on the lumbar disks and can be avoided by lying down or sometimes by walking.[5] Inversely, pain from a lumbar spinal canal stenosis can typically increase when walking and improve immediately upon bending forward.[8] In addition to the pain, the patients also often report paresthesia in the affected dermatome. The distribution of pain along a dermatome can be indicative in the determination of the level involved; however, there is a large variation in radiation pattern. The S1 dermatome seems the most reliable.[9] If present, the dermatomal distribution of paresthesia is more specific.[8]

Physical examination

The diagnostic value of anamnesis and physical examination has as yet been insufficiently studied. Only pain distribution is considered to be a meaningful parameter from anamnesis.[10] The clinical test described most often for the LSR is the Lasègue test.

Evidence-Based Interventional Pain Medicine: According to Clinical Diagnoses, First Edition. Edited by Jan Van Zundert, Jacob Patijn, Craig T. Hartrick, Arno Lataster, Frank J.P.M Huygen, Nagy Mekhail, Maarten van Kleef.

If radicular pain can be elicited under 60°, there is a large chance that a lumbar herniated disk is present. However, the sensitivity of this test for the detection of LSR due to a herniated disk varies sharply: the global sensitivity is 0.91 with a specificity of 0.26.[7,11] This specificity drops even more when the test is positive above 60°. The crossed Lasègue test is the only examination with good specificity (0.88), but this comes at the expense of the sensitivity (0.29).[11] Both tests are described in Table 11.1.

There is no consensus about the specificity of the other neurological signs (paresis, sensory loss, or loss of reflexes).[10] In practice, the presence of signs that are indicative of an L4 involvement (lessened patellar reflex, foot inversion) or an L5-S1 hernia (Achilles tendon reflex) are checked in a neurological examination. An L5 motor paresis will probably be characterized clinically by the "stomping foot," decreased ankle dorsiflexion and/or extension of the toes and an S1 paresis due to a decrease in plantar flexion, among other things[8] (Table 11.2).

In summary, a diagnosis of LSR appears to be justified if the patient reports radicular pain in one leg, combined with one or more positive neurological signs that indicate a nerve root irritation or neurological loss of function.[12]

Additional tests

Imaging studies

Given that the natural course of lumbosacral radicular pain is favorable in 60% to 80% of patients and that the pain improves spontaneously or even disappears completely after 6 to 12 weeks, additional examination has little value in the acute phase.[6,13]

Table 11.1. Lasègue and crossed Lasègue test.

The *Lasègue test* is performed by placing the patient in a supine position and having the patient lift up the affected leg (with a straight knee). The test is positive if this maneuver reproduces the symptoms. Rotation, abduction and adduction in the hip should be avoided, since these movements can have an effect on the result
The *crossed Lasègue test* is performed by a patient in the supine position lifting up the contralateral leg. The test is positive if lifting is accompanied by a pain reaction in the affected leg which follows the same pattern that appeared in the regular Lasègue test.

Medical imaging, primarily magnetic resonance imaging (MRI), can confirm the presence of a herniated disk; this technique is preferred because of the better visualization of soft tissues.[12] The specificity of MRI and computer tomography (CT) is very low given that a herniated disk was identified by CT or MRI in 20% to 36% of the asymptomatic population,[14] and there is little correlation between the severity of a possible radiculopathy and the magnitude of the spinal disk herniation. Incidentally, the symptoms can disappear after a conservative therapy without a corresponding decrease in the volume of the herniated disk.[15–17]

In addition to this, a hernia could not be demonstrated on the scans of some patients with clinical symptoms of a radicular syndrome.[18,19] In the event of an unclear clinical picture or in the absence of radiological arguments for radicular complaints, electromyography (EMG)/nerve conduction studies (NCS) can be performed to differentiate lumbar radicular syndrome from peripheral neuropathy (sensitivity 0.45 to 0.65).[20] Other common causes of lumbar radicular pain, such as stenosis of the foramen intervertebrale, may be revealed by MRI or CT. Entrapment of the sciatic nerve such as piriformis syndrome is not included in this chapter.

Selective segmental nerve blocks

Although the diagnostic nerve root block is a commonly used technique for determining the level of the radicular pain, there is uncertainty concerning its sensitivity and specificity. In a LSR without clear signs of a focal neurological deficit, there appears to have been a variable *hypoesthesia* already present in the majority of the patients before the execution of a diagnostic nerve root block.[21] These changes in sensory function can also vary in time and location.

With an intraforaminal block, there is also a real chance of a simultaneous block of the nervus sinuvertebralis. This nerve is responsible for the afferent input of the nearby disci intervertebrales (superficial annulus fibrosus), ligamentum longitudinale posterius, and the ventral dura mater and nerve root sleeve. In addition, the sensory fibers of the ramus dorsalis of the segmental nerve pass through the ganglion spinale (dorsal root ganglion, DRG) which is also blocked. This nerve innervates local back

Table 11.2. Neurological examination of the lumbosacral radicular syndrome.

Level	Pain	Sensory loss paresthesia	Motor disturbances or weakness	Disturbances in reflexes
L3	Front of the thigh to the knee	Medial portion thigh and knee	M. quadriceps femoris, m. iliopsoas, hip adductors	Patellar reflex, adductor reflex
L4	Medial portion leg	Medial portion leg	M. tibialis anterior, m. quadriceps femoris	Patellar reflex
L5	Lateral portion thigh and leg, dorsum of the foot	Lateral portion leg, dorsum of foot, first toe	Toe extensors and flexors, ankle dorsiflexors, eversion and inversion of the ankle, hip abductors	
S1	Posterior portion thigh, calf and heel	Sole of the foot, lateral portion foot and ankle, two most lateral toes	M. gastrocnemius, biceps femoris, m. gluteus maximus, toe flexors	Achilles reflexes

Adapted from: Tarulli AW, Raynor EM: Lumbosacral radiculopathy. Neurol Clin. 2007; 25 (2): 387–405. With permission of the publisher muscles and nearby facet joints. Furthermore, it is known that if the etiology of the pain is located proximally to a nerve block, this pain can be reduced by a peripheral nerve block. As a result, pain that originates from proximal spinal nerve root irritation with corresponding pain in the leg and back can in fact be influenced by a more peripheral block.[22] This was confirmed in a study by North[23] in which patients with radicular pain as their chief complaint had, in a randomized sequence, 4 different blocks with local anesthetic. Paraspinal lumbosacral root blocks and medial branch posterior primary ramus blocks (at the same level or proximally) as well as nervus ischiadicus (sciatic nerve) blocks (collaterally or distal to the pathology) with 3 mL bupivacaine 0.5% provide a temporary greater pain reduction in the majority of cases, in comparison with a lumbar subcutaneous administration of the same product in an identical volume. The specificity of a single-level diagnostic block is further influenced by the injected volume, as 0.5 mL of contrast already reaches the adjacent level in 30% of cases, and 1.0 mL even in 67% of cases.[24] As a result, it appears that the specificity of diagnostic nerve root blocks is limited: a negative block has a specific predictive value, but isolated positive blocks are nonspecific.[25]

An example of the variability of the effect of nerve root blocks in patients with LSR without neurological deficit is the incidence, location, and extent of the dermatomal areas with a hypoesthesia. Namely, the total area in which hypoesthesia can be found is very extensive, yet it is exceptional that in some patients, absolutely no hypoesthesia develops even though the technique performed is identical.[25] This pattern of hypoesthesia and radicular pain usually surpasses the boundaries of standard dermatomal charts, but is better understood if an overlap with the adjacent dermatomes is taken into account. The resulting adapted dermatomes are twice as large as those in standard dermatomal charts, but as a result, the sensory effects of diagnostic nerve root blocks lie more within the limits of the (adapted) dermatomal charts.[25]

Conversely, the variability of *paresthesia* as a result of electrostimulation appears to be much smaller; it is usually registered in the central sections of the standard dermatomes. The reproducibility of paresthesia by electrostimulation also appears to be high: 80% of the paresthesia can be traced to within the borders of the standard dermatomal charts, and 98% to within the borders of the adapted dermatomal charts. In spite of this, the relationship to pain remains unclear. When pain is reported in an "adapted" dermatome, in only 1/3 of cases can a corresponding reduction in pain, paresthesia, and hypoesthesia be induced by electrostimulation and nerve root blocks.

After a nerve root block, the average **muscle force** is reduced within the corresponding myotome, but the muscle force within the myotome is increased if the block has reduced the pain.[26] A possible explanation for the increase in muscle force in patients with a chronic lumbar radicular syndrome is the finding that pain has an inhibiting effect on the muscle force (diffuse noxious inhibitory control or DNIC).[27] After pain reduction, the inhibition lessens which results in a normalization of the muscle force.[28]

Table 11.3. Red Flags.

First appearance of back complaints before 20th or after the 55th year
Trauma
Constant progressive back pain
Malignant disorder in the medical history
Long-term use of corticosteroids
Drug use, immunosupression, HIV
(Frequent) general malaise
Unexplained weight loss
Structural deformities of the spinal column
Infectious disorders (eg, herpes zoster, epidural abscess, HIV, Lyme disease)
Neurological loss of function (motor weakness, sensory disturbances, and/or micturition disturbances)

In practice, the most rational method used to confirm the suspected level of radicular complaints is still the use of one or more selective diagnostic blocks. These selective infiltrations must occur with a limited amount of local anesthetic (max. 1 mL) per level and in separate sessions.

Differential diagnosis

In cases of acute low back pain, physical abnormalities, which can account for the complaints, are ruled out first on the basis of the so-called "red flags"; yet in cases of chronic low back pain, we recommend also checking whether there are signs which could indicate underlying pathology such as tumors and infections, among others (Table 11.3). When making a differential diagnosis, inflammatory/metabolic causes (diabetes, ankylosing spondylitis, Paget's disease, arachnoiditis, sarcoidosis) must also be taken into account; these must be ruled out first.[8]

The acute *cauda equina syndrome* is usually the result of a large, central disk herniation with compression of the low lumbar and sacral nerve roots, usually at the L4-L5 level. As a result of the sacral polyradiculopathy, a significant bowel and micturition dysfunction can arise with a characteristic saddle anesthesia. If the lumbar nerve roots are also involved, this leads to weakness in the legs that can possibly lead to paraplegia. Rapid recognition of these symptoms and referral for emergency surgery is recommended.[8]

Treatment options

Conservative management

(Sub)acute radicular complaints

Controversy exists concerning the conservative approach to LSR since there is no strong evidence of the effectiveness of most treatments.[29] Providing adequate *information to the patient* about the causes and prognosis of LSR can be a logical step in the management of this problem, but this has not yet been studied in randomized, controlled studies.[12]

There is no difference between the advice for *bed rest* when compared with the advice *to remain active.*[30]

The use of *Non-Steroidal Anti-Inflammatory Drugs or Cox-2 inhibitors* can have a significant effect on acute radicular pain compared with placebo.[31,32] There are however no long-term results on the evolution of LRS.

Exercise therapy can possibly have a beneficial effect. For this reason, it is often considered a first-line treatment. However, until now, evidential value for this is lacking.[10,29] A randomized study was able to demonstrate a better outcome after 52 weeks in patients who received physiotherapy in the form of exercise therapy combined with a conservative therapy from the general practitioner in comparison with patients who received only the conservative therapy (79% versus 56% Global Perceived Effect, respectively). However, this does not appear to be cost-effective.[33] For a selected population, a *surgical intervention* results in a more rapid lessening of the acute radicular complaints in comparison with a conservative approach, but the outcomes after 1 to 2 years are equivalent.[34–36] Furthermore, the effect of surgery on the natural course of the herniated disk disease is unclear and there are no proven arguments for an optimal time period for surgery.[37]

For patients with a neurological loss of function due to a herniated disk, immediate surgical treatment is usually recommended. From the available studies, it appears that this loss of function remains steady initially, but after surgery it can still regress (up to 50% of the patients).[38,39] It can therefore be stated that the outcome in cases of herniated disk with regard to neurological loss of function is determined by the severity of the lesion at the outset and not by whether an intervention occurs sooner or later.[40]

In patients with a spinal canal stenosis with secondary neurological loss of function on which surgery has been performed, reflex disturbances and sensory and motor deficits will be permanent or will only very slowly be partially restored. Up to 70% of the patients will continue to have residual neurological abnormalities after decompression[41] and the risk of permanent neuropathy is larger in central spinal canal stenosis in comparison with lateral spinal canal stenosis.[42]

Chronic radicular complaints

The place of physiotherapy in these cases is also unclear, since there are no randomized studies available.[43] For chronic LSR, a trial period with medication is indicated. Classically, neuropathic pain is treated by prescribing *tricyclic antidepressants* (TCAs) such as amitriptyline.[44] Although a medicinal treatment policy is still in the foreground, in practice, this is not always evident. Thus, for these neurogenic conditions, less than 1/3 of the patients will experience a reduction in pain that is better than "moderate".[44] Furthermore, various reviews were performed concerning the place of the TCAs[45] and anticonvulsants[4,44] in the treatment of neuropathic pain. It is striking that the included studies were mostly performed in patients with diabetic neuropathy and postherpetic neuralgia. The extension of these results to patients with LRS, with a physiopathology based more on compression and inflammation of the nerve root and the ganglion spinale (DRG) has not yet been scientifically proven.[3]

Anticonvulsants are a possible alternative for the treatment of neuropathic pain if tricyclic antidepressants cannot be tolerated or are contraindicated. Gabapentin has been studied most often in this indication and is supported by a randomized controlled trial (RCT).[46] The results are variable and optimization of the dosage is frequently hindered by side effects. The role of opioids in the treatment of neuropathic pain has long been considered controversial. Recent guidelines concerning the treatment of neuropathic pain mention tramadol and oxycodone as possible therapeutic options.[4] In an open-label trial using transdermal fentanyl in 18 patients with radicular pain, an average pain reduction of 32% was achieved.[47]

Interventional management

Anesthesiological treatment techniques are indicated for patients with radicular pain. Epidural administration of corticosteroids is generally indicated in cases of subacute radicular pain. In patients with chronic radicular complaints, corticosteroids will not provide any improvement in the outcome in comparison with local anesthetics alone. This indicates that epidural corticosteroids are more effective for (sub)acute radicular pain where a significant inflammatory pain component is present.[48] (Pulsed) radiofrequency (PRF) treatment is a treatment option for chronic radicular pain.

Epidural corticosteroid administration

The logic of epidural corticosteroid administration rests on the anti-inflammatory effect of the corticosteroids, which are administered directly onto the inflamed nerve root. There are three approaches: interlaminar, transforaminal, and caudal.

Interlaminar corticosteroids

The available evidence concerning interlaminar corticosteroid administration has been studied in systematic reviews. The conclusions of these reviews are divergent depending on the chosen evaluation parameters. McQuay and Moore calculated the Number Needed to Treat (NNT). To achieve 50% pain reduction in the short term (1 day to 3 months), an NNT of 3 is obtained and an NNT of 13 for long-term pain relief (3 months to 1 year).[49] A systematic review of RCTs concluded that there is insufficient proof of the efficacy of this technique. If there are benefits, then they are of short duration.[50] A recent systematic review of RCTs showed that among the 11 RCTs of interlaminar steroid injection for radiculopathy, four trials are rated high quality.[51] Three of the four trials used ligamantum interspinale (interspinous ligament) saline injection as control intervention. All three trials showed positive results for short-term benefits (≤1 months).[52–54] The other trial used epidural saline injection as control and did not show any benefit.[55]

Transforaminal corticosteroids

The variable results of corticosteroids administered interlaminarly are ascribed to the fact that there is no certainty that the needle reaches the epidural space and even if it did, there is no certainty that the medication reaches the ventral section of the epidural space.[56] Transforaminal administration allows a more precise application of the corticosteroids at the level of the inflamed nerve root. Three high quality, placebo controlled trials evaluating transforaminal approach reported mixed results.[51] One showed long-term benefits in one year,[57] one showed mixed short-term benefits,[58] and one showed no benefit.[48]

In a double-blind, randomized study, patients who were scheduled for surgical intervention received an epidural injection with local anesthetic only or local anesthetic with corticosteroid *at random*. By the follow-up (13 to 28 months), 20/28 patients in the local anesthetic with corticosteroid group had decided not to undergo surgery, while in the local anesthetic only group, 9/27 decided to forego a surgical intervention.[57] The majority (81%) of the patients who had not yet had surgery 1 year after infiltration were able to avoid the operation after 5 years.[59] There was no statistical difference between the treatment groups.

A prospective controlled study of transforaminal epidural corticosteroids showed superiority of this procedure over trigger-point injection in patients with disk herniation.[60] Karpinnen's group[58] carried out a randomized, controlled study in patients with radicular pain and disk herniation documented by MRI, in which the transforaminal administration of local anesthetic with corticosteroid was compared with transforaminal injections of normal saline solution. Two weeks after the treatment, the clinical result in the corticosteroid group was better than that of the group treated with normal saline solution. After 3 to 6 months, on the other hand, patients in the group with normal saline were in better condition owing to a rebound effect that was noted in the corticosteroid group. A subanalysis in which the results of patients with a "contained" herniation were compared with those of patients with an "extruded" herniation showed that in the first group, corticosteroid injections were superior to placebo while in the group with "extruded" herniation, the opposite was found.[61] In this study, "contained herniation" was defined as a herniation with a broad base, which is still contained within the ligamentum longitudinale posterius. "Extruded herniation" is a herniation that breaks through the ligamentum longitudinale posterius.

In a comparative study, the effectiveness of caudal, interlaminar, and transforaminal corticosteroid administration in the epidural space was compared in patients with radicular pain as a result of disk herniation. The transforaminal approach gave the best clinical results.[62] A double-blind, randomized study compared the efficacy of interlaminar and transforaminal corticosteroid administration in patients with lumbar radicular pain as a result of CT- or MRI-confirmed herniated disk that lasted less than 30 days. Six months after the treatment, the results in the transforaminal-treatment group was significantly better than that of the group that was treated interlaminarly in the areas of pain reduction, daily activity, free-time and work activities, and anxiety and depression.[63]

Caudal corticosteroids

Four placebo-controlled trials were conducted, but none were rated high quality.[51] The results are mixed and no definitive conclusions can be drawn from these studies.

In summary, one can state that the transforaminal epidural corticosteroid administration is preferable. In practice, due to the not-yet-completely elucidated, rare neurological complications associated with the transforaminal administration route, the interlaminar and caudal approaches can also still be considered.

PRF

The application of conventional RF treatment (at 67°C) adjacent to the lumbar ganglion spinale (DRG) has lost interest because no extra value could be shown in comparison with a sham procedure in a randomized, double-blind, sham-controlled study.[64]

PRF treatment adjacent to the lumbar ganglion spinale (DRG) was studied in a retrospective study. In a group of 13 patients for which a surgical intervention was planned, the PRF treatment adjacent to the ganglion spinale (DRG) of the nerve involved precluded the intervention in 11 patients. One patient had a disk operation and 1 underwent a spinal fusion 1 year after the treatment without having radicular pain at the time of the operation.[65] In another retrospective study, PRF treatments were carried out in patients with a radicular syndrome as a result of disk herniation, spinal canal stenosis, or failed back surgery syndrome (FBSS). A significant reduction in pain and in analgesic consumption was attained in the patients with a disk herniation (NNT: 1.38) and spinal canal stenosis (NNT: 1.19), but not in those with FBSS (NNT: 6.5).[66] An RCT aimed at identifying the potential additional effect of a conventional RF treatment directly after a PRF treatment adjacent to the lumbar ganglion spinale (DRG). Thirty-seven patients were treated with PRF and 39 patients with PRF and RF. A marked decrease in VAS pain score was observed in both groups, but no significant difference between groups in pain reduction and duration of action could be identified.[67]

Adhesiolysis and epiduroscopy

The goal of lysis of epidural adhesions is to remove barriers in the epidural space that may contribute to pain generation and prevent delivery of pain relieving drugs to target sites.

The development of a navigable, radio-opaque, kink- resistant, soft-tipped catheter has allowed placement at or near this target site in most patients. In the literature, adhesiolysis with or without endoscopic control is sometimes assessed together. There are 2 RCTs on fluoroscopic-guided adhesiolysis. Patients included in the RCTs suffered chronic low back pain and sciatica and might have undergone previous back surgery, furthermore the treatment protocols differed. Heavner et al.[68] compared the effect of mechanical adhesiolysis with (1) a combination of hyaluronidase and hypertonic saline; (2) hypertonic saline solution;

(3) isotonic saline solution; and (4) hyaluronidase and isotonic saline solution. The treatment consisted of a 3-day procedure where the catheter was inserted and the drugs were injected on three consecutive days. Manchikanti et al.[69] assessed a one-day procedure in 3 patient groups: a control group treated with injection of local anesthetic corticosteroid and normal saline without adhesiolysis; the second group consisting of patients undergoing adhesiolysis, with injection of local anesthetic, steroid, and normal saline; and the third group consisting of patients undergoing adhesiolysis, with an injection of 10% sodium chloride solution, in addition to local anesthetic and steroid. The third trial compared the effect of adhesiolysis and injection of corticosteroid and local anesthetic followed, 30 minutes later, by an injection of hypertonic saline (10%) with conservative treatment.[70] These trials and all the observational trials but one found positive short- and long-term outcome. The trial on the effect of adhesiolysis with hypertonic saline found only short-term positive outcome.[71]

Epiduroscopy, which is also called spinal endoscopy, is an alternative way to perform adhesiolysis under visual control. It couples the possibility of diagnostic and therapeutic interventions in one session. This technique was evaluated in 2 systematic reviews.[72,73]

A prospective randomized trial showed significant improvement without adverse effects in 80% of the patients receiving epiduroscopy at 3 months, 56% at 6 months, and 48% at 12 months, compared with 33% of the patients in the control group showing improvement at one month and none thereafter.[74] In an RCT, 60 patients with a 6-to-18-month history of sciatica received either targeted epidural local anesthetic and steroid placement with manipulation of the adhesions using a spinal endoscope or caudal epidural local anesthetic and steroid treatment. No significant differences were found between the groups for any of the measures at any time.[75] Observational studies showed good short- and long-term pain relief.[76–81]

Spinal cord stimulation in FBSS

FBSS is a persistent back pain that may or may not include pain radiating to the leg after one or more back operations. Spinal cord stimulation (SCS) consists of the percutaneous application of electrodes at the level of the spinal cord segment involved. These electrodes are then connected to a generator that delivers electrical pulses to stimulate the painful dermatome and to induce altered pain conductivity, transmissibility, and perception. A systematic review of the effectiveness of SCS for the treatment of chronic low back and leg pain in patients with FBSS included an RCT, a cohort study and 72 case reports. The RCT demonstrated clear advantage of SCS in comparison with repeat surgery. However, the results of the case reports are very heterogeneous.[82] A randomized study that compared SCS with conventional treatment in FBSS patients showed that fewer patients from the SCS group switched over to conventional treatment than did patients who initially received a conventional treatment and then switched over to SCS. The number of patients satisfied with the treatment was higher in the SCS group.[83]

Complications of interventional management

Complications and side effects of epidural corticosteroids

Interlaminar epidural corticosteroids

The most frequent side effect is a dural puncture (2.5%) with or without a transient headache (2.3%).[84] Minor side effects, such as transient increase in complaints or the appearance of new neurological symptoms more than 24 hours after the infiltration, occur in 4% of the patients; the median duration of the complaints was 3 days (1–20 days).[85] In a study examining side effects in 4,722 infiltrations with betamethasone dipropionate and betamethasone sodium phosphate, 14 (0.7%) serious side effects were reported (cardiovascular, gastrointestinal, allergy), 7 of which were attributed to the product.[86] More serious complications are cases of aseptic meningitis, arachnoiditis, and conus medullaris syndrome, but these typically occur after multiple accidental subarachnoidal injections. Two cases of epidural abscess, 1 case of bacterial meningitis, and 1 case of aseptic meningitis were also reported.[87]

Transforaminal epidural corticosteroids

At the time of preparing this manuscript, 7 publications report 9 cases of neurological complications such as paraplegia following lumbar transforaminal epidural corticosteroid administration.[88–94] The probable mechanism is an injury to an unusually low dominant radiculomedullary artery.[88] The largest radicular artery is the arteria radicularis magna (artery of Adamkiewicz); in 80% of the population, this artery is present in the spinal canal between T9 and L1. However, in a minority of cases, it can occur between T7 and L4, which results in the possibility that the artery is in the vicinity of the end position of the needle in a transforaminal infiltration. Depot injections can then mimic an embolism; if this occurs in a critical artery which supplies the anterior spinal artery, spinal cord ischemia may result.[95] Of the reported cases of neurologic complications, 1 occurred after Th12-L1, 1 case at L1-L2, 2 cases at L2-L3, 3 cases at L3-L4, 1 after simultaneous L3-L4 and L4-L5 injection, and finally, 1 case after an S1 injection.

A retroperitoneal hematoma was reported in a patient having anticoagulant therapy who received a transforaminal injection.[58] Two cases of dural puncture,[96] one disk entry,[97] one case of cauda equina[98] and one case of transient blindness attributed to the temporarily intra-epidural pressure increase.[99] Infectious complications such as epidural abscess caused by MRSA (1 case),[100] discitis (1 case)[101] and one case of vertebral osteomyelitis[102] are reported.

The recently reported cases of serious complication with the transforaminal approach warrant a cautious policy. It is recommended to only perform transforaminal infiltrations under the L3 level and to always administer the injection fluid during real-time imaging, the additional use of digital subtraction angiography may be of value. It is also recommended to first administer a test dosage of local anesthetic before infiltrating the depot corticosteroid after waiting 1 to 2 minutes to observe potential neurologic signs.[103] Neurological complications rarely occur when using the correct technique and when sedation is avoided. If a significant increase in pain is reported during the injection of contrast agent, local anesthetic and/or corticosteroids, the procedure must be immediately stopped in order to ascertain the cause of the pain.

Endocrine side effects

Cushing's syndrome was reported in the prospective study of the side effects of epidurally administered betamethasone dipropionate and betamethasone sodium phosphate.[86]

Side effects and complications of RF treatments

Conventional RF treatment

A burning pain was found to occur in 60% of RF-treated patients, and a hyposensitivity in the associated dermatome in 35% of RF-treated patients.[104] These side effects disappeared spontaneously after 6 weeks. However, in a later study, there was no difference in side effects and complications between a classic RF group and a sham group.[64]

PRF treatment

In an extensive review of the literature on the use of PRF covering over 1,200 patients no neurological complication was identified.[105] Twelve publications are currently available regarding PRF treatment adjacent to the ganglion spinale (DRG). Eight of those publications specifically report PRF treatment adjacent to the lumbar ganglion spinale (DRG).[65–67–106–110] In total information on 295 PRF procedures is listed and no side-effects or complications are mentioned.

Side effects and complications of epidural adhesiolysis and epiduroscopy

Four studies look specifically into the complications of epidural adhesiolysis.[111–114] The most commonly reported complications of percutaneous adhesiolysis are dural puncture, catheter shearing, and infection. Other potential complications include intravascular injection, vascular injury, cerebral vascular or pulmonary embolus, reaction to the steroids, hypertonic saline, or hyaluronidase, and administration of high volumes of fluids potentially, resulting in excessive epidural hydrostatic pressures, brain damage, and death.

Talu and Erdine[111] reviewed percutaneous adhesiolysis complications in 250 patients. Three patients (1.2%) developed epidural abscesses, and 1 patient developed a severe headache. Retained sheared adhesiolysis catheter was described in a patient who underwent percutaneous adhesiolysis to treat persistent back and leg pain after 2 previous lumbar surgeries.[112]

Unintended subarachnoid or subdural puncture with injection of local anesthetic or hypertonic saline is one of the major complications of the procedure with catheter adhesiolysis.

For epiduroscopy, side effects and complications are comparable to those of adhesiolysis without endoscopic control. There is however an additional potential of increased pressure in the epidural space due to the continuous pressurized liquid injection, necessary to obtain a clear image. Up till now, only one report of visual disturbances due to increased liquor pressure has been reported. Careful monitoring of pressure fluctuations is warranted to reduce the risk of prolonged increased liquor pressure and the duration of the procedure should be limited to maximum 60 minutes.

Side effects and complications of SCS

In a review of the complications of SCS, 18 studies on 112 patients receiving SCS for FBSS were identified. Forty-eight patients (42%) reported a side effect or complication. Complications can be subdivided in: technical, biological (postoperative), and others. The majority (>25%) of the complications are of technical order such as lead migration, lead breakage, hardware malfunction, battery failure, and loose connection. Postsurgical complications can be infection, cerebrospinal fluid leakage, and hematoma. Undesirable stimulation, pain over the implant, skin erosion, and allergy have also been reported.[115]

Evidence for interventional management

The summary of the evidence for interventional management of lumbosacral radicular pain is given in Table 11.4.

Recommendations

Based on the evidence available regarding effects and complications, we recommend the following techniques for the treatment of LRS:

- Since epidural corticosteroid injections have mainly short-term effects; these techniques are recommended for patients with subacute radicular pain symptoms.
- In patients with pain at the lumbosacral level (L4, L5, S1) as a result of a "contained herniation," a transforaminal epidural injection with local anesthetic and corticosteroids is recommended.

Table 11.4. Summary of the evidence for interventional management of lumbosacral radicular syndrome.

Technique	Assessment
Interlaminar corticosteroid administration	2 B±
Transforaminal corticosteroid administration in "contained herniation"	2 B+
Transforaminal corticosteroid administration in "extruded herniation"	2 B–
Radiofrequency lesioning at the level of the ganglion spinale (DRG)	2 A–
Pulsed radiofrequency treatment at the level of the ganglion spinale	2 C+
Spinal cord stimulation (Failed Back Surgery Syndrome only)	2 A+
Adhesiolysis—epiduroscopy	2 B±

A preference seems to exist for transforaminal epidural corticosteroid administration over caudal and interlaminar corticosteroids below level L3.

• RF treatment adjacent to the ganglion spinale (DRG) is not recommended. A PRF treatment adjacent to the ganglion spinale (DRG) can be considered.

• Spinal cord stimulation is recommended for patients with FBSS, but only in specialized centers.

• Epiduroscopy and adhesiolysis can be considered for patients with therapy resistant radicular syndrom in the context of a study and only in specialized centers.

Clinical practice algorithm

Figure 11.1 represents the treatment algorithm based on the available evidence.

Techniques

Practical recommendations epidural corticosteroid administration

There are 7 systematic reviews concerning epidural corticosteroid administration for the treatment of LRS. With regard to short-term effectiveness, 6 of the 7 systematic reviews give a positive assessment and 1 gives a negative assessment (conflicting evidence).[84–116–120] There are no comparative studies available for the effectiveness and/or complications of the various depot corticosteroids, which means that a distinction between these products cannot be verified.

It is possible that the particle size of the depot corticosteroid is related to the reported neurological complications, but the literature concerning this possibility is also inconclusive.[121] Up till now, no reported neurologic complications were noted with the nonparticulate corticosteroid dexamethasone. One abstract has prospectively compared the transforaminal use of triamcinolone with dexamethasone in 50 patients.[122] A significant greater reduction in pain was noted after 2 weeks in patients treated with triamcinolone, so this far evidence about its efficacy at the lumbar level is lacking. Currently, there is no evidence that a higher corticosteroid dosage produces a better clinical effect,[123] yet the risk of endocrine side effects is substantially higher. It is for this reason that the lowest dosage of depot corticosteroid is currently recommended.

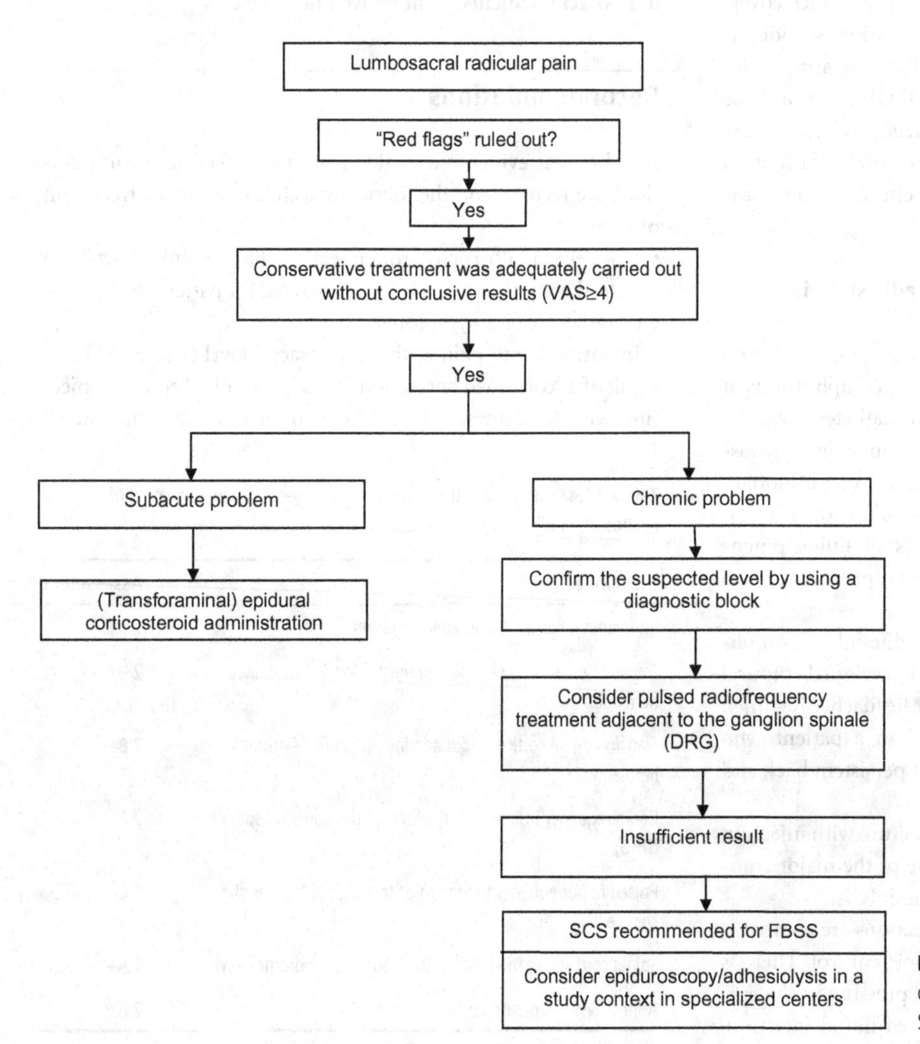

Figure 11.1. Practice algorithm for the treatment of lumbosacral radicular syndrome. FBSS, Failed Back Surgery Syndrome.

With regard to the number of infiltrations, there are no comparative studies that have shown that the systematic implementation of 3 infiltrations would result in superior outcome.[124] From the RCTs available concerning the transforaminal administration of corticosteroids, one finds an average of 1 to 2 infiltrations. Considering the potential endocrine side effects, adhering to an interval of at least 2 weeks between two infiltrations is recommended.

Interlaminar epidural corticosteroid administration

This technique can be carried out with the patient in a prone position, lying on the side or sitting; in the two latter postures, place the patient in flexion or in the "fetal" position.[125] The sitting posture is considered to be the most comfortable for the patient as well as for the pain physician. This position allows a correct assessment of the midline and avoids the rotation of a lateral decubitus position.

Determination of the correct level can occur with reference to the cresta iliaca (iliac crest) or via fluoroscopy. In the *medial approach*, first a local anesthetic will be infiltrated in the middle of two adjacent processus spinosi, thereafter, the subcutaneous tissue and the ligamentum supraspinale are approached with an epidural needle. The latter offers enough resistance to keep the epidural needle in position when the needle is released. Subsequently, the needle enters the ligamentum interspinale and the ligamentum flavum, which both provide additional resistance. A false sensation of loss of resistance may occur upon entering the space between the ligamentum interspinale and the ligamentum flavum. The ligamentum flavum provides the greatest resistance to the epidural needle since it is almost entirely composed of collagenous fibers. Breaking through this ligament to the epidural space is accompanied by a significant loss of resistance. When injecting medication into the epidural space, normally no resistance should be felt since it is filled with fat, blood vessels, lymph tissue and connective tissue. The epidural space is 5 to 6 mm wide at the L2-L3 level in a patient in a flexion position. In addition, the injection of contrast agent can verify the correct positioning in the epidural space.

In the case of aspiration of blood, the needle must be reoriented; in the case of aspiration of cerebrospinal fluid, the procedure must be repeated at another level. In the latter case, an overflow to the cerebrospinal fluid is possible; therefore, this procedure must be carried out with caution.

Classically, an infiltration consists of an injection of a local anesthetic with a corticosteroid. There is a tendency to perform this procedure under fluoroscopy, yet thus far, no advantages of fluoroscopic control have been demonstrated.[126,127]

Transforaminal epidural corticosteroid administration

In a transforaminal approach, the C-arm is adjusted in such a way that the X-rays run parallel to the cover plates of the relevant level. Thereafter, the C-arm is rotated until the processus spinosus projects over the contralateral facet column. With the C-arm in this projection, the injection point is found by projecting a metal ruler over the medial part of the foramen intervertebrale. If there is a superposition of the processus articularis superius (superior articular process) of the underlying joint, the C-arm must be rotated cranially.

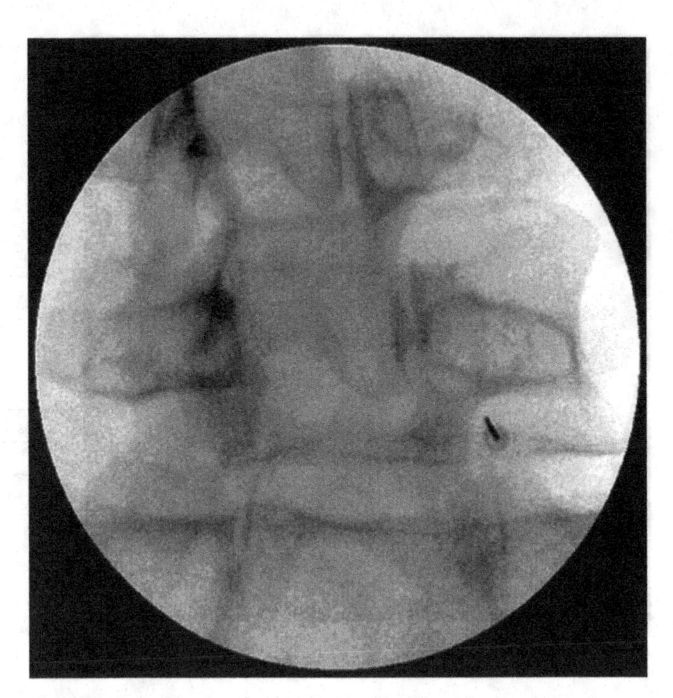

Figure 11.2. Lumbar transforaminal epidural injection: injection point (oblique insertion).

A 10-cm long, 25-G or 22-G needle with connection tubing that is first flushed with contrast medium is inserted here locally in the direction of the radiation beam. Thereafter, the direction is corrected such that the needle is projected as a point on the screen (Figure 11.2). Then, in a lateral view, the depth of the needle tip is checked. A classical approach is in the dorsocranial quadrant, care should be taken that no arterial/venous flow is noticed during real time imaging of contrast injection. We recommend avoiding needle elicitation of paresthesia in the patient. Paresthesia is considered unpleasant by the patient and, in addition, segmental medullary blood vessels may be hit.[89,128] Therefore, the "safe triangle" should be taken into account (Figure 11.3). This triangle is formed cranially by the underside of the upper pediculus, laterally by a line between the lateral edges of the upper and lower pediculus and medially by the spinal nerve root (as the tangential base of the triangle). This is considered to be a safe zone; if a radiating pain still occurs during the procedure, the needle must be pulled back several millimeters.

The direction of the radiation beam is now modified to forward-backward (A-P view); as a result, the point of the needle should be located between the lateral edge and the middle of the facet column. After the injection of a small quantity of contrast agent during real-time imaging, the course of the ramus ventralis (spinal nerve), in the epidural or laterocaudal direction becomes visible. If this image is not attained due to a position that is too

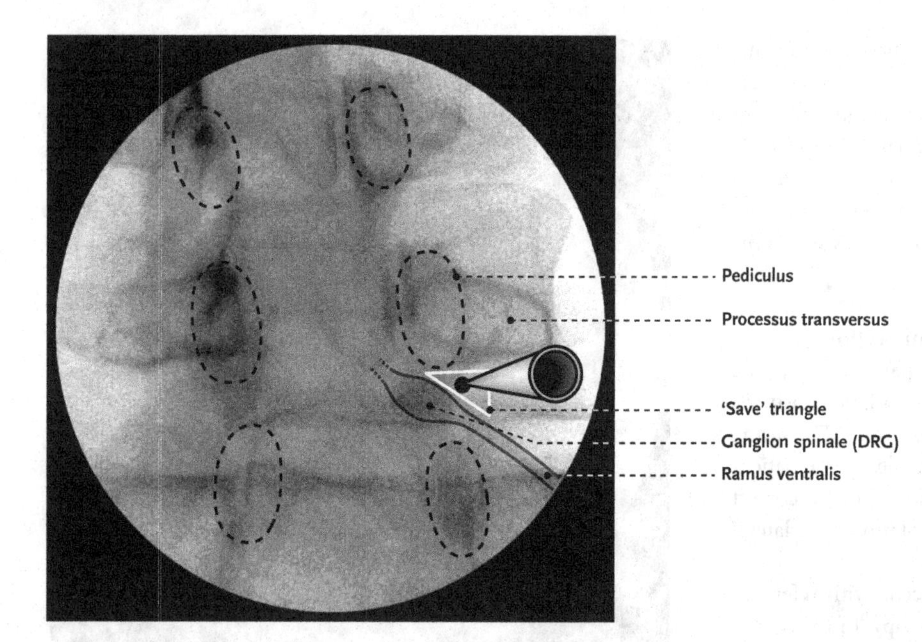

Figure 11.3. "Safe triangle" for the insertion of the needle in transforaminal epidural injection (illustration: Rogier Trompert Medical Art. www.medical-art.nl).

lateral, the needle must be more deeply inserted toward the ganglion spinale (DRG). The execution of this procedure during real-time imaging allows the distinction to be made between an accidental intrathecal, intra-arterial or intravenous injection.

After a correct visualization of the ramus ventralis (spinal nerve), a test is carried out with 1 mL bupivacaine 0.5% or xylocaine, 1 to 2 minutes thereafter, the patient is asked to move the legs to rule out a sudden paresthesia based on medullary ischemia.[89,95] The corticosteroid dosage can then be injected.

S1 transforaminal epidural procedure

The technique used at the S1 level is analogous with that used for the lumbar levels; however, this time the needle is positioned through the foramen sacrale dorsale of S1 on the S1 pedicle. For this, the target lies on the caudal edge of the S1 pediculus on a location homologous to that in the case of the lumbar transforaminal infiltrations. Radiologically, this foramen cannot be that clearly distinguished, but by reorienting the C-arm cephalocaudally and rotating it ipsilaterally, one can cause the foramen sacrale ventrale and the foramen sacrale dorsale of S1 to overlap. The puncture point is chosen at the level of the lateral edge of the foramen sacrale dorsale of S1. In an optimal position, the needle point is positioned at 5 mm from the floor of the canalis sacralis in a lateral view.

PRF treatment

Diagnostic block

In a diagnostic block, the C-arm is adjusted in such a way that the X-rays run parallel to the end plates of the relevant level. Thereafter, the C-arm is rotated until the processus spinosus projects over the contralateral facet column. With the C-arm in this projection, the injection point is found by projecting a metal ruler over the *lateral part* of the foramen intervertebrale. A 10-cm long, 22-G needle is inserted here locally in the direction of the rays. Thereafter, the direction is corrected such that the needle is projected as a point on the screen (Figure 11.4). The direction of the radiation beam is now modified to a profile (lateral) view, and the needle inserted until the point is located in the craniodorsal part of the foramen intervertebrale (Figure 11.5).

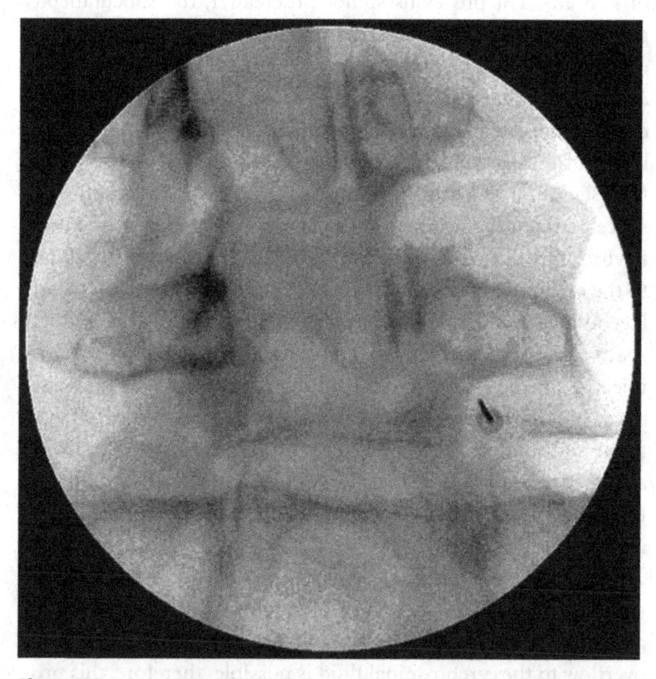

Figure 11.4. Lumbar diagnostic block ganglion spinale (DRG): oblique view.

In an AP view, the course of a small amount of contrast agent is followed with "real-time imaging"; it spreads out laterocaudally

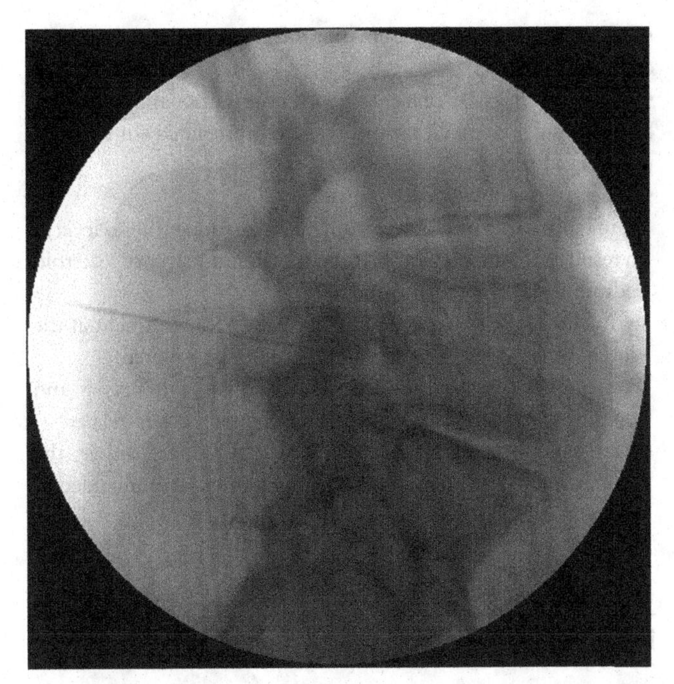

Figure 11.5. Lumbar diagnostic block ganglion spinale (DRG) lateral view.

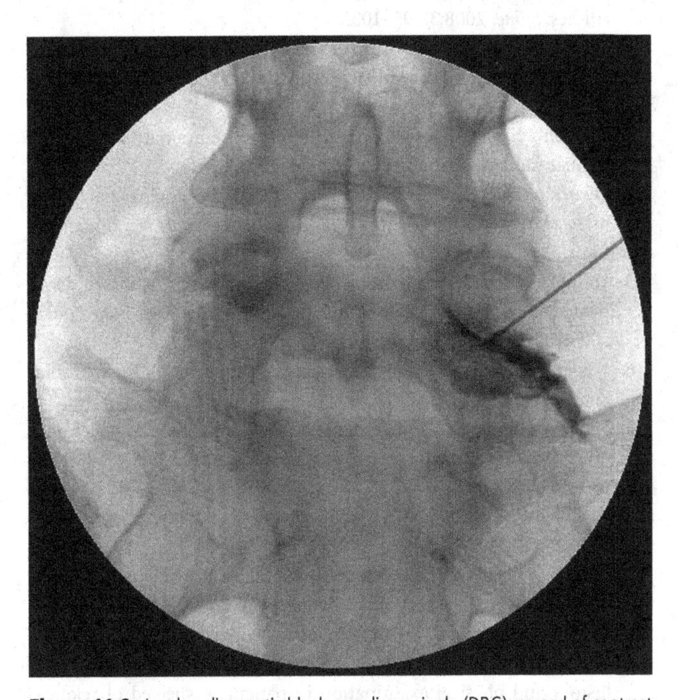

Figure 11.6. Lumbar diagnostic block ganglion spinale (DRG): spread of contrast fluid along the segmental nerve.

along the spinal nerve (Figure 11.6). Finally, a maximum of 1 mL lidocaine 2% or bupivacaine 0.5% is injected.

A prognostic block is considered positive if there is a 50% reduction in symptoms 20 to 30 minutes after the intervention. The level that best satisfies the aforementioned criteria is chosen for PRF treatment.

Lumbar percutaneous PRF

The insertion point for PRF treatment is determined in the same way as for the diagnostic block; this time, the projection is kept as *medial* as possible in order to maximally reach the ganglion spinale (DRG). The cannula is inserted in the direction of the radiation beam. While the cannula is still located in the superficial layers, the direction is corrected so that the cannula is projected as a point on the screen. Thereafter, the cannula is carefully inserted further until the point is located in the middle on the foramen intervertebrale in lateral view.

The stylet is removed and exchanged for the RF probe. The impedance is checked, and thereafter, stimulation at 50 Hz is done. The patient should now feel tingling at a voltage of <0.5 V.

If these criteria are met, the position of the cannula is recorded in two directions on a video printer. Thereafter, a pulsed current (routinely 20 ms current and 480 ms without current) is applied for 120 s with an output of 45 V; during this procedure, the temperature at the tip of the electrode may not surpass 42°C. The output may need to be reduced.

The target is an impedance of less than 500 Ω. If it is higher, fluid injection can reduce this value. There are reports that the injection of a contrast agent can paradoxically increase the impedance. After repositioning, one can search for a lower stimulation threshold for additional treatment.

Adhesiolysis[129]

Under fluoroscopic control the target level is identified. The C-arm is then rotated 15 to 20° oblique to the ipsilateral side of the targeted foramen intervertebrale. Once a "Scotty dog" image is obtained, the fluoroscope is rotated in a caudal-cephalad direction for 15 to 20°. A caudal-cephalad rotation elongates the superior articular process ("ear of the Scotty dog"). The tip of the ear, or processus articularis superior, in the "gun barrel" technique is marked on the skin as entry point. An 18-G needle is used to make a puncture wound. Through this wound, a 16-G Epimed R-K epidural needle is advanced anteriorly until bone is contacted. A lateral fluoroscopic image is obtained before further introduction of the needle. To facilitate passage of the needle past the processus articularis superior, the epidural needle is turned laterally to slide past the bone and stop just after a "pop" is felt. The needle tip on a lateral view should be in the posterior aspect of the foramen intervertebrale. An Epimed Tun-L-XL epidural catheter is then inserted through the epidural needle. Occasionally, the epidural needle must be tilted at the hub laterally to aid entry of the epidural catheter into the anterior epidural space. The catheter is advanced medial to the pediculus. After catheter placement is confirmed to be in the anterior epidural space under anteroposterior and lateral views, the stylet is removed from the catheter and a connector is placed on the proximal end of the epidural catheter.

Aspiration should be negative before 3 mL radiographic contrast is injected. The contrast injection should show opening of the entered foramen intervertebrale, with contrast exiting along the path of the nerve root.

Lysis is commonly performed with hypertonic saline but remains controversial due to its potential neurotoxocity should intrathecal spread occur.

After performing the lysis, local anesthetic and corticosteroid is injected.

When performing adhesiolysis according to the Racz procedure, the catheter is kept in place and lysis is repeated on 3 consecutive days.[130] Manchikanti on the other hand advocates a one-day procedure.[131]

Epiduroscopy[77]

Epiduroscopy is performed with the patient in the prone position on a translucent table. Intravenous access, electrocardiographic, blood pressure, and oxygen saturation monitoring must be established. The patient is lightly sedated, making sure that communication is possible throughout the procedure.

The sacral cornua are identified. When this proves to be difficult, internal rotation of the feet will widen the gluteal cleft, thus facilitating the identification of the hyatus sacralis. After anesthesia of the skin and underlying tissues, an 18-G Tuohy needle is advanced 2 to 3 cm into the canalis sacralis. Care must be taken not to exceed the level of S3 to prevent intradural placement of the needle and subsequent equipment. Through the Tuohy needle a guide-wire is directed cranially, as close as possible to the target area. The Manchikanti group recommends not to position the guidewire beyond the S3 level. In this case, however, there is an increased risk of dislocation when placing the introducer and performing dilation. A small incision is made at the introduction site and after removal of the Tuohy needle, a dilator is passed over the guide wire followed by the introducer sheath. The side arm of the introducer sheath is left open to allow drainage of excess saline. A flexible 0.9 mm (outer diameter) fiberoptic endocscope (magnification ×45) is introduced through one of two main access ports of a disposable 2.2 mm (outer diameter) steering catheter. The steering catheter also contains 2 side channels for fluid instillation. One side channel of the steering catheter is used for the intermittent flush of normal saline. The other side channel is connected to an automatic monitoring system by means of a standard arterial pressure monitoring system, to allow for continuous monitoring of epidural/saline delivery pressure. After distention of the sacral epidural space with normal saline, the steering catheter with the fiberoptic endoscope is slowly advanced to the target area. The epidural space is kept distended with normal saline, but the pressure should be limited to minimize the risks of compromised perfusion. Total saline volume ranges between 50 and 250 mL. When fibrosis or adhesions become visible during epiduroscopy, these can be mobilized with the tip of the endoscope. It is recommended to limit the duration of the procedure to maximum 60 minutes

Summary

There is no gold standard for the diagnosis of lumbosacral radicular pain.

- History and clinical examination are the cornerstones of the diagnostic process.
- In case red flags are present or if an interventional treatment is being considered, medical imaging is recommended with a slight preference for MRI.
- When conservative treatment fails:
  - in (sub)acute lumbosacral radicular pain under the L3 level as a result of a contained herniation, transforaminal corticosteroid administration is recommended.
  - In chronic lumbosacral radicular pain, PRF treatment at the level of the ganglion spinale (DRG) can be considered.
  - For refractory lumbosacral radicular pain, adhesiolysis and epiduroscopy can be considered, preferentially study-related.
  - In patients with a therapy-resistant radicular pain in the context of an FBSS, spinal cord stimulation is recommended in a study design.

References

1. Dionne CE, Dunn KM, Croft PR, et al. A consensus approach toward the standardization of back pain definitions for use in prevalence studies. *Spine.* 2008;33:95–103.
2. Konstantinou K, Dunn KM. Sciatica: review of epidemiological studies and prevalence estimates. *Spine (Phila Pa 1976).* 2008;33:2464–2472.
3. Khoromi S, Patsalides A, Parada S, et al. Topiramate in chronic lumbar radicular pain. *J Pain.* 2005;6:829–836.
4. Dworkin RH, O'Connor AB, Backonja M, et al. Pharmacologic management of neuropathic pain: evidencebased recommendations. *Pain.* 2007;132:237–251.
5. Younes M, Bejia I, Aguir Z, et al. Prevalence and risk factors of disk-related sciatica in an urban population in Tunisia. *Joint Bone Spine.* 2006;73:538–542.
6. Weber H. The natural course of disc herniation. *Acta Orthop Scand Suppl.* 1993;251:19–20.
7. Peul WC, Brand R, Thomeer RT, Koes BW. Influence of gender and other prognostic factors on outcome of sciatica. *Pain.* 2008;138: 180–191.
8. Tarulli AW, Raynor EM. Lumbosacral radiculopathy. *Neurol Clin.* 2007;25:387–405.
9. Murphy DR, Hurwitz EL, Gerrard JK, Clary R. Pain patterns and descriptions in patients with radicular pain: does the pain necessarily follow a specific dermatome? *Chiropr Osteopat.* 2009;17:9.
10. Vroomen PC, de Krom MC, Knottnerus JA. Diagnostic value of history and physical examination in patients suspected of sciatica due to disc herniation: a systematic review. *J Neurol.* 1999;246: 899–906.
11. Deville WL, van der Windt DA, Dzaferagic A, Bezemer PD, Bouter LM. The test of Lasegue: systematic review of the accuracy in diagnosing herniated discs. *Spine.* 2000;25:1140–1147.
12. Koes BW, van Tulder MW, Peul WC. Diagnosis and treatment of sciatica. *BMJ.* 2007;334:1313–1317.
13. Hofstee DJ, Gijtenbeek JM, Hoogland PH, et al. Westeinde sciatica trial: randomized controlled study of bed rest and physiotherapy for acute sciatica. *J Neurosurg.* 2002;96:45–49.

14. Jensen MC, Brant-Zawadzki MN, Obuchowski N, et al. Magnetic resonance imaging of the lumbar spine in people without back pain. *N Engl J Med.* 1994;331:69–73.
15. Delauche-Cavallier MC, Budet C, Laredo JD, et al. Lumbar disc herniation. Computed tomography scan changes after conservative treatment of nerve root compression. *Spine.* 1992;17:927–933.
16. Wiesel SW, Tsourmas N, Feffer HL, Citrin CM, Patronas N. A study of computer-assisted tomography. I. The incidence of positive CAT scans in an asymptomatic group of patients. *Spine.* 1984;9: 549–551.
17. Maigne JY, Rime B, Deligne B. Computed tomographic follow-up study of forty-eight cases of nonoperatively treated lumbar intervertebral disc herniation. *Spine.* 1992;17:1071–1074.
18. Modic MT, Obuchowski NA, Ross JS, et al. Acute low back pain and radiculopathy: MR imaging findings and their prognostic role and effect on outcome. *Radiology.* 2005;237:597–604.
19. Modic MT, Ross JS, Obuchowski NA, et al. Contrast-enhanced MR imaging in acute lumbar radiculopathy: a pilot study of the natural history. *Radiology.* 1995;195:429–435.
20. Tullberg T, Svanborg E, Isaccsson J, Grane P. A preoperative and postoperative study of the accuracy and value of electrodiagnosis in patients with lumbosacral disc herniation. *Spine.* 1993;18: 837–842.
21. Wolff AP, Groen GJ, Wilder-Smith OH. Influence of needle position on lumbar segmental nerve root block selectivity. *Reg Anesth Pain Med.* 2006;31:523–530.
22. Xavier AV, Farrell CE, McDanal J, Kissin I. Does antidromic activation of nociceptors play a role in sciatic radicular pain? *Pain.* 1990;40:77–79.
23. North RB, Kidd DH, Zahurak M, Piantadosi S. Specificity of diagnostic nerve blocks: a prospective, randomized study of sciatica due to lumbosacral spine disease. *Pain.* 1996;65:77–85.
24. Furman MB, Lee TS, Mehta A, Simon JI, Cano WG. Contrast flow selectivity during transforaminal lumbosacral epidural steroid injections. *Pain Physician.* 2008;11:855–861.
25. Wolff AP, Groen GJ, Crul BJ. Diagnostic lumbosacral segmental nerve blocks with local anesthetics: a prospective double-blind study on the variability and interpretation of segmental effects. *Reg Anesth Pain Med.* 2001;26:147–155.
26. Wolff AP, Wilder Smith OH, Crul BJ, van de Heijden MP, Groen GJ. Lumbar segmental nerve blocks with local anesthetics, pain relief, and motor function: a prospective double-blind study between lidocaine and ropivacaine. *Anesth Analg.* 2004;99:496–501, table of contents.
27. Le Bars D. The whole body receptive field of dorsal horn multireceptive neurones. *Brain Res Brain Res Rev.* 2002;40:29–44.
28. Wolff A, Wilder-Smith O. Diagnosis in patients with chronic radiating low back pain without overt focal neurological deficits: what is the value of segmental nerve root blocks? *Therapy.* 2005;2:577–585.
29. Luijsterburg PA, Lamers LM, Verhagen AP, et al. Cost-effectiveness of physical therapy and general practitioner care for sciatica. *Spine.* 2007;32:1942–1948.
30. Hagen KB, Jamtvedt G, Hilde G, Winnem MF. The updated cochrane review of bed rest for low back pain and sciatica. *Spine.* 2005;30:542–546.
31. Amlie E, Weber H, Holme I. Treatment of acute low-back pain with piroxicam: results of a double-blind placebo-controlled trial. *Spine (Phila Pa 1976).* 1987;12:473–476.
32. Dreiser RL, Le Parc JM, Velicitat P, Lleu PL. Oral meloxicam is effective in acute sciatica: two randomised, double-blind trials versus placebo or diclofenac. *Inflamm Res.* 2001;50(suppl 1): S17–S23.
33. Luijsterburg PA, Verhagen AP, Ostelo RW, et al. Physical therapy plus general practitioners' care versus general practitioners' care alone for sciatica: a randomised clinical trial with a 12-month follow-up. *Eur Spine J.* 2008;17:509–517.
34. Atlas SJ, Keller RB, Wu YA, Deyo RA, Singer DE. Long-term outcomes of surgical and nonsurgical management of lumbar spinal stenosis: 8–10 year results from the maine lumbar spine study. *Spine.* 2005;30:936–943.
35. Weinstein JN, Tosteson TD, Lurie JD, et al. Surgical vs nonoperative treatment for lumbar disk herniation: the Spine Patient Outcomes Research Trial (SPORT): a randomized trial. *JAMA.* 2006;296: 2441–2450.
36. Peul WC, van Houwelingen HC, van den Hout WB, et al. Surgery versus prolonged conservative treatment for sciatica. *N Engl J Med.* 2007;356:2245–2256.
37. Gibson JN, Waddell G. Surgical interventions for lumbar disc prolapse: updated Cochrane Review. *Spine.* 2007;32:1735–1747.
38. Jonsson B, Stromqvist B. Clinical characteristics of recurrent sciatica after lumbar discectomy. *Spine.* 1996;21:500–505.
39. Postacchini F, Giannicola G, Cinotti G. Recovery of motor deficits after microdiscectomy for lumbar disc herniation. *J Bone Joint Surg Br.* 2002;84:1040–1045.
40. CBO. Het Lumbosacrale radiculaire syndroom. In: Toetsing CbvdI, ed. *Consensus Richtlijnen*. Utrecht: CBO; 1996.
41. Guigui P, Cardinne L, Rillardon L, et al. Per- and postoperative complications of surgical treatment of lumbar spinal stenosis. Prospective study of 306 patients. *Rev Chir Orthop Reparatrice Appar Mot.* 2002;88:669–677.
42. Jonsson B, Stromqvist B. Motor affliction of the L5 nerve root in lumbar nerve root compression syndromes. *Spine.* 1995;20: 2012–2015.
43. Hahne AJ, Ford JJ. Functional restoration for a chronic lumbar disk extrusion with associated radiculopathy. *Phys Ther.* 2006;86: 1668–1680.
44. Finnerup NB, Otto M, McQuay HJ, Jensen TS, Sindrup SH. Algorithm for neuropathic pain treatment: an evidence based proposal. *Pain.* 2005;118:289–305.
45. Saarto T, Wiffen PJ. Antidepressants for neuropathic pain. *Cochrane Database Syst Rev.* 2007;4: CD005454.
46. Yildirim K, Kataray S. The effectiveness of gabapentin n patients with chronic radiculopathy. *Pain Clin.* 2003;15:213–218.
47. Dellemijn PL, van Duijn H, Vanneste JA. Prolonged treatment with transdermal fentanyl in neuropathic pain. *J Pain Symptom Manage.* 1998;16:220–229.
48. Ng L, Chaudhary N, Sell P. The efficacy of corticosteroids in periradicular infiltration for chronic radicular pain: a randomized, double-blind, controlled trial. *Spine.* 2005;30:857–862.
49. McQuay HJ, Moore RA. *Epidural Corticosteroids for Sciatica.* Oxford, New York, Tokyo: Oxford University Press; 1998.
50. Koes BW, Scholten RJPM, Mens JMA, Bouter LM. Epidural steroid injections for low back pain and sciatica: an updated systematic review of randomized clinical trials. *Pain Digest.* 1999;9: 241–247.
51. Chou R, Atlas SJ, Stanos SP, Rosenquist RW. Nonsurgical interventional therapies for low back pain: a review of the evidence for an

American Pain Society clinical practice guideline. *Spine (Phila Pa 1976)*. 2009;34:1078–1093.

52. Arden NK, Price C, Reading I, et al. A multicentre randomized controlled trial of epidural corticosteroid injections for sciatica: the WEST study. *Rheumatology (Oxford)*. 2005;44:1399–1406.
53. Dilke TF, Burry HC, Grahame R. Extradural corticosteroid injection in management of lumbar nerve root compression. *Br Med J.* 1973;2:635–637.
54. Wilson-MacDonald J, Burt G, Griffin D, Glynn C. Epidural steroid injection for nerve root compression. A randomised, controlled trial. *J Bone Joint Surg Br.* 2005;87:352–355.
55. Carette S, Leclaire R, Marcoux S, et al. Epidural corticosteroid injections for sciatica due to herniated nucleus pulposus. *N Engl J Med.* 1997;336:1634–1640.
56. Bogduk N. Epidural steroids. *Spine.* 1995;20:845–848.
57. Riew KD, Yin Y, Gilula L, et al. The effect of nerveroot injections on the need for operative treatment of lumbar radicular pain. A prospective, randomized, controlled, doubleblind study. *J Bone Joint Surg Am.* 2000;82-A:1589–1593.
58. Karppinen J, Malmivaara A, Kurunlahti M, et al. Periradicular infiltration for sciatica: a randomized controlled trial. *Spine.* 2001;26:1059–1067.
59. Riew KD, Park JB, Cho YS, et al. Nerve root blocks in the treatment of lumbar radicular pain. A minimum five-year follow-up. *J Bone Joint Surg Am.* 2006;88:1722–1725.
60. Vad VB, Bhat AL, Lutz GE, Cammisa F. Transforaminal epidural steroid injections in lumbosacral radiculopathy: a prospective randomized study. *Spine.* 2002;27:11–16.
61. Karppinen J, Ohinmaa A, Malmivaara A, et al. Cost effectiveness of periradicular infiltration for sciatica: subgroup analysis of a randomized controlled trial. *Spine.* 2001;26:2587–2595.
62. Ackerman WE, 3rd, Ahmad M. The efficacy of lumbar epidural steroid injections in patients with lumbar disc herniations. *Anesth Analg.* 2007;104:1217–1222, tables of contents.
63. Thomas E, Cyteval C, Abiad L, et al. Efficacy of transforaminal versus interspinous corticosteroid injectionin discal radiculalgia—a prospective, randomised, double-blind study. *Clin Rheumatol.* 2003;22:299–304.
64. Geurts JW, van Wijk RM, Wynne HJ, et al. Radiofrequency lesioning of dorsal root ganglia for chronic lumbosacral radicular pain: a randomised, double-blind, controlled trial. *Lancet.* 2003;361:21–26.
65. Teixeira A, Grandinson M, Sluijter M. Pulsed radiofrequency for radicular pain due to a herniated intervertebral disc—an initial report. *Pain Prac.* 2005;5:111–115.
66. Abejon D, Garcia-del-Valle S, Fuentes ML, et al. Pulsed radiofrequency in lumbar radicular pain: clinical effects in various etiological groups. *Pain Pract.* 2007;7:21–26.
67. Simopoulos TT, Kraemer J, Nagda JV, Aner M, Bajwa ZH. Response to pulsed and continuous radiofrequency lesioning of the dorsal root ganglion and segmental nerves in patients with chronic lumbar radicular pain. *Pain Physician.* 2008;11:137–144.
68. Heavner JE, Racz GB, Raj P. Percutaneous epidural neuroplasty: prospective evaluation of 0.9% NaCl versus 10% NaCl with or without hyaluronidase. *Reg Anesth Pain Med.* 1999;24:202–207.
69. Manchikanti L, Rivera JJ, Pampati V, et al. One day lumbar epidural adhesiolysis and hypertonic saline neurolysis in treatment of chronic low back pain: a randomized, doubleblind trial. *Pain Physician.* 2004;7:177–186.
70. Veihelmann A, Devens C, Trouillier H, et al. Epidural neuroplasty versus physiotherapy to relieve pain in patients with sciatica: a prospective randomized blinded clinical trial. *J Orthop Sci.* 2006;11: 365–369.
71. Manchikanti L, Pakanati R, Bakhit CE, Pampati V. Role of adhesiolysis and hypertonic saline neurolysis in management of low back pain. Evaluation of modification of Racz protocol. *Pain Digest.* 1999;9:91–96.
72. Gillespie G, MacKenzie P. Epiduroscopy—a review. *Scott Med J.* 2004;49:79–81.
73. Boswell MV, Trescot AM, Datta S, et al. Interventional techniques: evidence-based practice guidelines in the management of chronic spinal pain. *Pain Physician.* 2007;10:7–111.
74. Manchikanti L, Boswell MV, Rivera JJ, et al. [ISRCTN 16558617] A randomized, controlled trial of spinal endoscopic adhesiolysis in chronic refractory low back and lower extremity pain. *BMC Anesthesiol.* 2005;5:10.
75. Dashfield AK, Taylor MB, Cleaver JS, Farrow D. Comparison of caudal steroid epidural with targeted steroid placement during spinal endoscopy for chronic sciatica: a prospective, randomized, double-blind trial. *Br J Anaesth.* 2005;94:514–519.
76. Manchikanti L, Pampati V, Bakhit CE, Pakanati RR. Non-endoscopic and endoscopic adhesiolysis in postlumbar laminectomy syndrome: a one-year outcome study and cost effectiveness analysis. *Pain Physician.* 1999;2:52–58.
77. Geurts JW, Kallewaard JW, Richardson J, Groen GJ. Targeted methylprednisolone acetate/hyaluronidase/clonidine injection after diagnostic epiduroscopy for chronic sciatica: a prospective, 1-year follow-up study. *Reg Anesth Pain Med.* 2002;27:343–352.
78. Ruetten S, Meyer O, Godolias G. Endoscopic surgery of the lumbar epidural space (epiduroscopy): results of therapeutic intervention in 93 patients. *Minim Invasive Neurosurg.* 2003;46:1–4.
79. Igarashi T, Hirabayashi Y, Seo N, et al. Lysis of adhesions and epidural injection of steroid/local anaesthetic during epiduroscopy potentially alleviate low back and leg pain in elderly patients with lumbar spinal stenosis. *Br J Anaesth.* 2004;93:181–187.
80. Raffaeli W, Righetti D. Surgical radio-frequency epiduroscopy technique (R-ResAblator) and FBSS treatment: preliminary evaluations. *Acta Neurochir Suppl.* 2005;92:121–125.
81. Sakai T, Aoki H, Hojo M, et al. Adhesiolysis and targeted steroid/ local anesthetic injection during epiduroscopy alleviates pain and reduces sensory nerve dysfunction in patients with chronic sciatica. *J Anesth.* 2008;22:242–247.
82. Taylor RS, Van Buyten JP, Buchser E. Spinal cord stimulation for chronic back and leg pain and failed back surgery syndrome: a systematic review and analysis of prognostic factors. *Spine.* 2005;30:152–160.
83. Kumar K, Taylor RS, Jacques L, et al. Spinal cord stimulation versus conventional medical management for neuropathic pain: a multicentre randomised controlled trial in patients with failed back surgery syndrome. *Pain.* 2007;132:179–188.
84. Watts RW, Silagy CA. A Meta-Analgysis on the efficacy of epidural corticosteroids in the treatment of sciatica. *Anaesth Intensive Care.* 1995;23:564–569.
85. Armon C, Argoff CE, Samuels J, Backonja MM. Assessment: use of epidural steroid injections to treat radicular lumbosacral pain: report of the Therapeutics and Technology Assessment Subcommittee of the American Academy of Neurology. *Neurology.* 2007;68: 723–729.

86. Van Zundert J, le Polain de Waroux B. Safety of epidural steroids in daily practice: evaluation of more than 4,000 administrations. In: Monitor TI, ed. *XX Annual ESRA Meeting*. Rome: ESRA; 2000:122.
87. Abram SE, O'Connor TC. Complications associated with epidural steroid injections. *Reg Anesth.* 1996;21:149–162.
88. Houten JK, Errico TJ. Paraplegia after lumbosacral nerve root block: report of three cases. *Spine J.* 2002;2:70–75.
89. Huntoon MA, Martin DP. Paralysis after transforaminal epidural injection and previous spinal surgery. *Reg Anesth Pain Med.* 2004;29:494–495.
90. Glaser SE, Falco F. Paraplegia following a thoracolumbar transforaminal epidural steroid injection. *Pain Physician.* 2005;8:309–314.
91. Somayaji HS, Saifuddin A, Casey AT, Briggs TW. Spinal cord infarction following therapeutic computed tomography-guided left L2 nerve root injection. *Spine (Phila Pa 1976).* 2005;30:E106–E108.
92. Quintero N, Laffont I, Bouhmidi L, et al. Transforaminal epidural steroid injection and paraplegia: case report and bibliographic review. *Ann Readapt Med Phys.* 2006;49:242–247.
93. Kennedy DJ, Dreyfuss P, Aprill CN, Bogduk N. Paraplegia following image-guided transforaminal lumbar spine epidural steroid injection: two case reports. *Pain Med.* 2009;10:1389–1394.
94. Lyders EM, Morris PP. A case of spinal cord infarction following lumbar transforaminal epidural steroid injection: MR imaging and angiographic findings. *AJNR Am J Neuroradiol.* 2009;30:1691–1693.
95. Rathmell JP, Benzon HT. Transforaminal injection of steroids: should we continue? *Reg Anesth Pain Med.* 2004;29:397–399.
96. Goodman BS, Bayazitoglu M, Mallempati S, Noble BR, Geffen JF. Dural puncture and subdural injection: a complication of lumbar transforaminal epidural injections. *Pain Physician.* 2007;10:697–705.
97. Finn KP, Case JL. Disk entry: a complication of transforaminal epidural injection—a case report. *Arch Phys Med Rehabil.* 2005;86:1489–1491.
98. Bilir A, Gulec S. Cauda equina syndrome after epidural steroid injection: a case report. *J Manipulative Physiol Ther.* 2006;29:492 e1–3.
99. Young WF. Transient blindness after lumbar epidural steroid injection: a case report and literature review. *Spine.* 2002;27:E476–E477.
100. Kabbara A, Rosenberg SK, Untal C. Methicillinresistant Staphylococcus aureus epidural abscess after transforaminal epidural steroid injection. *Pain Physician.* 2004;7:269–272.
101. Hooten WM, Mizerak A, Carns PE, Huntoon MA. Discitis after lumbar epidural corticosteroid injection: a case report and analysis of the case report literature. *Pain Med.* 2006;7:46–51.
102. Simopoulos TT, Kraemer JJ, Glazer P, Bajwa ZH. Vertebral osteomyelitis: a potentially catastrophic outcome after lumbar epidural steroid injection. *Pain Physician.* 2008;11:693–697.
103. Bogduk N. Lumbar transforaminal injections of corticosteroids. In: Bogduk N, ed. *International Spine Intervention Society Practice Guidelines for Spinal Diagnoses and Treatment*. San Francisco, USA: ISIS; 2004.
104. van Kleef M, Spaans F, Dingemans W, et al. Effects and side effects of a percutaneous thermal lesion of the dorsal root ganglion in patients with cervical pain syndrome. *Pain.* 1993;52:49–53.
105. Cahana A, Van Zundert J, Macrea L, van Kleef M, Sluijter M. Pulsed radiofrequency: current clinical and biological literature available. *Pain Med.* 2006;7:411–423.
106. Sluijter ME, Cosman ER, Rittman IIWB, van Kleef M. The effects of pulsed radiofrequency field applied to the dorsal root ganglion—a preliminary report. *Pain Clin.* 1998;11:109–117.
107. Munglani R. The longer term effect of pulsed radiofrequency for neuropathic pain. *Pain.* 1999;80:437–439.
108. Pevzner E, David R, Leitner Y, et al. Pulsed radiofrequency treatment of severe radicular pain. *Harefuah.* 2005;144:178–180, 231.
109. Ramanavarapu V, Simopoulos TT. Pulsed radiofrequency of lumbar dorsal root Ganglia for chronic postamputation stump pain. *Pain Physician.* 2008;11:561–566.
110. Chao SC, Lee HT, Kao TH, et al. Percutaneous pulsed radiofrequency in the treatment of cervical and lumbar radicular pain. *Surg Neurol.* 2008;70:59–65.
111. Talu G, Erdine S. Complications of epidural neuroplasty: a retrospective evaluation. *Neuromodulation.* 2003;6:237–347.
112. Perkins WJ, Davis DH, Huntoon MA, Horlocker TT. A retained Racz catheter fragment after epidural neurolysis: implications during magnetic resonance imaging. *Anesth Analg.* 2003;96:1717–1719, table of contents.
113. Wagner KJ, Sprenger T, Pecho C, et al. Risks and complications of epidural neurolysis—a review with case report. *Anasthesiol Intensivmed Notfallmed Schmerzther.* 2006;41:213–222.
114. Richter H. Is the so-called epidural neuroplasty (Racz catheter) a harmless procedure? In: Neurochirurgie DGf, ed. *Deutsche Gesellschaft Fur Neurochirurgie.* Strasbourg, Germany: Deutsche Gesellschaft fur Neurochirurgie; 2005.
115. Kumar K, Buchser E, Linderoth B, Meglio M, Van Buyten JP. Avoiding Complications from spinal cord stimulation: practical recommendations from an international panel of experts. *Neuromodulation.* 2007;10:24–33.
116. Luijsterburg PA, Verhagen AP, Ostelo RW, et al. Effectiveness of conservative treatments for the lumbosacral radicular syndrome: a systematic review. *Eur Spine J.* 2007;16:881–899.
117. Abdi S, Datta S, Trescot AM, et al. Epidural steroids in the management of chronic spinal pain: a systematic review. *Pain Physician.* 2007;10:185–212.
118. DePalma MJ, Bhargava A, Slipman CW. A critical appraisal of the evidence for selective nerve root injection in the treatment of lumbosacral radiculopathy. *Arch Phys Med Rehabil.* 2005;86: 1477–1483.
119. Vroomen PC, de Krom MC, Slofstra PD, Knottnerus JA. Conservative treatment of sciatica: a systematic review. *J Spinal Disord.* 2000;13:463–469.
120. Koes B, Scholten RJ, Mens JMA, Bouter LM. Efficacy of epidural steroid injections for low-back pain and sciatica: a systematic review of randomized clinical trials. *Pain.* 1995;63:279–288.
121. Benzon HT, Chew TL, McCarthy RJ, Benzon HA, Walega DR. Comparison of the particle sizes of different steroids and the effect of dilution: a review of the relative neurotoxicities of the steroids. *Anesthesiology.* 2007;106:331–338.
122. O'Donnell C, Cano W, D'Eramo G. Comparison of triamcinolone to dexamethasone in the treatment of low back and leg pain via lumbar transforaminal epidural steroid injection. In: ISIS, ed. *North American Spine Society 23rd Annual Meeting.* Toronto: ISIS; 2008.
123. Owlia MB, Salimzadeh A, Alishiri G, Haghighi A. Comparison of two doses of corticosteroid in epidural steroid injection for lumbar radicular pain. *Singapore Med J.* 2007;48:241–245.
124. Novak S, Nemeth WC. The basis for recommending repeating epidural steroid injections for radicular low back pain: a literature review. *Arch Phys Med Rehabil.* 2008;89:543–552.
125. Waldman SD. *Waldman Interventional Pain Management.* Philadelphia, PA: W.B. Saunders; 2001.

126. Merrill DG, Rathmell JP, Rowlingson JC. Epidural steroid injections. *Anesth Analg.* 2003;96:907–908, author reply 8.
127. Cluff R, Mehio AK, Cohen SP, et al. The technical aspects of epidural steroid injections: a national survey. *Anesth Analg.* 2002;95:403–408, table of contents.
128. Botwin K, Gruber R, Bouchlas C, et al. Complications of fluoroscopically guided transforaminal lumbar epidural injections. *Arch Phys Med Rehabil.* 2000;81:1045–1050.
129. Lou L, Racz G. Spinal decompressive neuroplasty via the caudal and cervical approaches. In: Beltrutti D, Benzon HT, Erdine S, et al., eds. *Raj: Textbook of Regional Anesthesia.* 1st ed. Philadelphia, Pennsylvania, US: Churchill Livingstone; 2002.
130. Heavner J, Chokhavatia S, Kizelshteyn G. Percutaneous evaluation of the epidural and subarachnoid space with a flexible fiberscope. *Reg Anesth.* 1991;15:85.
131. Manchikanti L, Pampati V. Role of one day epidural adhesiolysis in managemnt of chronic low back pain: a radomized clinical trial. *Pain Physician.* 2001;4:153–166.

12 Pain Originating from the Lumbar Facet Joints

Maarten van Kleef, Pascal Vanelderen, Steven P. Cohen, Arno Lataster, Jan Van Zundert and Nagy Mekhail

Introduction

Pain emanating from the lumbar facet joints (zygapophysial joints) is a common cause of low back pain in the adult population. Golthwaite was the first to describe the syndrome in 1911, and Ghormley is generally credited with coining the term "facet syndrome" in 1933. Facet pain is defined as pain that arises from any structure that is part of the facet joints, including the fibrous capsule, synovial membrane, hyaline cartilage, and bone.[1–3]

The reported prevalence rate varies widely in different studies from less than 5% to as high as 90%, being heavily dependent on diagnostic criteria and selection methods.[4–11] Based on information from studies that were done on well-selected patient populations, we estimate the prevalence to range between 5% and 15% of the population with axial low back pain.[12–15] Because arthritis is a prominent cause of facetogenic pain, the prevalence rate increases with age.[16,17]

Although some experts have expressed doubts about the validity of "facet syndrome," studies conducted in patients and volunteers have confirmed its existence.[18–23] In rare cases, facet joint pain can result from a specific traumatic event (ie, high-energy trauma associated with a combination of hyperflexion, extension, and distraction).[24] More commonly, it is the result of repetitive stress and/or cumulative low-level trauma. This leads to inflammation, which can cause the facet joint to be filled with fluid and swell, which in turn results in stretching of the joint capsule and subsequent pain generation.[25] Inflammatory changes around the facet joint can also irritate the spinal nerve via foraminal narrowing, resulting in sciatica. In addition, Igarashi et al.[26] found that inflammatory cytokines released through the ventral joint capsule in patients with zygapophysial joint degeneration may be partially responsible for the neuropathic symptoms in individuals with spinal stenosis. Predisposing factors for zygapophysial joint pain include spondylolisthesis/lysis, degenerative disc disease, and advanced age.[3]

The treatment of facet pain is the subject of great controversy. In 1963, Hirsch et al.[19] were the first group to describe the technique of facet joint injections, and in the mid-1970s, Shealy published the first reports of radiofrequency (RF) treatment of the zygapophysial joints under radiographic guidance.[27,28] Because each facet joint receives dual innervation from adjacent levels and most individuals have multilevel pathology, several levels usually need to be treated[29–31] (Figure 12.1).

Diagnosis

History

A number of researchers have attempted to elucidate the clinical entity "facetogenic pain," mostly through provocation of pain in volunteers.[21–32–37]

The most frequent complaint is axial low back pain. Although bilateral symptoms are more common than for sacroiliac joint pain, centralization of pain is less predictive of response to analgesic blocks than it is for discogenic pain.[38,39] Sometimes, pain may be referred into the groin or thigh.[21] Pain originating from the upper facet joints often extends into the flank, hip, and lateral thigh regions, whereas pain from the lower facet joints typically radiates into the posterior thigh. Pain distal to the knee is rarely associated with facet pathology (Figure 12.2).

Physical examination

There are no physical examination findings that are pathognomonic for diagnosis. Because facet pain originates from the mobile elements of the back, examination of motion seems

Evidence-Based Interventional Pain Medicine: According to Clinical Diagnoses, First Edition. Edited by Jan Van Zundert, Jacob Patijn, Craig T. Hartrick, Arno Lataster, Frank J.P.M Huygen, Nagy Mekhail, Maarten van Kleef.

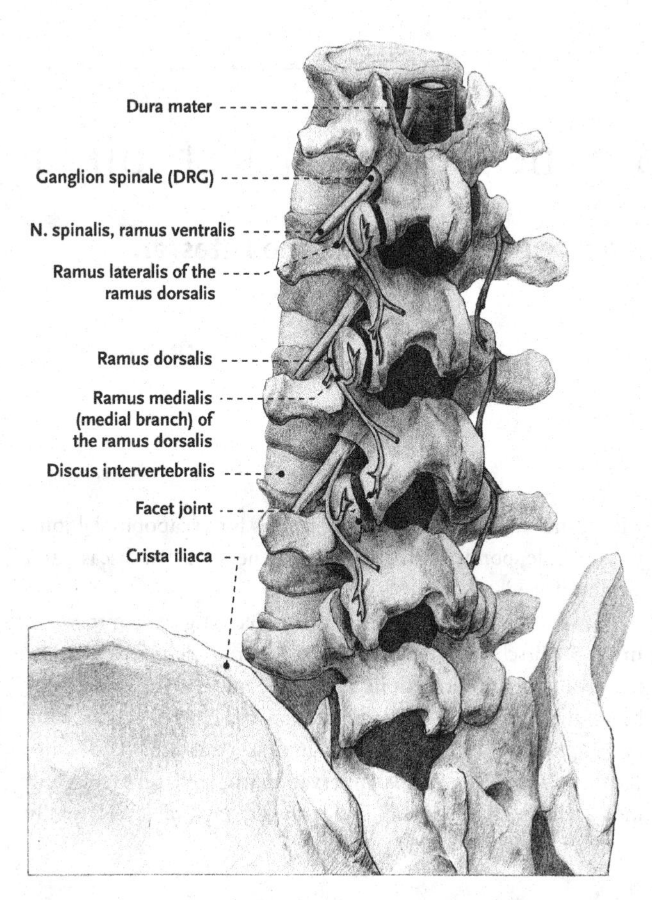

Figure 12.1. Anatomy of the lumbar spinal column. "Illustration: Rogier Trompert Medical Art. www.medical-art.nl." DRG, dorsal root ganglion.

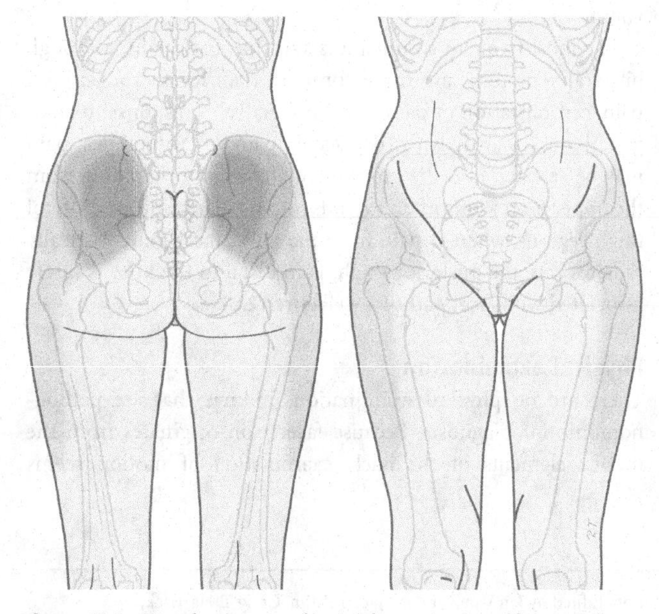

Figure 12.2. Pain referral pattern of lumbar facet pain adapted from McCall et al.[21] "Illustration: Rogier Trompert Medical Art. www.medical-art.nl."

relevant. In a series of cadaveric studies, Ianuzzi et al.[40] determined that the largest strain on the lower lumbar facet joints occurred during flexion and lateral bending, with extension also stressing L5/S1. It is therefore possible that pain worsened by flexion and extension is suggestive of pathology originating from the lowest lumbar segment(s).

Revel was the first to correlate symptoms and physical exam signs with the response to placebo-controlled blocks.[12,37]

The Revel criteria for lumbar facet joint pain are as follows:

- Pain not worsened by coughing.
- Pain not worsened by straightening from flexion.
- Pain not worsened by extension–rotation.
- Pain not worsened by hyperextension.
- Pain improved in the supine position.

However, previous and subsequent studies have failed to corroborate these findings.[41–43] It is widely acknowledged that lumbar paravertebral tenderness is indicative of facetogenic pain, which is a claim supported by clinical trials.[44] Recently, indicators of facet pain have been described based on a survey of an expert panel. They specified a panel of 12 indicators that create the framework for a diagnosis of facet pain.[45] These indicators are not in line with previous studies.[37,44,46]

Additional tests

The prevalence rate of pathological changes in the facet joints on radiological examination depends on the mean age of the subjects, the radiological technique used, and the definition of "abnormality." Degenerative facet joints can be best visualized via computed tomography (CT) examination.[47]

CT studies conducted in patients with low back pain show a prevalence rate of facet joint degeneration ranging between 40% and 80%.[10,48] Magnetic resonance imaging scans may be somewhat less sensitive in the detection of facet pathology.[5,47] Interestingly, the number of studies demonstrating a positive correlation between radiological abnormalities and the response to diagnostic blocks is roughly equivalent to the number showing no correlation.[5–9–12,30,34,35,41–48–50]

Differential diagnosis

As earlier indicated in the literature on guidelines for chronic nonspecific low back complaints, supplementary radiological examination may also be necessary to rule out so-called "red flags" such as malignancy, compression fracture, or spinal infection.[16,51]

Other causes of predominantly axial low back pain that must be considered in the differential diagnosis include discogenic pain, sacroiliac joint pathology, ligamentous injury, and myofascial pain. Within the context of facet pathology, inflammatory arthritides, such as rheumatoid arthritis, ankylosing spondylitis, gout, psoriatic arthritis, reactive arthritis, and other spondylarthropathies, as well as osteoarthrosis and synovitis, must also be considered.

Diagnostic blocks

Diagnostic blocks are most frequently performed under radiographic guidance but can also be done under ultrasound.[52,53]

Although intra-articular injection and medial branch (facet joint nerve) blocks are often described as "equivalent," this has yet to be demonstrated in a comparative, crossover study design.[3] Neither of these approaches have been shown to be superior.[20] Both medial branch and intra-articular blocks are associated with significant false-positive and false-negative rates. For both techniques, the rate of false positives is most often cited as ranging between 15% and 40%.[3] Regarding the false-negative rate, Kaplan et al. found that 11% of volunteers retained the ability to perceive capsular distension after appropriately performed medial branch blocks, which was attributed to aberrant innervation.[54] Other causes of false-negative blocks include inappropriate needle placement, failure to detect vascular uptake, and inability of the patient to discern baseline from procedure-related pain.[55]

False-positive results can be ascribed to several phenomena including placebo response, use of sedation, and/or the excessive use of superficial local anesthesia, which can obscure myofascial pain.[56,57] In addition, the local anesthetic can spread to surrounding pain generating structures. Over 70 years ago, Kellegren noted that an intramuscular injection of 0.5 mL of fluid spreads over an area encompassing 6 cm^2 of tissue, and this was later confirmed by Cohen and Raja.[3,58] Dreyfuss et al.[55] found that either epidural or intervertebral foraminal spread occurred in 16% of blocks using the traditional target point at the superior junction of the processus transversus and processus articularis superior. Given the close proximity of the ramus lateralis and intermedius to the ramus medialis (medial branch) of the primary ramus dorsalis, it is not possible to selectively block one without the others. During intra-articular facet blocks, the capsule can rupture after the injection of 1 to 2 mL of injection fluid with the resultant spread of the local anesthetic to other potential pain generating structures.

Perhaps because of their safety, simplicity, and prognostic value, diagnostic medial branch blocks are done more frequently than intra-articular injections. Dreyfuss et al.[55] researched the ideal needle position for diagnostic medial branch blocks. They compared 2 different target sites—one with the needle tip positioned on the upper edge of the processus transversus and the other with the needle tip located halfway between the upper edge of the processus transversus and the ligamentum mammilloaccessorium. The authors found that the lower (i.e., latter) target position was associated with a lower incidence of inadvertent injectate spread to the segmental nerves and epidural space when a volume of 0.5 mL was used. It is thus recommended to use the lower target site when performing diagnostic medial branch blocks.

After the procedure, the patient is given a pain diary with instructions to discount procedure-related discomfort and engage in normal activities in order to permit adequate assessment of effectiveness. Failure to properly discriminate between baseline pain and that related to the procedure is a common cause of false negative blocks.

In general, a definitive treatment is carried out if a patient experiences 50% or greater pain reduction lasting for the duration of action of the local anesthetic (e.g., >30 minutes with lidocaine and 3 hours with bupivacaine). Because double, comparative blocks are associated with a significant false-negative rate and have not been shown to be cost-effective, the "double-block" paradigm is not advisable at this time.[59–61]

Treatment options

Conservative management

The treatment of facet pain should ideally occur in a multidisciplinary fashion and include conservative (pharmacological treatment, cognitive behavioral therapy, manual medicine, exercise therapy and rehabilitation, and, if necessary, a more detailed psychological evaluation) as well as interventional pain management techniques.

Because there are no clinical studies evaluating pharmacological or non-interventional treatments for patients with injection-confirmed facet joint pain, one must extrapolate from studies that have been conducted on patients with chronic nonspecific low back complaints. Although nonsteroidal anti-inflammatory drugs are often used, scientific evidence supporting their long-term use for low back complaints is scant.[51] Antidepressants appear to be effective, though the treatment effect is small.[62] Manipulation can also be effective,[63,64] although 1 study showed no difference with "sham" therapy.[65]

Interventional management

Currently, the gold standard for treating facetogenic pain is RF treatment. The major advantage of temperature-controlled RF treatment compared with voltage-controlled and other "neurolytic" techniques is that it produces controlled and reproducible lesion dimensions.[66] RF facet treatment can also be repeated without a loss of efficacy, which is important because the duration of benefit is limited by the inexorable rate of nerve regeneration.[67] There are currently no randomized studies comparing RF facet treatment with intra-articular injections.[3]

Intra-articular corticosteroid injections

The use of intra-articular corticosteroid injections in the facet joints is controversial. Uncontrolled studies have mostly demonstrated transient beneficial effects, but the results of controlled studies have been mostly disappointing. Lilius et al.[68] performed the largest randomized study, involving 109 patients. They found no difference among large-volume (8 mL) intra-articular saline injections, intra-articular corticosteroid, and local anesthetic, and the same mixture injected around 2 facet joints. In a randomized, controlled study, Carette et al.[69] found only a small difference between the injection of saline (10% good effect) and depot corticosteroid (22% good effect) up to 6 months after treatment. One caveat with placebo-controlled trials that is not commonly recognized is that the intra-articular injection of saline may itself provide therapeutic benefit.[70] Observational studies involving intra-articular local anesthetic and corticosteroid typically show symptom palliation lasting for up to 3 months.[49,71] Based on the literature, one can conclude that intra-articular corticosteroid injections are of very limited value in the treatment of unscreened patients with suspected facetogenic pain. However, subgroup analyses have revealed that patients with positive single photon emission CT scans may be more likely to respond than patients without an acute inflammatory process.[71,72]

RF treatment

RF treatment is frequently performed for various forms of spinal pain, though the scientific evidence for this intervention remains controversial. The first controlled study was published by Gallagher et al. in 1994.[73] The authors selected 41 patients with chronic low back complaints who responded with some pain relief to diagnostic intra-articular injections and randomized them to receive either "sham" or true RF treatment of the rami mediales (medial branches). The 2 study groups were then subdivided into patients who obtained "good" and "equivocal" relief after the diagnostic block. After 6 months, a significant difference was found only between treatment and control subjects who had experienced good relief from the test blocks. In a well-designed placebo-controlled study, van Kleef et al.[74] demonstrated good results after RF treatment lasting up to 12 months after treatment. Leclaire et al.[75] did not establish a therapeutic effect for RF treatment in a placebo-controlled trial, but this study has been criticized because the criterion for a positive "diagnostic" block was ≥24 hours of pain relief after lidocaine infiltration, which is inconsistent with the drug's pharmacokinetics. In addition, 94% of the screened patients with back pain were selected for participation, which is much greater than the presumed prevalence for lumbar facetogenic pain (17% to 30%) in this cohort. For this reason, this study is judged to have major methodological flaws. van Wijk et al.[76] also found no difference between the treatment and control groups with regard to visual analog scale pain score, medication usage, and function. However, the RF group in this study did report ≥50% reduction in complaints significantly more often (62% vs. 39%) than those who received a sham procedure. The evaluation method was, however, subject to discussion. Finally, in the most recent randomized placebo-controlled trial undertaken in 40 patients who obtained significant pain relief following 3 diagnostic blocks, a significantly greater improvement in pain symptoms, global perception of improvement, and quality of life was observed after 6 months in those subjects allocated to RF treatment.[15] In 2 randomized studies comparing pulsed and conventional RF treatment for facetogenic pain, both showed conventional RF to be superior.[77,78]

From these 7 controlled studies, one can conclude that RF treatment of the facet joints can provide intermediate-term benefit in carefully selected patients.

However, in a recent review, the value of this intervention was questioned.[79] In a letter to the editor, the methodology was questioned, and a meta-analysis was performed. When including the 6 randomized controlled trials, RF was significantly better than placebo. Even when only the 2 trials without shortcomings were included, the difference in favor of RF treatment remained significant.[80]

Complications of interventional management

Complications of diagnostic blocks

The most prevalent complication of a diagnostic block results from an overflow of local anesthetic to the segmental nerves. This can cause temporary paresthesias in the legs and loss of motor function.

Complications of RF treatment

The complications and side effects of RF treatment have been previously described in a small retrospective study by Kornick et al.[81] Out of 116 procedures, the 2 most commonly occurring complications were transient, localized burning pain and self-limiting back pain lasting longer than 2 weeks, each occurring with a frequency of 2.5% per procedure. In this study, no infections, motor, or new sensory deficits were identified.

Unlike diagnostic blocks, which, in rare instances, have been complicated by spinal infection(s), RF treatment has never been associated with infectious complications.[82] This may be because heat lesioning serves a protective function. In rare instances, local burns and motor weakness have been reported.[3,83]

Other treatment options

There is presently no evidence to support the use of operative interventions for injection-confirmed facetogenic pain.[3] Although several devices have been used and advocated for percutaneous facet joint fusion, none have been evaluated in rigorous trials.

Evidence for interventional management

A summary of the available evidence is given in Table 12.1.

Recommendations

In patients with chronic low back pain putatively originating from the facet joints, RF treatment of the rami mediales (medial branches) arising from rami dorsales of lumbar segmental nerves can be recommended after a positive diagnostic block.

Clinical practice algorithm

A practice algorithm for the management of lumbar facet pain is illustrated in Figure 12.3.

Table 12.1. Summary of evidence for interventional management of lumbar facetogenic pain.

Technique	Assessment
Intra-articular injections	2 B±
Radiofrequency treatment of the rami mediales (medial branches) and L5 primary rami dorsales	1 B+

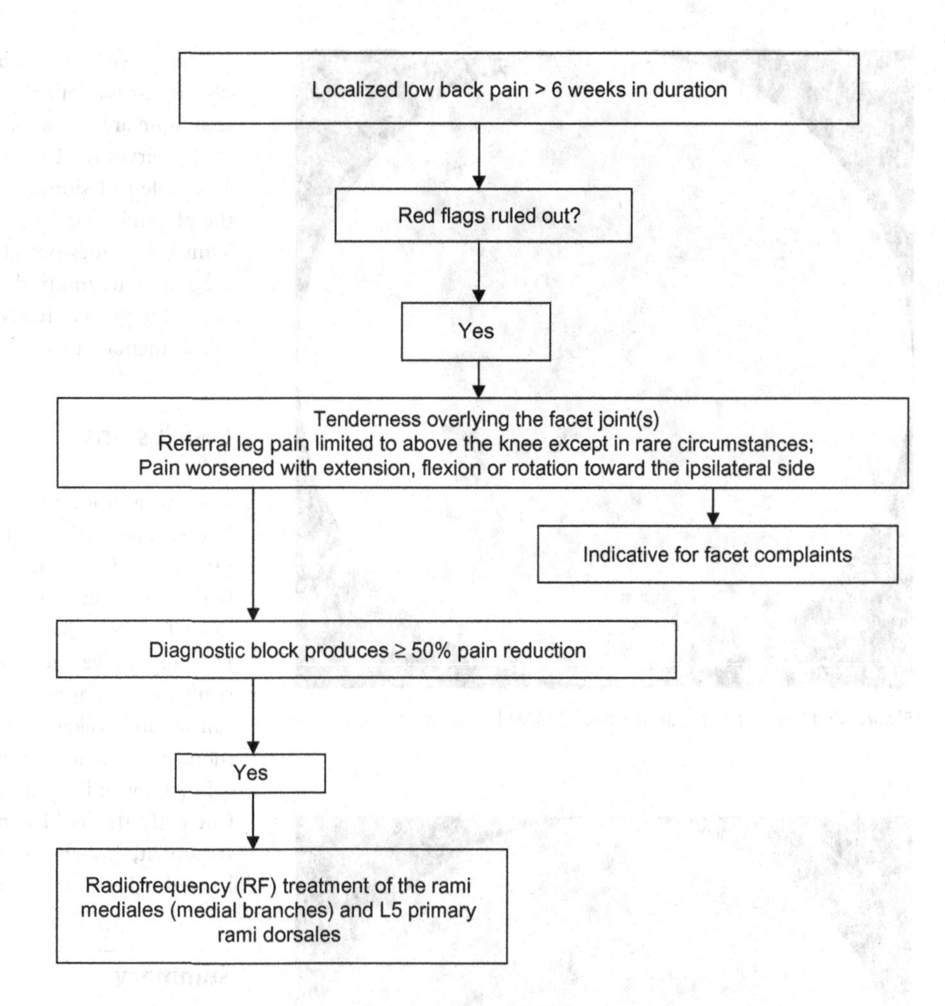

Figure 12.3. Clinical practice algorithm for the treatment of lumbar facet pain.

Techniques

Procedure for RF treatment of the lumbar facet joints

There are several ways to perform lumbar facet RF treatment, and comparative studies between different techniques are lacking. This section describes just 1 technique. RF treatment is a procedure that requires continuous feedback from the patient during the procedure. Therefore, if sedation is used, it should be light enough to enable conversation. The patient is placed in a prone position on an examination table. A cushion is placed under the abdomen to straighten the physiological lumbar lordosis. First, the anatomical structures are identified with an anterior-posterior examination. Next, the C-arm is rotated axially to align the X-ray beam parallel with the L4–L5 disc to remove parallax of the end plates. The C-arm is then rotated approximately 15° obliquely to the ipsilateral side so that the junction between the processus articularis superior and the processus transversus, the traditional target point, is more easily accessible. Several preclinical studies have demonstrated that placing the active tip parallel to the course of the nerve maximizes lesion size.[84,85] Hence, if the practitioner desires to orient the electrode parallel to the targeted nerve in a co-axial view to facilitate placement, the image intensifier can be further angled in the caudad direction.

The injection point is then marked on the skin. The traditional target is the cephalad junction between the processus articularis superior and the processus transversus. However, 1 cadaveric study and literature review determined the optimal needle position to be with the electrode tip lying across the lateral neck of the processus articularis superior.[84]

When inserting the electrode, one should first make contact with the processus transversus as close as possible to the processus articularis superior. After contacting bone, the needle is advanced slightly in a cranial direction so that the tip slides over the processus transversus (Figure 12.4). In the lateral fluoroscopic view, the electrode tip should now lie at the base of the processus articularis superior in the plane formed by the so-called facet column at the lower aspect of the foramen intervertebrale, approximately 1 mm dorsal to its posterior border (Figure 12.5). When proper needle position is confirmed in multiple views, the impedance is checked and a sensory stimulus current of 50 Hz is applied. The electrode position is generally deemed adequate if concordant stimulation is obtained at ≤0.5 V. Motor stimulation at 2 Hz serves to confirm correct needle placement via contraction of the musculus multifidus and to ensure the absence of distal muscle contraction in the leg, which indicates improper placement. Local muscle contractions in the back can generally be observed and palpated by

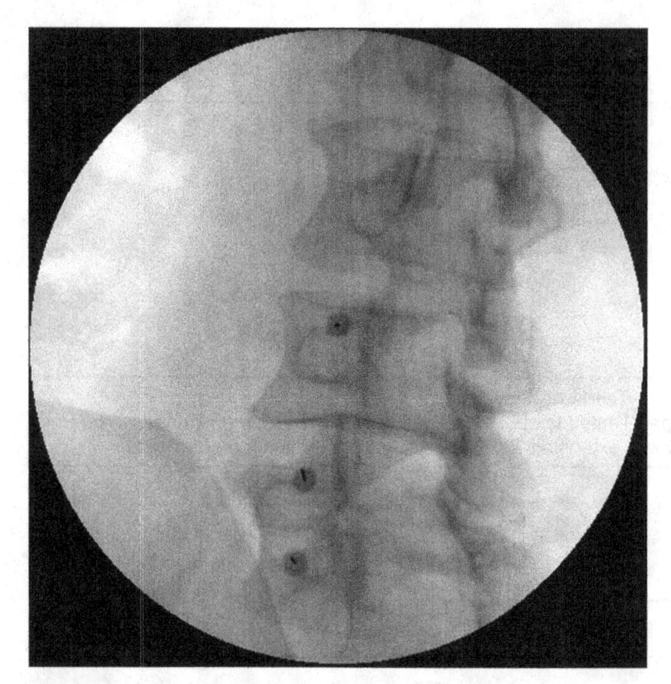

Figure 12.4. Radiofrequency treatment of L3, L4, and L5 dorsal rami/facet, oblique view.

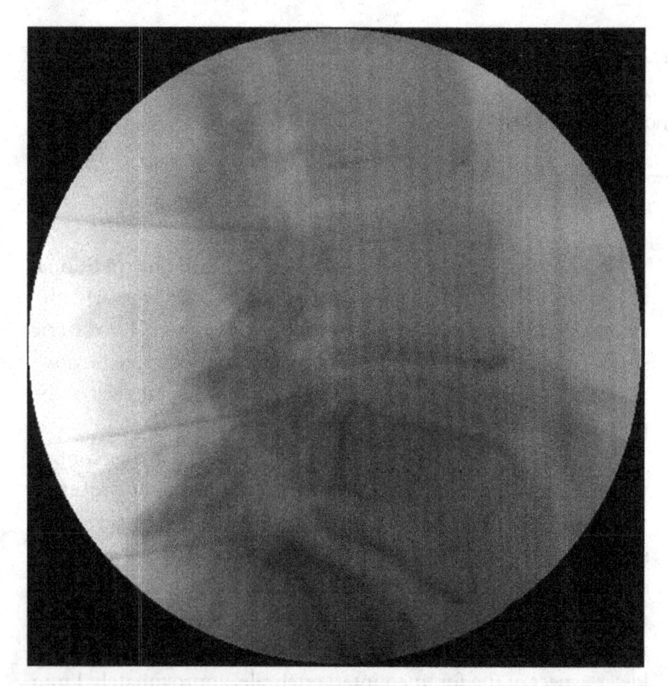

Figure 12.5. Radiofrequency treatment of L3, L4, and L5 dorsal rami/facet, lateral view.

the practitioner, though this is not always detectable. If leg movement is observed or the patient feels contractions in the leg, the needle must be repositioned. When the practitioner is confident that the needle is properly positioned, 0.5 mL of local anesthetic is injected.

After a brief interval in which the local anesthetic takes effect, a ≥67° lesion is applied for at least 1 minute. The nerve location and technique are the same for the ramus medialis (medial branch) of the nerves L1–L4. For L5, it is the ramus dorsalis itself that is amenable to lesioning, as it courses along the junction between the ala and processus articularis ossis sacri. At this level, 2 Hz stimulation does not always produce prominent contraction of the musculus multifidus, yet motor stimulation should be performed to prevent inadvertent lesioning too close in proximity to the segmental nerve.

Conclusions

Lumbar facet joint pain is a common yet controversial source of low back pain. Although the diagnosis is generally made by either ramus medialis (medial branch) or intra-articular injections, both are subject to high false-positive and, possibly, false-negative rates. To date, superiority or equivalence has yet to be established in comparative crossover studies. In patients with injection-confirmed zygapophysial joint pain, procedural interventions can be undertaken in the context of a multidisciplinary, multimodal treatment regimen that includes pharmacotherapy, physical therapy and regular exercise, and, if indicated, psychotherapy. Currently, the "gold standard" for treating facetogenic pain is RF treatment, though the effect size is moderate, and the duration is limited to less than a year.

Summary

There is no gold standard for making the diagnosis of low back complaints originating from the facet joints.

Unilateral localized back pain without radicular referral and pain in a movement examination together with paravertebral pressure pain appear to support this diagnosis.

However, the diagnosis must be confirmed by a diagnostic block of the suspected painful facet joints. If this treatment produces a pain reduction of at least 50%, moving to a RF treatment seems justified. If RF treatment is contraindicated, a 1-time intra-articular injection with local anesthetic can be considered.

References

1. Goldthwaite J. The lumbosacral articulation: an explanation of many cases of lumbago, sciatica, and paraplegia. *Boston Med Surg J.* 1911;365–372.
2. Ghormley R. Low back pain with special reference to the articular facets, with presentation of an operative procedure. *JAMA.* 1933;1773–1777.
3. Cohen SP, Raja SN. Pathogenesis, diagnosis, and treatment of lumbar zygapophysial (facet) joint pain. *Anesthesiology.* 2007;106:591–614.

4. Long DM, BenDebba M, Torgerson WS, et al. Persistent back pain and sciatica in the United States: patient characteristics. *J Spinal Disord.* 1996;9:40–58.
5. Murtagh FR. Computed tomography and fluoroscopy guided anesthesia and steroid injection in facet syndrome. *Spine.* 1988;13:686–689.
6. Destouet JM, Gilula LA, Murphy WA, Monsees B. Lumbar facet joint injection: indication, technique, clinical correlation, and preliminary results. *Radiology.* 1982;145:321–325.
7. Lau LS, Littlejohn GO, Miller MH. Clinical evaluation of intra-articular injections for lumbar facet joint pain. *Med J Aust.* 1985;143:563–565.
8. Moran R, O'Connell D, Walsh MG. The diagnostic value of facet joint injections. *Spine.* 1988;13:1407–1410.
9. Raymond J, Dumas JM. Intraarticular facet block: diagnostic test or therapeutic procedure? *Radiology.* 1984;151:333–336.
10. Carrera GF. Lumbar facet joint injection in low back pain and sciatica: description of technique. *Radiology.* 1980;137:661–664.
11. Lewinnek GE, Warfield CA. Facet joint degeneration as a cause of low back pain. *Clin Orthop Relat Res.* 1986;213:216–222.
12. Revel ME, Listrat VM, Chevalier XJ, et al. Facet joint block for low back pain: identifying predictors of a good response. *Arch Phys Med Rehabil.* 1992;73:824–828.
13. Dreyfuss P, Halbrook B, Pauza K, Joshi A, McLarty J, Bogduk N. Efficacy and validity of radiofrequency neurotomy for chronic lumbar zygapophysial joint pain. *Spine.* 2000;25:1270–1277.
14. Manchikanti L, Boswell MV, Singh V, Pampati V, Damron KS, Beyer CD. Prevalence of facet joint pain in chronic spinal pain of cervical, thoracic, and lumbar regions. *BMC Musculoskelet Disord.* 2004;5:15.
15. Nath S, Nath CA, Pettersson K. Percutaneous lumbar zygapophysial (facet) joint neurotomy using radiofrequency current, in the management of chronic low back pain: a randomized double-blind trial. *Spine.* 2008;33:1291–1297, discussion 8.
16. Hicks GE, Morone N, Weiner DK. Degenerative lumbar disc and facet disease in older adults: prevalence and clinical correlates. *Spine (Phila Pa 1976).* 2009;34:1301–1306.
17. Manchikanti L, Manchikanti KN, Cash KA, Singh V, Giordano J. Age-related prevalence of facet-joint involvement in chronic neck and low back pain. *Pain Physician.* 2008;11:67–75.
18. Cavanaugh JM, Ozaktay AC, Yamashita HT, King AI. Lumbar facet pain: biomechanics, neuroanatomy and neurophysiology. *J Biomech.* 1996;29:1117–1129.
19. Hirsch C, Ingelmark BE, Miller M. The anatomical basis for low back pain. Studies on the presence of sensory nerve endings in ligamentous, capsular and intervertebral disc structures in the human lumbar spine. *Acta Orthop Scand.* 1963;33:1–17.
20. Marks RC, Houston T, Thulbourne T. Facet joint injection and facet nerve block: a randomised comparison in 86 patients with chronic low back pain. *Pain.* 1992;49:325–328.
21. McCall IW, Park WM, O'Brien JP. Induced pain referral from posterior lumbar elements in normal subjects. *Spine.* 1979;4:441–446.
22. Kuslich SD, Ulstrom CL, Michael CJ. The tissue origin of low back pain and sciatica: a report of pain response to tissue stimulation during operations on the lumbar spine using local anesthesia. *Orthop Clin North Am.* 1991;22:181–187.
23. Mooney V, Robertson J. The facet syndrome. *Clin Orthop Relat Res.* 1976;115:149–156.
24. Song KJ, Lee KB. Bilateral facet dislocation on L4-L5 without neurologic deficit. *J Spinal Disord Tech.* 2005;18:462–464.
25. Yang KH, King AI. Mechanism of facet load transmission as a hypothesis for low-back pain. *Spine.* 1984;9:557–565.
26. Igarashi A, Kikuchi S, Konno S. Correlation between inflammatory cytokines released from the lumbar facet joint tissue and symptoms in degenerative lumbar spinal disorders. *J Orthop Sci.* 2007;12:154–160.
27. Shealy CN. Facet denervation in the management of back and sciatic pain. *Clin Orthop Relat Res.* 1976;115:157–164.
28. Shealy CN. Percutaneous radiofrequency denervation of spinal facets. *J Neurosurg.* 1975;43:448–451.
29. Bogduk N, Long DM. The anatomy of the so-called "articular nerves" and their relationship to facet denervation in the treatment of low-back pain. *J Neurosurg.* 1979;51:172–177.
30. Schwarzer AC, Aprill CN, Derby R, Fortin J, Kine G, Bogduk N. The false-positive rate of uncontrolled diagnostic blocks of the lumbar zygapophysial joints. *Pain.* 1994;58:195–200.
31. Schwarzer AC, Wang SC, Bogduk N, McNaught PJ, Laurent R. Prevalence and clinical features of lumbar zygapophysial joint pain: a study in an Australian population with chronic low back pain. *Ann Rheum Dis.* 1995;54:100–106.
32. Marks R. Distribution of pain provoked from lumbar facet joints and related structures during diagnostic spinal infiltration. *Pain.* 1989;39:37–40.
33. Fukui S, Ohseto K, Shiotani M, Ohno K, Karasawa H, Naganuma Y. Distribution of referred pain from the lumbar zygapophyseal joints and dorsal rami. *Clin J Pain.* 1997;13:303–307.
34. Fairbank JC, Park WM, McCall IW, O'Brien JP. Apophyseal injection of local anesthetic as a diagnostic aid in primary low-back pain syndromes. *Spine.* 1981;6:598–605.
35. Helbig T, Lee CK. The lumbar facet syndrome. *Spine.* 1988;13:61–64.
36. Schwarzer AC, Aprill CN, Derby R, Fortin J, Kine G, Bogduk N. The relative contributions of the disc and zygapophyseal joint in chronic low back pain. *Spine.* 1994;19:801–806.
37. Revel M, Poiraudeau S, Auleley GR, et al. Capacity of the clinical picture to characterize low back pain relieved by facet joint anesthesia. Proposed criteria to identify patients with painful facet joints. *Spine.* 1998;23:1972–1976, discussion 7.
38. Cohen SP. Sacroiliac joint pain: a comprehensive review of anatomy, diagnosis, and treatment. *Anesth Analg.* 2005;101:1440–1453.
39. Laslett M, McDonald B, Aprill CN, Tropp H, Oberg B. Clinical predictors of screening lumbar zygapophyseal joint blocks: development of clinical prediction rules. *Spine J.* 2006;6:370–379.
40. Ianuzzi A, Little JS, Chiu JB, Baitner A, Kawchuk G, Khalsa PS. Human lumbar facet joint capsule strains: I. During physiological motions. *Spine J.* 2004;4:141–152.
41. Jackson RP, Jacobs RR, Montesano PX. 1988 Volvo award in clinical sciences. Facet joint injection in low-back pain. A prospective statistical study. *Spine.* 1988;13:966–971.
42. Schwarzer AC, Aprill CN, Derby R, Fortin J, Kine G, Bogduk N. Clinical features of patients with pain stemming from the lumbar zygapophysial joints. Is the lumbar facet syndrome a clinical entity? *Spine.* 1994;19:1132–1137.
43. Laslett M, Oberg B, Aprill CN, McDonald B. Zygapophysial joint blocks in chronic low back pain: a test of Revel's model as a screening test. *BMC Musculoskelet Disord.* 2004;5:43.

44. Cohen SP, Hurley RW, Christo PJ, Winkley J, Mohiuddin MM, Stojanovic MP. Clinical predictors of success and failure for lumbar facet radiofrequency denervation. *Clin J Pain.* 2007;23:45–52.
45. Wilde VE, Ford JJ, McMeeken JM. Indicators of lumbar zygapophyseal joint pain: survey of an expert panel with the Delphi technique. *Phys Ther.* 2007;87:1348–1361.
46. Cohen SP, Argoff CE, Carragee EJ. Management of low back pain. *BMJ.* 2008;337:a2718.
47. Weishaupt D, Zanetti M, Boos N, Hodler J. MR imaging and CT in osteoarthritis of the lumbar facet joints. *Skeletal Radiol.* 1999;28: 215–219.
48. Carrera GF, Williams AL. Current concepts in evaluation of the lumbar facet joints. *Crit Rev Diagn Imaging.* 1984;21:85–104.
49. Dolan AL, Ryan PJ, Arden NK, et al. The value of SPECT scans in identifying back pain likely to benefit from facet joint injection. *Br J Rheumatol.* 1996;35:1269–1273.
50. Schwarzer AC, Wang SC, O'Driscoll D, Harrington T, Bogduk N, Laurent R. The ability of computed tomography to identify a painful zygapophysial joint in patients with chronic low back pain. *Spine.* 1995;20:907–912.
51. Airaksinen O, Brox JI, Cedraschi C, et al. Chapter 4. European guidelines for the management of chronic nonspecific low back pain. *Eur Spine J.* 2006;15(suppl 2):S192–S300.
52. Greher M, Kirchmair L, Enna B, et al. Ultrasound-guided lumbar facet nerve block: accuracy of a new technique confirmed by computed tomography. *Anesthesiology.* 2004;101:1195–1200.
53. Shim JK, Moon JC, Yoon KB, Kim WO, Yoon DM. Ultrasound-guided lumbar medial-branch block: a clinical study with fluoroscopy control. *Reg Anesth Pain Med.* 2006;31:451–454.
54. Kaplan M, Dreyfuss P, Halbrook B, Bogduk N. The ability of lumbar medial branch blocks to anesthetize the zygapophysial joint. A physiologic challenge. *Spine (Phila Pa 1976).* 1998;23: 1847–1852.
55. Dreyfuss P, Schwarzer AC, Lau P, Bogduk N. Specificity of lumbar medial branch and L5 dorsal ramus blocks. A computed tomography study. *Spine.* 1997;22:895–902.
56. Ackerman WE, Munir MA, Zhang JM, Ghaleb A. Are diagnostic lumbar facet injections influenced by pain of muscular origin? *Pain Pract.* 2004;4:286–291.
57. Cohen SP, Larkin TM, Chang AS, Stojanovic MP. The causes of false-positive medial branch (facet joint) blocks in soldiers and retirees. *Mil Med.* 2004;169:781–786.
58. Kellegren J. On the distribution of pain arising from deep somatic structures with charts of segmental pain areas. *Clin Sci.* 1939;4: 35–46.
59. Lord SM, Barnsley L, Bogduk N. The utility of comparative local anesthetic blocks versus placebo-controlled blocks for the diagnosis of cervical zygapophysial joint pain. *Clin J Pain.* 1995;11:208–213.
60. O'Neill C, Owens DK. Lumbar facet joint pain: time to hit the reset button. *Spine J.* 2009;9:619–622.
61. Bogduk N, Holmes S. Controlled zygapophysial joint blocks: the travesty of cost-effectiveness. *Pain Med.* 2000;1:24–34.
62. Schnitzer TJ, Ferraro A, Hunsche E, Kong SX. A comprehensive review of clinical trials on the efficacy and safety of drugs for the treatment of low back pain. *J Pain Symptom Manage.* 2004;28:72–95.
63. Andersson GB, Lucente T, Davis AM, Kappler RE, Lipton JA, Leurgans S. A comparison of osteopathic spinal manipulation with standard care for patients with low back pain. *N Engl J Med.* 1999; 341:1426–1431.
64. Giles LG, Muller R. Chronic spinal pain: a randomized clinical trial comparing medication, acupuncture, and spinal manipulation. *Spine.* 2003;28:1490–1502, discussion 502–503.
65. Licciardone JC, Stoll ST, Fulda KG, et al. Osteopathic manipulative treatment for chronic low back pain: a randomized controlled trial. *Spine.* 2003;28:1355–1362.
66. Silvers HR. Lumbar percutaneous facet rhizotomy. *Spine (Phila Pa 1976).* 1990;15:36–40.
67. Schofferman J, Kine G. Effectiveness of repeated radiofrequency neurotomy for lumbar facet pain. *Spine.* 2004;29:2471–2473.
68. Lilius G, Laasonen EM, Myllynen P, Harilainen A, Salo L. [Lumbar facet joint syndrome. Significance of nonorganic signs. A randomized placebo-controlled clinical study]. *Rev Chir Orthop Reparatrice Appar Mot.* 1989;75:493–500.
69. Carette S, Marcoux S, Truchon R, et al. A controlled trial of corticosteroid injections into facet joints for chronic low back pain. *N Engl J Med.* 1991;325:1002–1007.
70. Egsmose C, Lund B, Bach Andersen R. Hip joint distension in osteoarthrosis. A triple-blind controlled study comparing the effect of intra-articular indoprofen with placebo. *Scand J Rheumatol.* 1984;13:238–242.
71. Pneumaticos SG, Chatziioannou SN, Hipp JA, Moore WH, Esses SI. Low back pain: prediction of short-term outcome of facet joint injection with bone scintigraphy. *Radiology.* 2006;238: 693–698.
72. Holder LE, Machin JL, Asdourian PL, Links JM, Sexton CC. Planar and high-resolution SPECT bone imaging in the diagnosis of facet syndrome. *J Nucl Med.* 1995;36:37–44.
73. Gallagher J, Vadi PLP, Wesley JR. Radiofrequency facet joint denervation in the treatment of low back pain—a prospective controlled double-blind study to assess its efficacy. *Pain Clinic.* 1994;7:193–198.
74. van Kleef M, Barendse GA, Kessels F, Voets HM, Weber WE, de Lange S. Randomized trial of radiofrequency lumbar facet denervation for chronic low back pain. *Spine.* 1999;24:1937–1942.
75. Leclaire R, Fortin L, Lambert R, Bergeron YM, Rossignol M. Radiofrequency facet joint denervation in the treatment of low back pain: a placebo-controlled clinical trial to assess efficacy. *Spine.* 2001;26:1411–1416, discussion 7.
76. van Wijk RM, Geurts JW, Wynne HJ, et al. Radiofrequency denervation of lumbar facet joints in the treatment of chronic low back pain: a randomized, double-blind, sham lesion-controlled trial. *Clin J Pain.* 2005;21:335–344.
77. Tekin I, Mirzai H, Ok G, Erbuyun K, Vatansever D. A comparison of conventional and pulsed radiofrequency denervation in the treatment of chronic facet joint pain. *Clin J Pain.* 2007;23:524–529.
78. Kroll HR, Kim D, Danic MJ, Sankey SS, Gariwala M, Brown M. A randomized, double-blind, prospective study comparing the efficacy of continuous versus pulsed radiofrequency in the treatment of lumbar facet syndrome. *J Clin Anesth.* 2008;20:534–537.
79. Chou R, Atlas SJ, Stanos SP, Rosenquist RW. Nonsurgical interventional therapies for low back pain: a review of the evidence for an American Pain Society clinical practice guideline. *Spine (Phila Pa 1976).* 2009;34:1078–1093.
80. Van Zundert J, Vanelderen P, Kessels A. Re: Chou R, Atlas SJ, Stanos SP, et al. Nonsurgical interventional therapies for low back pain: a review of the evidence for an American Pain Society clinical practice guideline. *Spine* (Phila Pa 1976) 2009;34:1078–1093. *Spine* (Phila Pa 1976) 2010;35:841; author reply 841–842.

81. Kornick C, Kramarich SS, Lamer TJ, Todd Sitzman B. Complications of lumbar facet radiofrequency denervation. *Spine.* 2004;29: 1352–1354.
82. Cheng J, Abdi S. Complications of joint, tendon, and muscle injections. *Tech Reg Anesth Pain Manag.* 2007;11:141–147.
83. Ogsbury JS 3rd, Simon RH, Lehman RA. Facet "denervation" in the treatment of low back syndrome. *Pain.* 1977;3:257–263.
84. Lau P, Mercer S, Govind J, Bogduk N. The surgical anatomy of lumbar medial branch neurotomy (facet denervation). *Pain Med.* 2004;5:289–298.
85. Bogduk N, Macintosh J, Marsland A. Technical limitations to the efficacy of radiofrequency neurotomy for spinal pain. *Neurosurgery.* 1987;20:529–535.

13 Sacroiliac Joint Pain

Pascal Vanelderen, Karolina Szadek, Steven P. Cohen, Jan De Witte, Arno Lataster, Jacob Patijn, Nagy Mekhail, Maarten van Kleef and Jan Van Zundert

Introduction

The sacroiliac (SI) joint has long been considered an important source of low back pain because of the empirical finding that treatment targeting the SIJ can relieve pain. The International Association for the Study of Pain (IASP) has formulated criteria for the diagnosis of SI joint pain.[1] SI joint pain is defined as pain localized in the region of the SI joint, reproducible by stress and provocation tests of the SI joint, and reliably relieved by selective infiltration of the SI joint with a local anesthetic. Depending on the diagnostic criteria employed (clinical examination, intra-articular test blocks, medical imaging), the reported prevalence of SI pain among patients with axial low back pain varies between 16% and 30%.[2–4]

The SI joint is a diarthrodial synovial joint. Only the anterior part is a true synovial joint. The posterior part is a syndesmosis consisting of the ligamenta sacroiliaca, the musculus gluteus medius and minimus, and the musculus piriformis. The SI joint cannot function independently because all of these muscles are shared with the hip joint. The ligamentous structures and the muscles they support influence the stability of the SI joint. The SI joint is innervated mainly by the sacral rami dorsales.[5]

SI joint pain can be divided into intra-articular causes (infection, arthritis, spondyloarthropathies, malignancies) and extra-articular causes (enthesopathy, fractures, ligamentous, and myofascial injuries). Frequently, no specific cause can be identified. Unidirectional pelvic shear stress, repetitive torsional forces, and inflammation can all cause pain. Risk factors include leg length discrepancy, abnormal gait pattern, trauma, scoliosis, lumbar fusion surgery with fixation of the sacrum, heavy physical exertion, and pregnancy.[6–11] In patients who suffer from persistent low back pain after a technically successful lumbar arthrodesis, a prevalence rate between 32% and 35% has been demonstrated by means of diagnostic intra-articular blocks.[9]

Diagnosis

History

Pain from the SI joint is generally localized in the gluteal region (94%). Referred pain may also be perceived in the lower lumbar region (72%), groin (14%), upper lumbar region (6%), or abdomen (2%). Pain referred to the lower limb occurs in 28% of patients; 12% report pain in the foot[12] (Figure 13.1).

Physical examination

Solitary provocative maneuvers have little diagnostic value. Because of the size and the immobility of the SI interface, large forces are needed to stress the joint (causing false negatives). In addition, if forces are exerted incorrectly, pain can be provoked in neighboring structures, resulting in false-positive tests. However, both the sensitivity and specificity of the clinical examination increase as a direct function of the number of positive tests. Two studies found that 3 or more positive provocative tests resulted in a specificity and sensitivity of 79% and 85%, and 78% and 94%, respectively.[13,14] This was confirmed by a meta-analysis, which showed that 3 or more positive stress tests have discriminative power for diagnosing SI joint pain.[15] Young et al.[16] found a positive correlation between SI joint pain and worsening of symptoms when rising from a sitting position, when symptoms are unilateral, and with 3 positive provocative tests.

The 7 most important clinical tests, which are positive when they reproduce a patient's typical pain, are listed below.

1 Compression test (approximation test): The patient lies on his or her side with the affected side up; the patient's hips are flexed 45°, and the knees are flexed 90°. The examiner stands behind the patient and places both hands on the front side of the crista iliaca and then exerts downward, medial pressure.

Evidence-Based Interventional Pain Medicine: According to Clinical Diagnoses, First Edition. Edited by Jan Van Zundert, Jacob Patijn, Craig T. Hartrick, Arno Lataster, Frank J.P.M Huygen, Nagy Mekhail, Maarten van Kleef.

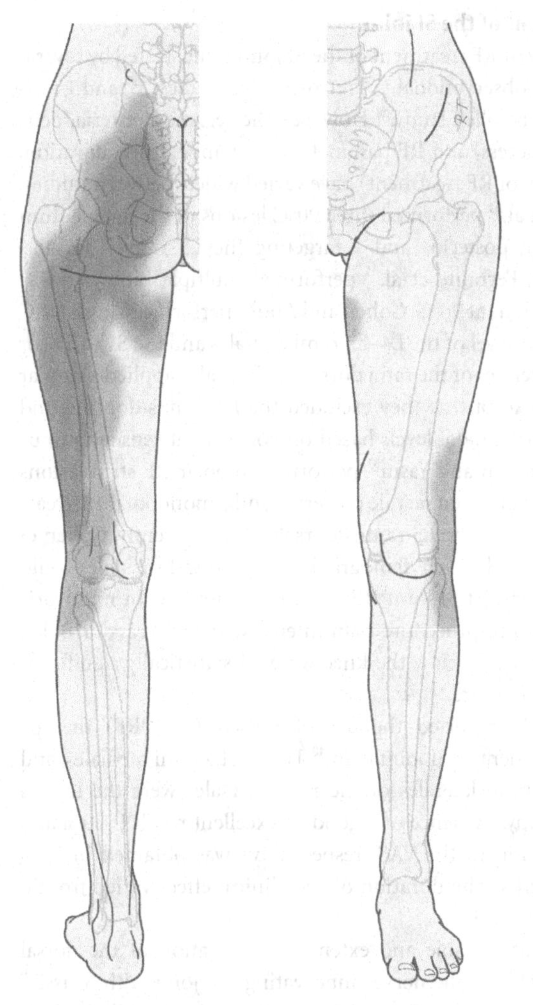

Figure 13.1. Typical pain referral pattern of sacroiliac joint pain (illustration: Rogier Trompert Medical Art www.medicalart.nl).

2 Distraction test (gapping test): The examiner stands on the affected side of the supine patient and places his/her hands on the ipsilateral spinae iliacae anteriores superiores. The examiner then applies pressure in the dorso-lateral direction.
3 Patrick's sign (flexion abduction external rotation test): The patient is positioned supine with the examiner standing next to the affected side. The leg of the affected side is bent at the hip and knee, with the foot positioned under the opposite knee. Downward pressure is then applied to the knee of the affected side.
4 Gaenslen test (pelvic torsion test): The patient lies in a supine position with the affected side on the edge of the examination table. The unaffected leg is bent at both the hip and knee, and maximally flexed until the knee is pushed against the abdomen. The contralateral leg (affected side) is brought into hyperextension, and light pressure is applied to that knee.
5 Thigh thrust test (posterior shear test): The patient lies in the supine position with the unaffected leg extended. The examiner stands next to the affected side and flexes the extremity at the hip to an angle of approximately 90° with slight adduction while applying light pressure to the bent knee.
6 Fortin's finger test: The patient can consistently indicate the location of the pain with 1 finger inferomedially to the spinae iliacae posteriores superiores.
7 Gillet test: The patient stands on one leg and pulls the other leg up to his or her chest.

Additional tests

Medical imaging is indicated only to rule out so-called "red flags."[17] In various studies, the use of radiography, computed tomography (CT), single photon emission CT, bone scans, and other nuclear imaging techniques have been used to identify specific disorders of the SI joint. However, no correlation has been consistently demonstrated between the imaging findings and injection-confirmed SI joint pain.[18] Magnetic resonance imaging (MRI) does not allow evaluation of normal anatomy. However, in the presence of spondylarthropathy, MRI can detect inflammation and destruction of cartilage despite normal clinical presentation.[19,20]

Diagnostic blocks

The IASP criteria mandate that pain should disappear after intra-articular SI joint infiltration with local anesthetic in order to confirm the diagnosis. A number of authors have used a single diagnostic block for clinical studies.[3,5,12,21] Others advocate confirmatory (double) diagnostic blocks using 2 different local anesthetics containing different durations of action.[4,13,14,22–25] Yet, the diagnostic value of SI joint infiltration with local anesthetic remains controversial in light of the potential for false-positive and false-negative results. Potential causes of inaccurate blocks include dispersal of the local anesthetic to adjacent pain-generating structures (muscles, ligaments, nerve roots), the over-zealous use of superficial anesthesia or sedation, and failure to achieve infiltration throughout the entire SI joint complex. The use of fluoroscopy or other imaging to guide needle placement during SI joint blocks is strongly recommended; in 1 study, only 22% of blind procedures resulted in intra-articular injectate spread.[26] CT-monitored injections are useful when the SI joint cannot be accessed using fluoroscopy.[27]

Differential diagnosis

- Spondyloarthropathy (ankylosing spondylitis, reactive arthritis, psoriatic arthritis . . .).
- Lumbar nerve root compression.
- Facetogenic pain.
- Hip pain.
- Endometriosis.
- Myofascial pain.
- Piriformis syndrome.

Treatment options

Treatment of SI joint pain best consists of a multidisciplinary approach and must include conservative (pharmacological treatment, cognitive–behavioral therapy, manual medicine, exercise therapy and rehabilitation treatment, and, if necessary, psychiatric evaluation) as well as interventional pain management techniques.

Conservative management

The conservative treatments primarily address the underlying cause. In SI joint pain attributed to postural and gait disturbances, exercise therapy and manipulation can reduce pain and improve mobility. However, there are no controlled studies evaluating patients with injection-confirmed SI joint pain.[28]

Ankylosing spondylitis (Morbus Bechterew) is an inflammatory rheumatological disorder that affects the vertebral column and the SI joint. Controlled studies have demonstrated analgesic efficacy for immunomodulating agents in ankylosing spondylitis and other spondylarthropathies. However, no conclusions can be drawn with respect to their specific efficacy in SI joint pain.[28]

Interventional management

Patients with SI joint pain resistant to conservative treatment are eligible for intra-articular injections or radiofrequency (RF) treatment.

Intra-articular injections

SI joint injections with local anesthetic and corticosteroids may provide good pain relief for periods of up to 1 year. It is assumed that intra-articular injections would produce better results than peri-articular infiltrations. Yet, peri-articular infiltrations were demonstrated to provide good pain relief in short-term follow-up in 2 double-blind studies,[24,25] indicating the importance of extra-articular sources of SI pathology.[29–31] Controlled studies support the assertion that both intra- and extra-articular injections may be beneficial. Luukkainen et al.[30] randomized 24 patients to receive either peri-articular corticosteroid with local anesthetic ($n = 13$), or local anesthetic and saline ($n = 11$). One month after the intervention, visual analog scale (VAS) pain scores had decreased significantly in the corticosteroid group compared with the control patients. Maugars et al.[32] treated 13 SI joints in 10 patients. Intra-articular corticosteroids were injected into 6 SI joints, while the remaining 7 joints received physiological saline solution. After 1 month, pain reduction of >70% was noted in 5 of the 6 SI joints treated with corticosteroid, whereas no benefit was noted in the placebo group. In all control patients and 2 in the treatment group who had short-term symptom palliation, a repeat corticosteroid injection was performed. After 1, 3, and 6 months, significant pain reduction was observed in 86%, 62%, and 58% of patients, respectively.

RF treatment of the SI joint

The efficacy of RF treatment of the SI joint is illustrated by several prospective observational,[33,34] retrospective studies[35–37] and 1 randomized controlled study.[38] However, the selection criteria, definition of success, and RF parameters (ie, temperature, duration, and location of RF treatment) have varied widely between studies. Gevargez et al.[34] performed three 90°C lesions in the ligamentum sacroiliacum posterius and 1 targeting the L5 ramus dorsalis. In contrast, Ferrante et al.[35] performed multiple bipolar intra-articular lesions at 90°C. Cohen and Abdi[36] performed single 80°C lesions at the level of the L4–L5 rami dorsales and the S1 to S3 (or S4) rami laterales of the rami dorsales. Yin et al.[37] applied a similar technique, except that they excluded the L4 ramus dorsalis, and selected more caudal levels based on concordant sensory stimulation. Burnham and Yasui[33] performed bipolar RF strip lesions lateral to the foramen sacrale posterius and a monopolar RF treatment at the level the L5 ramus dorsalis. More recently, Cohen et al.[39] investigated which demographic and clinical variables could be used to predict SI joint RF treatment outcome. In multivariate analysis, pre-procedure pain intensity, age 65 years or older, and pain referral below the knee were all statistically significant predictors of failure.

One study reported the use of pulsed RF (PRF) therapy for the treatment of SI joint pain.[40] The L4, L5 rami mediales, and the S1, S2 rami laterales of the rami dorsales were the targets of the therapy. Evidence of a good or excellent result (>50% and 80% reduction in the VAS, respectively) was obtained in 73% of the patients. The duration of the clinical effect varied from 6 weeks to 32 weeks.

Because of variable and extensive innervation of the dorsal SI joint, targeting the nerves innervating the joint with "classic" RF methods is sometimes difficult. In 2 double-blind randomized, controlled studies, Dreyfuss et al.[41,42] demonstrated the superiority of multisite, multi-depth sacral lateral branch blocks over single-site, single-depth blocks to anesthetize the SI joint ligaments. However, these studies also demonstrated that lateral branch blocks do not reliably interrupt nociceptive information emanating from the intra-articular portion of the SI joint complex (ie, capsular distension). To circumvent anatomical variations in innervations, some investigators have employed internally cooled RF electrodes, which increase the ablative area by minimizing the effect of tissue charring to limit lesion expansion. In 2008, a retrospective case series[43] and a randomized controlled trial[38] concerning cooled RF treatment of the SI joint were published. In the retrospective trial 3 to 4 months post-treatment, a mean VAS pain score improvement of 2.9 points was noted (7.1 to 4.2).[43] Eighteen patients rated their improvement in pain as either improved or much improved, while 8 reported minimal or no improvement. Cohen et al.[38] performed a randomized placebo-controlled study in which a "classic" RF procedure was performed on the L4 and L5 rami dorsales, and a cooled RF treatment of the S1 to S3 rami laterales. One, 3, and 6 months post-treatment, 79%, 64%, and 57% of patients reported ≥50% pain relief, respectively. In the placebo group, only 14%

experienced significant improvement at 1 month follow-up, and none experienced significant benefit 3 months post-procedure. The additional cost of disposable components needed for a cooled RF procedure should be taken into consideration, because in some countries, no reimbursement exists for this procedure.

Complications of interventional management

Although potential complications of articular injections and RF procedures include infection, hematoma formation, neural damage, trauma to the sciatic nerve, gas and vascular particulate embolism, weakness secondary to extra-articular extravasation, and complications related to drug administration, the reported rate of these complications in SI joint treatment is low.[44]

Luukkainen et al.[29,30] reported no complications from peri-articular SI joint injections. For intra-articular injections, Maugars et al.[32] reported only transient perineal anesthesia lasting a few hours and mild sciatalgia (sciatica) lasting 3 weeks, but no information was given as to the number of patients that reported these side effects.

For RF treatment of the SI joint, Cohen et al.[38] noted that the majority of 28 patients experienced temporary worsening of pain 5 to 10 days after the procedure that was attributed to procedure-related tissue trauma and temporary neuritis. In a follow-up study, Cohen et al. reported 5 complications out of 77 treated patients.[39] These included 3 cases of temporary paresthesia, 1 superficial skin infection that resolved with antibiotics, and 1 case of hyperglycemia in a diabetic patient requiring increased insulin use for 3 days. The latter was caused by the corticoid used to prevent procedure-related neuritis; this is a relatively common practice that is, however, not supported by improved outcome in the literature. In their study evaluating PRF of the SI joint, Vallejo et al. observed no complications or worsening of pain.[40,43] Transient buttock dysesthesia or hypoesthesia, and temporary worsening of pain have also been commonly reported in other studies evaluating heat RF.[33,34,37]

Evidence for interventional management

A summary of the available evidence for interventional treatment of SIJ pain is given in Table 13.1.

Table 13.1. Summary of evidence of interventional pain management for SI joint pain.

Technique	Assessment
Therapeutic intra-articular injections with corticosteroids and local anesthetic	1 B+
Radiofrequency (RF) treatment of rami dorsales and laterales	2 C+
Pulsed RF treatment of rami dorsales and rami laterales	2 C+
Cooled/RF treatment of the rami laterales	2 B+

SI, sacroiliac.

Recommendations

In patients with chronic aspecific low back complaints possibly originating from the SI joint, an intra-articular injection with a local anesthetic and corticosteroids can be recommended. If the latter fail or produce only short-term effects, cooled/RF treatment of the lateral branches of S1 to S3 (S4) is recommended if available. When this procedure cannot be used, (pulsed) RF procedures targeted at L5 dorsal ramus and lateral branches of S1 to S3 may be considered.

Clinical practice algorithm

The practice algorithm is illustrated in Figure 13.2.

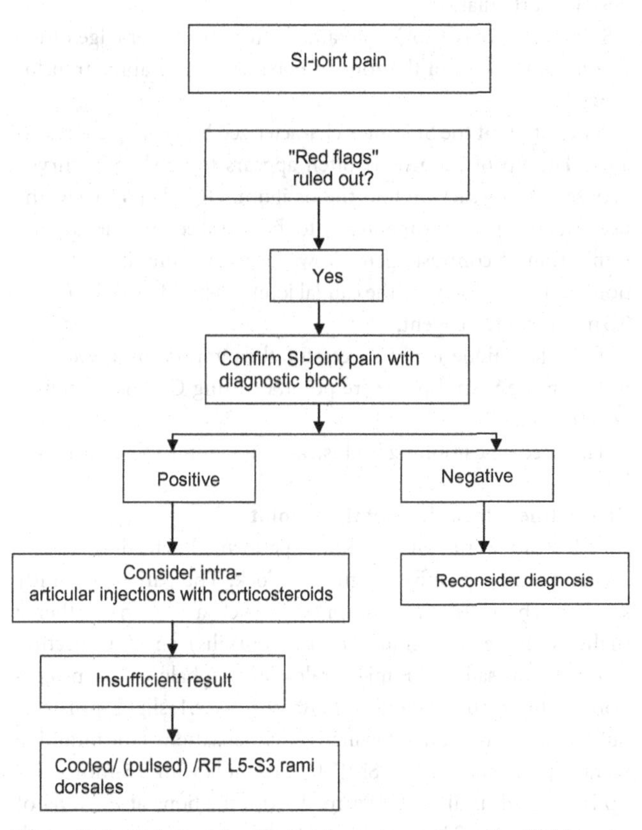

Figure 13.2. Clinical practice algorithm for treatment of sacroiliac (SI) joint pain. RF, radiofrequency.

Techniques

Classical SI joint infiltration technique

- The patient lies in a prone position.
- In anterior-posterior (AP) fluoroscopic projection, the medial SI joint line is formed by the posterior joint articulation.
- Next, the C-arm is rotated contralaterally until the medial cortical line of the posterior articulation is in focus. Tilting the C-arm longitudinally in relation to the patient (cephalo-caudally) can

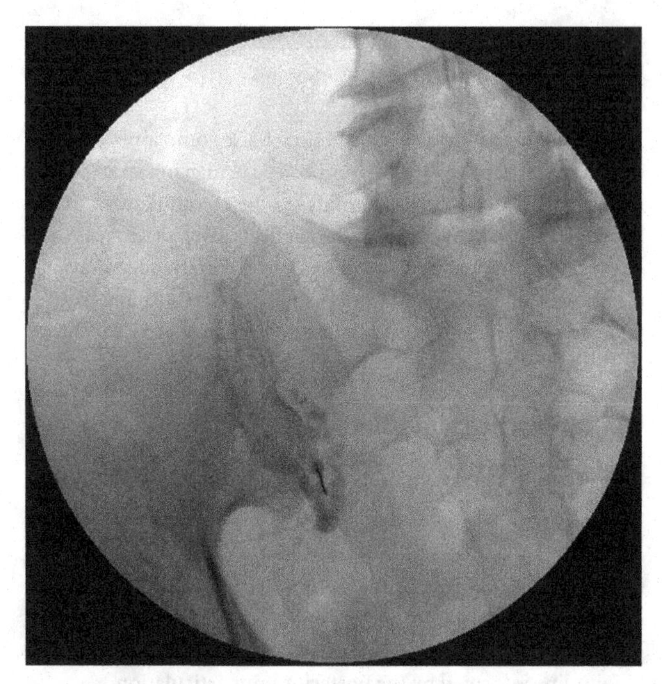

Figure 13.3. Intra-articular injection of sacroiliac joint with contrast in anterior-posterior view.

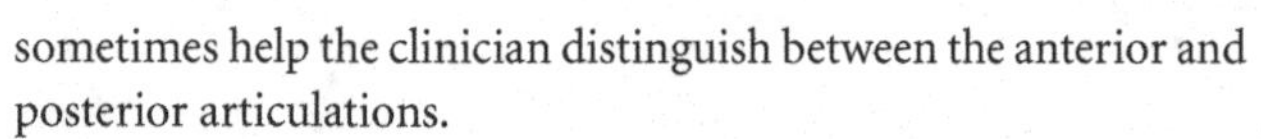

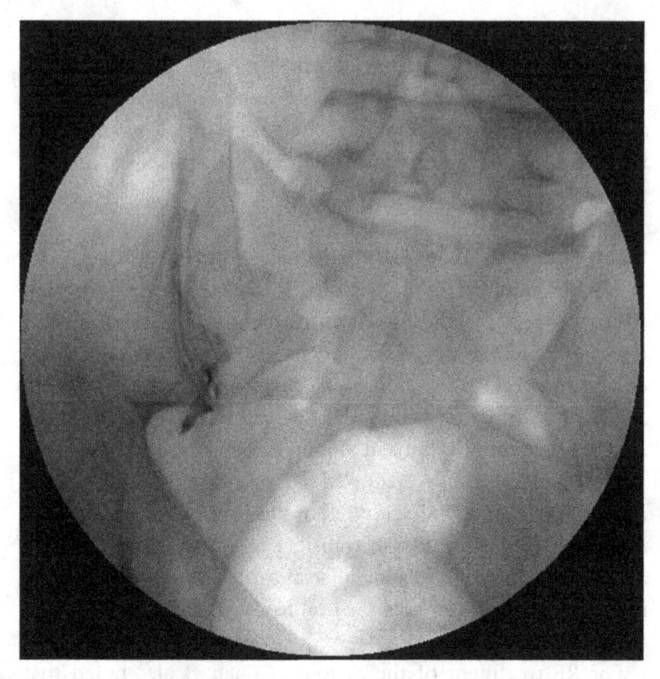

Figure 13.4. Intra-articular injection of sacroiliac joint with contrast in anterior-posterior view.

sometimes help the clinician distinguish between the anterior and posterior articulations.

• Skin puncture is 1 to 2 cm cranially from the lower edge of the SI joint at the level of the zone of maximal radiographic translucency.

• Penetration of the SI joint is characterized by a change in resistance. The tip of the needle often appears to be slightly curved between the os sacrum and the os ilium. On a lateral view, the needle tip should appear anterior to the dorsal edge of the sacrum.

• Injection of contrast agent shows dispersal along the articulations and also a filling of the caudal joint capsule. Use only 0.25 to 0.5 mL of contrast agent.

• If this technique is not successful, then approaching the joint from a more rostral puncture point, or using CT, may facilitate penetration.

The needle positioning is illustrated in Figures 13.3 and 13.4.

RF treatment technique of the SI joint

An RF treatment of the SI joint is performed with fluoroscopic imaging after a positive diagnostic block. The patient is lightly sedated. The C-arm is positioned in such a way that either a slightly oblique projection (L4 ramus dorsalis), an AP projection (L5 ramus dorsalis and rami laterales), or a cephalo-caudal projection (S1 to S3 rami laterales) is attained. For S1, slight ipsilateral oblique angulation can often increase visualization of the foramina sacralia posteriora. A 22G SMK-C10 cannula with a 5-mm active tip is inserted until contact is made with the bone at the level of the target nerve. The correct needle position is confirmed with electrostimulation at 50 Hz, at which point paresthesia should be felt in the painful area with thresholds <0.5 V. Right S1 and S2 rami laterales are usually found between "1 o'clock and 5 o'clock" positions on the lateral side of the foramina sacralia posteriora. For the left S1 and S2 rami laterales, the locations correspond to between "7 o'clock and 11 o'clock." In view of the small lesion size created by conventional electrodes, and the wide-spread variability in the location and number of nerves converging on each foramina sacralia posteriora, multiple lesions may be necessary. Before performing the RF treatment, motor stimulation should be performed to ensure the absence of leg or sphincter contraction. If present, the needle position is incorrect, and repositioning is needed. After correct positioning of the electrode, the RF probe is inserted, and a 90-second RF treatment at 80°C is made.[36]

Another technique, which has been successfully implemented, targets the S1, S2, and S3 (S4) rami laterales.[45]

Cooled RF of the SI joint

A cooled RF treatment of the SI joint is performed after a positive diagnostic block. The patient is lightly sedated. C-arm fluoroscopy is used to visualize the sacrum by imaging through the L5/S1 disk space. The L5 ramus dorsales and S1 to S3 rami laterales are targeted. An introducer with stylet is inserted onto the bone endpoint of the posterior sacrum. When inserted, the stylet extends 6 mm beyond the tip of the introducer. The RF probe, which is subsequently inserted via the same introducer, extends only 4 mm beyond the tip of the introducer. To maximize encasement of the rami laterales of the S1 to S3 (S4) nerves, the electrode is placed 8 to 10 mm from the lateral edge of the foramina sacralia posteriora, with the tip positioned approximately 2 mm proximal to the surface (because of the 2 mm longer introducer). Two or 3 lesions are created at each sacral level. Typically, these lesions are spaced about 1 cm apart from one another, creating a continuous strip of ablated tissue lateral to each foramen sacrale. RF energy is delivered for 2 minutes (30 seconds per lesion) with a target electrode temperature of 60°C. The ramus dorsalis of the L5 nerve is targeted in a classical manner.

Summary

The SI joint is responsible for 16% to 30% of axial low back complaints and can be difficult to distinguish from other forms of low back pain. Clinical examination and radiological imaging is of limited diagnostic value. The result of diagnostic blocks must be interpreted with caution, because false-positive as well as false-negative results occur frequently. Currently, the majority of scientific evidence points toward intra-articular SI joint infiltrations for short-term improvement. If the latter fail or produce only short-term effects, a combination of cooled and conventional RF treatment of the rami laterales of S1 to S3 (S4) is recommended (2 B+) if available. When this procedure cannot be used, (pulsed) RF procedures targeted at L5 ramus dorsalis and rami laterales of S1 to S3 may be considered (2 C+).

References

1. Merskey H, Bogduk N. *Classification of Chronic Pain: Descriptions of Chronic Pain Syndromes and Definitions of Pain Terms.* 2nd ed. Seattle, WA: IASP Press; 1994.
2. Bernard TN Jr, Kirkaldy-Willis WH. Recognizing specific characteristics of nonspecific low back pain. *Clin Orthop Relat Res.* 1987; 266–280.
3. Schwarzer AC, Aprill CN, Bogduk N. The sacroiliac joint in chronic low back pain. *Spine.* 1995;20:31–37.
4. Maigne JY, Aivaliklis A, Pfefer F. Results of sacroiliac joint double block and value of sacroiliac pain provocation tests in 54 patients with low back pain. *Spine.* 1996;21:1889–1892.
5. Fortin JD, Kissling RO, O'Connor BL, Vilensky JA. Sacroiliac joint innervation and pain. *Am J Orthop.* 1999;28:687–690.
6. Schuit D, McPoil TG, Mulesa P. Incidence of sacroiliac joint malalignment in leg length discrepancies. *J Am Podiatr Med Assoc.* 1989;79:380–383.
7. Herzog W, Conway PJ. Gait analysis of sacroiliac joint patients. *J Manipulative Physiol Ther.* 1994;17:124–127.
8. Schoenberger M, Hellmich K. Sacroiliac dislocation and scoliosis. *Hippokrates.* 1964;476–479.
9. Katz V, Schofferman J, Reynolds J. The sacroiliac joint: a potential cause of pain after lumbar fusion to the sacrum. *J Spinal Disord Tech.* 2003;16:96–99.
10. Marymont JV, Lynch MA, Henning CE. Exercise-related stress reaction of the sacroiliac joint. An unusual cause of low back pain in athletes. *Am J Sports Med.* 1986;14:320–323.
11. Albert H, Godskesen M, Westergaard J. Prognosis in four syndromes of pregnancy-related pelvic pain. *Acta Obstet Gynecol Scand.* 2001;80:505–510.
12. Slipman CW, Jackson HB, Lipetz JS, et al. Sacroiliac joint pain referral zones. *Arch Phys Med Rehabil.* 2000;81:334–338.
13. Laslett M, Aprill CN, McDonald B, Young SB. Diagnosis of sacroiliac joint pain: validity of individual provocation tests and composites of tests. *Man Ther.* 2005;10:207–218.
14. van der Wurff P, Buijs EJ, Groen GJ. A multitest regimen of pain provocation tests as an aid to reduce unnecessary minimally invasive sacroiliac joint procedures. *Arch Phys Med Rehabil.* 2006;87:10–14.
15. Szadek KM, van der Wurff P, van Tulder MW, Zuurmond WW, Perez RS. Diagnostic validity of criteria for sacroiliac joint pain: a systematic review. *J Pain.* 2009;10:354–368.
16. Young S, Aprill C, Laslett M. Correlation of clinical examination characteristics with three sources of chronic low back pain. *Spine J.* 2003;3:460–465.
17. Bigos S, Bowyer O, Braen G, et al. Acute low back pain problems in adults. Clinical Practice Guideline No. 14. AHCPR Publication No. 95-0642. Rockville, MD: Agency for Healthcare Policy and Research, Public Health Service, U.S. Department of Health and Human Services; December 1994.
18. Hansen HC, McKenzie-Brown AM, Cohen SP, et al. Sacroiliac joint interventions: a systematic review. *Pain Physician.* 2007;10: 165–184.
19. Puhakka KB, Jurik AG, Schiottz-Christensen B, et al. MRI abnormalities of sacroiliac joints in early spondylarthropathy: a 1-year follow-up study. *Scand J Rheumatol.* 2004;33:332–338.
20. Puhakka KB, Melsen F, Jurik AG, et al. MR imaging of the normal sacroiliac joint with correlation to histology. *Skeletal Radiol.* 2004;33: 15–28.
21. Dreyfuss MD. Practice guidelines and protocols for sacroiliac joint blocks. In: International Spine Intervention Society, ed. *ISIS 9th Annual Scientific Meeting.* San Francisco, CA: ISIS; 2001:35–49.
22. Laslett M, Young SB, Aprill CN, McDonald B. Diagnosing painful sacroiliac joints: a validity study of a McKenzie evaluation and sacroiliac provocation tests. *Aust J Physiother.* 2003;49:89–97.
23. Maigne JY, Boulahdour H, Chatellier G. Value of quantitative radionuclide bone scanning in the diagnosis of sacroiliac joint syndrome in 32 patients with low back pain. *Eur Spine J.* 1998;7:328–331.
24. Manchikanti L, Singh V, Pampati V, et al. Evaluation of the relative contributions of various structures in chronic low back pain. *Pain Physician.* 2001;4:308–316.
25. van der Wurff P, Buijs EJ, Groen GJ. Intensity mapping of pain referral areas in sacroiliac joint pain patients. *J Manipulative Physiol Ther.* 2006;29:190–195.
26. Rosenberg JM, Quint TJ, de Rosayro AM. Computerized tomographic localization of clinically-guided sacroiliac joint injections. *Clin J Pain.* 2000;16:18–21.
27. Bollow M, Braun J, Taupitz M, et al. CT-guided intraarticular corticosteroid injection into the sacroiliac joints in patients with spondyloarthropathy: indication and follow-up with contrast-enhanced MRI. *J Comput Assist Tomogr.* 1996;20:512–521.
28. Cohen SP. Sacroiliac joint pain: a comprehensive review of anatomy, diagnosis, and treatment. *Anesth Analg.* 2005;101:1440–1453.
29. Luukkainen R, Nissila M, Asikainen E, et al. Periarticular corticosteroid treatment of the sacroiliac joint in patients with seronegative spondylarthropathy. *Clin Exp Rheumatol.* 1999;17:88–90.
30. Luukkainen RK, Wennerstrand PV, Kautiainen HH, Sanila MT, Asikainen EL. Efficacy of periarticular corticosteroid treatment of the sacroiliac joint in non-spondylarthropathic patients with chronic low

back pain in the region of the sacroiliac joint. *Clin Exp Rheumatol.* 2002;20:52–54.

31. Borowsky CD, Fagen G. Sources of sacroiliac region pain: insights gained from a study comparing standard intraarticular injection with a technique combining intra- and peri-articular injection. *Arch Phys Med Rehabil.* 2008;89:2048–2056.
32. Maugars Y, Mathis C, Berthelot JM, Charlier C, Prost A. Assessment of the efficacy of sacroiliac corticosteroid injections in spondylarthropathies: a double-blind study. *Br J Rheumatol.* 1996;35:767–770.
33. Burnham RS, Yasui Y. An alternate method of radiofrequency neurotomy of the sacroiliac joint: a pilot study of the effect on pain, function, and satisfaction. *Reg Anesth Pain Med.* 2007;32:12–19.
34. Gevargez A, Groenemeyer D, Schirp S, Braun M. CT-guided percutaneous radiofrequency denervation of the sacroiliac joint. *Eur Radiol.* 2002;12:1360–1365.
35. Ferrante FM, King LF, Rochë EA, et al. Radiofrequency sacroiliac joint denervation for sacroiliac syndrome. *Reg Anesth Pain Med.* 2001;26:137–142.
36. Cohen SP, Abdi S. Lateral branch blocks as a treatment for sacroiliac joint pain: a pilot study. *Reg Anesth Pain Med.* 2003;28:113–119.
37. Yin W, Willard F, Carreiro J, Dreyfuss P. Sensory stimulation-guided sacroiliac joint radiofrequency neurotomy: technique based on neuroanatomy of the dorsal sacral plexus. *Spine.* 2003;28:2419–2425.
38. Cohen SP, Hurley RW, Buckenmaier CC 3rd, et al. Randomized placebo-controlled study evaluating lateral branch radiofrequency denervation for sacroiliac joint pain. *Anesthesiology.* 2008;109:279–288.
39. Cohen SP, Strassels SA, Kurihara C, et al. Outcome predictors for sacroiliac joint (lateral branch) radiofrequency denervation. *Reg Anesth Pain Med.* 2009;34:206–214.
40. Vallejo R, Benyamin RM, Kramer J, Stanton G, Joseph NJ. Pulsed radiofrequency denervation for the treatment of sacroiliac joint syndrome. *Pain Med.* 2006;7:429–434.
41. Dreyfuss P, Snyder BD, Park K, et al. The ability of single site, single depth sacral lateral branch blocks to anesthetize the sacroiliac joint complex. *Pain Med.* 2008;9:844–850.
42. Dreyfuss P, Henning T, Malladi N, Goldstein B, Bogduk N. The ability of multi-site, multi-depth sacral lateral branch blocks to anesthetize the sacroiliac joint complex. *Pain Med.* 2009;10:679–688.
43. Kapural L, Nageeb F, Kapural M, et al. Cooled radiofrequency system for the treatment of chronic pain from sacroiliitis: the first case-series. *Pain Pract.* 2008;8:348–354.
44. Manchikanti L, Boswell MV, Singh V, et al. Comprehensive evidence-based guidelines for interventional techniques in the management of chronic spinal pain. *Pain Physician.* 2009;12:699–802.
45. Buijs EJ, Kamphuis E, Groen GJ. Radiofrequency treatment of sacroiliac joint-related pain aimed at the first three sacral dorsal rami: a minimal approach. *Pain Clin.* 2004;16:139–146.

14 Coccygodynia

Jacob Patijn, Markus Janssen, Salim Hayek, Nagy Mekhail, Jan Van Zundert and Maarten van Kleef

Introduction

Coccygodynia is a painful disorder of the tailbone (os coccygis) localized just above the anus, for which a traumatic as well as an idiopathic form can be differentiated. Precise incidence and prevalence figures for the traumatic and idiopathic forms of this condition are not available. However, it is known that the idiopathic form comprises less than 1% of all nontraumatic disorders of the vertebral column.[1] In rare cases a precoccygeal epidermal inclusion cyst can present as coccygodynia.[2] A clear relationship exists between coccygodynia and the female gender; the female/male incidence ratio is 5:1.[3] Moreover, a relationship exists between weight and the occurrence of coccygodynia; a body-mass index (BMI) of >27.4 in females and >29.4 in males increases the chance of developing coccygodynia.[4]

In the acute form of coccygodynia, a trauma (usually a fall into the sitting position) is the cause of the complaints in the majority of the cases.[4,5] Repetitive microtrauma resulting from an inadequate sitting posture or from activities such as cycling or motor sports can also give rise to coccygodynia.[6,7] In females, parturition can be regarded as a trauma for the development of coccygodynia.[8] The coccygeal joints are involved in 70% of traumatic childbirth cases.[5] Dynamic, radiological examination of function (os coccygis stressed and unstressed) and discography indicate that the following five causes may play a role in these traumatic and idiopathic coccygodynias: anterior luxation, hypermobility, coccygeal spicules, subluxation, and luxation.[5,8] MRI studies show that mobility during tightening of the muscles of the pelvic floor and defecation is independent of age, gender, and the presence or absence of coccygodynia.

The os coccygis usually consists of four bony segments that are attached cranially to the os sacrum at the sacrococcygeal joint. Between the first two segments, a rudimentary discus intervertebralis may be present and can form a potential localization point for post-traumatic hypermobility.[4] The other segments are synarthroses and have no mobility.[9] Due to a more posteriorly situated os sacrum and os coccygis,[10] and a longer os coccygis relative to men,[11] females have a greater chance of developing coccygodynia.

Diagnosis

Diagnosis is usually made on the basis of the typical anamnesis in which the symptoms are generally related to a trauma (including parturition). The chance of developing coccygodynia may be increased by repetitive microtrauma from sitting in females with a BMI > 27.4 and in males with a BMI > 29.4.[4]

History

Most patients with coccygodynia complain anamnestically about pain at the site of the tailbone, usually provoked by sitting.[12] Due to the direct pressure of the saddle on the os coccygis, cycling is usually impossible in these patients.

Physical examination

In addition to standard physical and neurological examination, manual examination of the os coccygis is also very important.[11] The presence or absence of pain during mobilization of the os coccygis can differentiate between a nociceptive pain of the os coccygis with the ligamentous and muscular structures and a referred pain due to pathology in the lower pelvic region. In addition, the Valsalva maneuver should be positive in the case of coccygodynia based on disorders of the neural structures, and negative in the case of primary involvement of the os coccygis.[11]

Additional tests

First of all, lateral images of the os coccygis are indicated. Dynamic radiological images of these patients can also be made. In this instance, the angle is measured according to the Maigne

Evidence-Based Interventional Pain Medicine: According to Clinical Diagnoses, First Edition. Edited by Jan Van Zundert, Jacob Patijn, Craig T. Hartrick, Arno Lataster, Frank J.P.M Huygen, Nagy Mekhail, Maarten van Kleef.

method[4,5,8] in the standing and sitting (stressful for the os coccygis) positions. Coccygeal mobility between 2° and 25° is considered normal. The position of discography is unclear. No specificity or sensitivity studies have been published for all diagnostics.

Given the relationship to the patient being overweight, BMI determination is useful: a body mass index of >27.4 in females and >29.4 in males increases the chance of developing coccygodynia.[4] As in the case of all chronic pain symptoms (>3 months), exploratory psycho-cognitive examination is indicated, during which kinesiophobia, catastrophizing, and depression should particularly be evaluated. If there is any suspicion of other causes, and in particular of idiopathic coccygodynia, more detailed diagnostic techniques such as MRI and/or referral should definitely take place in order to be able to rule out infections, precoccygeal cysts and malignancies.

Differential diagnosis

Three groups of diagnoses can be determined in the differential diagnosis of coccygodynia: a nociceptive (from the os coccygis) diagnosis, a neuropathic diagnosis, or a visceral diagnosis. In the case of a nociceptive differential diagnosis, the Levator Ani Syndrome[10] should be considered, in which mobilization of the os coccygis is not painful as it is in the case of a traumatic etiology. Furthermore, to make the differential diagnosis, osteomyelitis, arthritis and intraossal lipoma, intraossal chondroma, avascular necrosis and precoccygeal cysts should be considered.[2,13]

In the case of a neuropathic differential diagnosis, a lumbar disk herniation should primarily be considered.[10] In this case, the symptoms are usually not related to provocation by sitting and manipulation of the os coccygis. Other diagnoses that can be the cause of referred neuropathic pain in the os coccygis region are neural tumors in this area, such as Schwannomas, neurinomas, arachnoid cysts of the cauda equina, sacrococcygeal meningeal cysts, chordomas, and very rarely, paragangliomas at the caudal end of the os coccygis.[10]

Coccygodynia can also be the result of pain referred from visceral structures due to conditions such as disorders of the rectum, the colon sigmoideum, and the urogenital system. In these cases, infections as well as primary tumors and metastases can mimic the clinical appearance of coccygodynia.[11]

Treatment options

In general, there have been few controlled studies showing the efficacy of any known coccygodynia treatments. Most treatments have been evaluated in retrospective studies.

Conservative management

In the acute phase of a post-traumatic coccygodynia, a conservative policy has been proposed. This conservative approach includes nonsteroidal anti-inflammatory drugs (NSAIDs) and an adapted sitting posture.[11] In a controlled pilot study, conservative treatment, in the sense of mobilization of the os coccygis, has been shown to have a long-term effect in 25% of patients.[13] A subsequent randomized controlled study, by the same group, compared intrarectal manipulation (applied in three 5-minute sessions over a period of 10 days) to short-wave magnetic field physiotherapy (delivered in three sessions over a period of 10 days). Intrarectal manipulation was more effective than the control treatment in improving visual analog scale (VAS) scores as well as functional and pain questionnaires. However, the efficacy was modest.[14] Infrared thermography before and after manual therapy and diathermy in patients with coccygodynia objectively showed decrement of surface temperature correlating ($r = 0.67$, $P < 0.01$) with changes of subjective pain intensity after treatment.[15]

Interventional management

In a prospective study, the combination of local injections of corticosteroids/local anesthetic with mobilization was shown to have a positive effect in 85% of cases, while local injections of corticosteroids/local anesthetic alone produced a 60% success rate.[1] In this study, it was indicated that the infiltration occurred next to the os coccygis and at the level of the caudal end of the spinal column, but that no attempt was made to infiltrate the sacrococcygeal joint. The effect of intradiscal corticosteroid injections into the os coccygis has yet to be demonstrated.[5] The same is true for dextrose prolotherapy in case of recalcitrant coccygodynia.[16]

In addition to local injections of corticosteroids/local anesthetic, interventional pain management techniques include radiofrequency (RF) treatment of the sacral roots. However, there are no studies available that prove the utility of RF. The same is true of the caudal block. Only one study of mediocre quality has described the long-term effects of rhizotomy of the S5 and S6 roots. Based on the results and complications reported, this treatment is not recommended.[17]

Blocking of the ganglion impar with local anesthetic was described in a case report as well as in a case series. The series consisted of six patients who were subjected to 20 blocks with 0.5% bupivacaine. Each injection produced pain relief which was scored by the majority of patients as being more than a 75% reduction in pain. The beneficial effect was retained with repeated injections.[18] The case report refers to a patient with 100% pain relief that continued for more than one year.[19]

Reig et al.[20] performed a prospective study on 13 patients, four of whom had been diagnosed with coccygodynia in which an RF thermic lesion of the ganglion impar was performed using two needles. The thermic lesion was only performed if a positive result (pain reduction >50% in a test block with corticosteroids/local anesthetic) had been attained beforehand. Reig describes significant pain reduction of more than 50% in the entire group (all forms of non-oncological pain in the pelvis) with an average duration of effectiveness of 2.2 months. Given the small size of the group of patients with coccygodynia who were studied, and the relatively short duration of its effectiveness, as well as the risk of puncture of the rectum inherent to this method, this technique can only be recommended in a study context. The authors recommend the technique with two needles since the position of the

Table 14.1. Summary of evidence for interventional management of coccygodynia.

Technique	Assessment
Local injections corticosteroids/local anesthetic	2 C+
Intradiscal corticosteroid injections, ganglion impar block, RF ganglion impar, caudal block	0
Neurostimulation	0

ganglion impar is extremely variable. This corresponds with the results of an anatomical study performed by Oh.[21]

Surgical treatment

In the subacute and chronic phases, many forms of treatment for coccygodynia are advised, up to and including surgical removal of the os coccygis. Although retrospective studies are still being published concerning coccygectomy,[22] there are strong contraindications to this surgical intervention due to the long-term moderate results and the chance of major complications.[11,16]

Neurostimulation

Few case reports suggest a possible beneficial effect for spinal cord stimulation at the conus medullaris level[23] or peripheral nerve stimulation in the caudal space[24] or subcutaneously.[25] However, given the paucity of experience and reports, this treatment modality may be considered with much caution only after other more established therapies have failed.

Complications of interventional management

Local anesthetic injection with corticosteroids always carries the risk of going through the disc and penetrating the rectum. The same is true for the ganglion impar block.

Evidence for interventional management

A summary of the available evidence is given in Table 14.1.

Recommendations

In the chronic stage of coccygodynia, a combination of manual mobilization of the sacrococcygeal articular capsule or the first intercoccygeal joint and a local injection of corticosteroids with anesthetic should be the first choice of treatment. Other interventional pain treatments should only be considered for research purposes.

Clinical practice algorithm

The practice algorithm is illustrated in Figure 14.1.

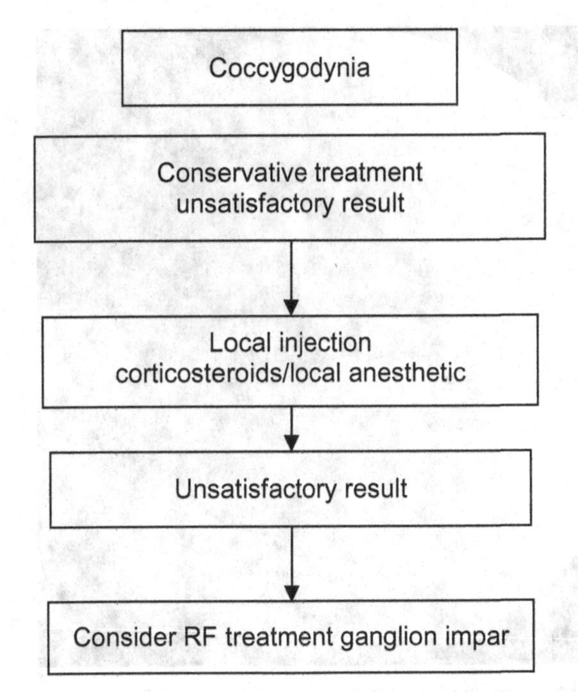

Figure 14.1. Clinical practice algorithm for the treatment of coccygodynia.

Technique(s)

Radiofrequency treatment (RF) of the ganglion impar

For this technique, the patient lies face down in the prone position. During radiographic examination, one needle is inserted *trans*-sacrococcygeally (through the ligamentum sacrococcygeum posterius and anterius), while the second needle is inserted through a coccygeal disk (Figure 14.2). Using a lateral projection, the positions of the needles are checked while contrast agent is administered (Figure 14.3). After stimulation at 50 Hz (up to 1 V) and 2 Hz (no motor reaction up to 3 V), each needle is warmed up to 80°C for 80 seconds by means of RF.

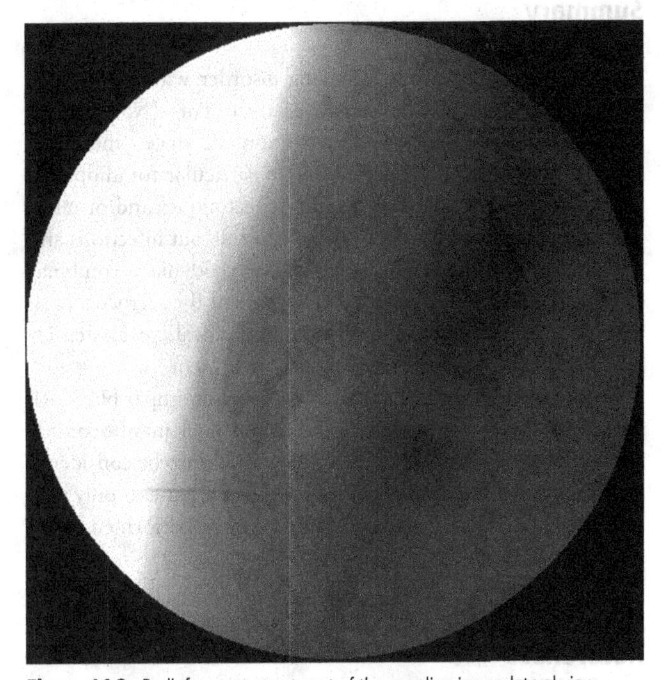

Figure 14.2. Radiofrequency treatment of the ganglion impar: lateral view.

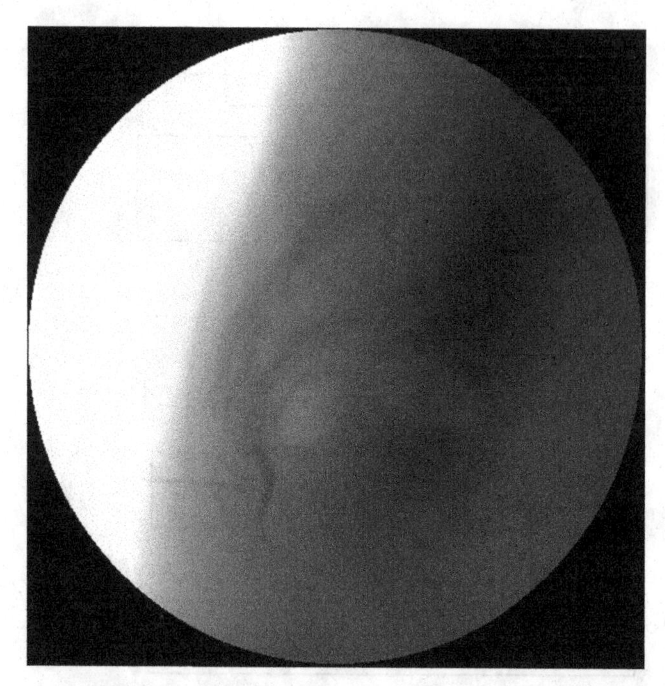

Figure 14.3. RF ganglion impar: Lateral view with contrast agent in place.

Summary

Coccygodynia is a serious, disabling disorder with few proven therapeutic options. Conservative treatment (NSAIDs) is always—especially in the acute posttraumatic stage—indicated. When other causes are suspected, and in particular, for idiopathic coccygodynia, more detailed diagnostic techniques and/or referral must take place in order to be able to rule out infections and malignancies. In the chronic stage of coccygodynia, a combination of manual mobilization of the capsule of the sacrococcygeal joint or the first intercoccygeal joint and a local corticosteroid/anesthetic injection is the first choice of treatment.

Intradiscal corticosteroid injections, ganglion impar block, RF treatment of the ganglion impar, and caudal block may be considered for research purposes. Neuromodulation may be considered in appropriately selected, psychologically stable patients only if all other modalities have failed and should only be performed under research conditions.

References

1. Wray CC, Easom S, Hoskinson J. Coccydynia. Aetiology and treatment. *J Bone Joint Surg Br.* 1991;73:335–338.
2. Jaiswal A, Shetty AP, Rajasekaran S. Precoccygeal epidermal inclusion cyst presenting as coccygodynia. *Singapore Med J.* 2008;49:e212–e214.
3. Peyton FW. Coccygodynia in women. *Indiana Med.* 1988;81:697–698.
4. Maigne JY, Doursounian L, Chatellier G. Causes and mechanisms of common coccydynia: role of body mass index and coccygeal trauma. *Spine.* 2000;25:3072–3079.
5. Maigne JY, Guedj S, Straus C. Idiopathic coccygodynia. Lateral roentgenograms in the sitting position and coccygeal discography. *Spine.* 1994;19:930–934.
6. Frazier LM. Coccydynia: a tail of woe. *N C Med J.* 1985;46:209–212.
7. van Kleef M, Barendse G, Wilmink JT, et al. Percutaneous intradiscal radio-frequency thermocoagulation in chronic non-specific low back pain. *Pain Clin.* 1996;9:259–268.
8. Maigne JY, Tamalet B. Standardized radiologic protocol for the study of common coccygodynia and characteristics of the lesions observed in the sitting position. Clinical elements differentiating luxation, hypermobility, and normal mobility. *Spine.* 1996;21:2588–2593.
9. Moore K, Delley A. *Clinically Oriented Anatomy.* Philadelphia, PA: Lippincott Williams and Wilkins; 1999.
10. CL N. Levator ani syndrome—a case study and literature review. *Aust Fam Physician.* 2007;36:449–452.
11. De Andres J, Chaves S. Coccygodynia: a proposal for an algorithm for treatment. *J Pain.* 2003;4:257–266.
12. Lourie J, Young S. Avascular necrosis of the coccyx: a cause of coccydynia? Case report and histological findings in 16 patients. *Br J Clin Pract.* 1985;39:247–248.
13. Maigne JY, Chatellier G. Comparison of three manual coccydynia treatments: a pilot study. *Spine.* 2001;26:E479–E483; discussion E84.
14. Maigne JY, Chatellier G, Faou ML, Archambeau M. The treatment of chronic coccydynia with intrarectal manipulation: a randomized controlled study. *Spine.* 2006;31:E621–E627.
15. Wu CL, Yu KL, Chuang HY, Huang MH, Chen TW, Chen CH. The application of infrared thermography in the assessment of patients with coccygodynia before and after manual therapy combined with diathermy. *J Manipulative Physiol Ther.* 2009;32:287–293.
16. Khan SA, Kumar A, Varshney MK, Trikha V, Yadav CS. Dextrose prolotherapy for recalcitrant coccygodynia. *J Orthop Surg (Hong Kong).* 2008;16:27–29.
17. Albrektsson B. Sacral rhizotomy in cases of anococcygeal pain. A follow-up of 24 cases. *Acta Orthop Scand.* 1981;52:187–190.
18. Buttaci C, Foye PM, Stitik TP. Coccygodynia succesfully treated with ganglion Impar blocks: a case series. *Am J Phys Med Rehabil.* 2005;84:218.
19. Foye PM, Buttaci CJ, Stitik TP, Yonclas PP. Successful injection for coccyx pain. *Am J Phys Med Rehabil.* 2006;85:783–784.
20. Reig E, Abejon D, del Pozo C, Insausti J, Contreras R. Thermocoagulation of the ganglion impar or ganglion of Walther: description of a modified approach. Preliminary results in chronic, nononcological pain. *Pain Pract.* 2005;5:103–110.
21. Oh CS, Chung IH, Ji HJ, Yoon DM. Clinical implications of topographic anatomy on the ganglion impar. *Anesthesiology.* 2004;101:249–250.
22. Traub S, Glaser J, Manino B. Coccygectomy for the treatment of therapy-resistant coccygodynia. *J Surg Orthop Adv.* 2009;18:147–149.
23. Nittner K. Stimulation of conus-epiconus with pisces. Further indications. *Acta Neurochir Suppl (Wien).* 1980;30:311–316.
24. Haider N, Ali R. Coccygodynia treated with spinal cord stimulation: a case report. *Pain Med.* 2008;9:107.
25. Kothari S. Neuromodulatory approaches to chronic pelvic pain and coccygodynia. *Acta Neurochir Suppl.* 2007;97:365–371.

15 Discogenic Low Back Pain

Jan Willem Kallewaard, Michel A. M. B. Terheggen, Gerbrand J. Groen, Menno E. Sluijter, Richard Derby, Leonardo Kapural, Nagy Mekhail and Maarten van Kleef

Introduction

Each year, many people become disabled as a result of back complaints. Back pain is a multifactorial ailment. In approximately 45% of the cases, low back pain appears to be of discogenic origin.[1,2] The sacroiliac joint or the facet joints are indicated as the cause of the pain in 13% and 15% to 40% of the cases, respectively.[2] Furthermore, in clinical practice, often, more than one cause can be found simultaneously that might be held responsible for the patients' pain. Discogenic pain shares clinical signs with lumbosacral radicular pain characterized by radiating pain in one or more lumbar or sacral dermatomes with or without neurological deficits. Disk herniation in patients under the age of 50 and spine degeneration in older patients are often associated with chronic low back pain. The development of interventional techniques to treat discogenic pain has stimulated the refinement of diagnostic procedures with a high specificity and sensitivity, to confirm or refute the hypothesis that the patients' pain is primarily due to a painful internally disrupted discus intervertebralis.

Anatomy of the discus intervertebralis

The discus intervertebralis is composed of the nucleus pulposus (NP), the annulus fibrosus (AF), and the vertebral end-plates (VE). The corpora vertebrae lie above and below the disk. On the posterior side, the disk is supported by two facet joints. Together, the weightbearing joints provide support and stability, especially by limiting movement of the spine in all directions.[3] The healthy disk is avascular, and its nutrition depends on diffusion via the AF and the VE. The nucleus pulposus itself has no blood supply.

Nerve supply

The nerve supply of the discus intervertebralis is complex. The sensory innervation of the discus intervertebralis occurs via branches of the truncus sympathicus.[4] The dorsal circumference of the AF is innervated via branches of the nervi sinuvertebrales (or recurrentes meningei) (Figure 15.1), which stem from rami communicantes. The nervus sinuvertebralis runs ventral to the nerve root, back to the canalis spinalis, where the nerve splits into finer branches, which form nerve networks—one in the ligamentum longitudinale posterius (LLP) and the other in the ventral dura.[4] The nerve plexus is characterized by many left-right connections and many cranio-caudal connections. Ultimately, the posterior discus intervertebralis and corpus vertebrae are innervated via this nerve network in the LLP. The same accounts for the ventral dura. The ligamentum longitudinale anterius (LLA) also contains a network of nerves with many left-right and high-low connections of branching nerves. It is formed by branches from the trunci sympathici from both sides. The ventral and lateral sides of the discus intervertebralis are supplied by branches of the rami communicantes, direct branches of the truncus sympathicus, and by the LLA nerve plexus[4] (Figure 15.1).

Because many of the afferent fibers from the discus intervertebralis travel along with nervi sympathici, some investigators have sought to prove the disk has a sympathetic innervation and that both nerve networks consist of interconnected nerves with somatic and autonomic branches from various lumbar spinal nerves.[4] This assumption has been endorsed by Suseki et al.[5]

Evidence-Based Interventional Pain Medicine: According to Clinical Diagnoses, First Edition. Edited by Jan Van Zundert, Jacob Patijn, Craig T. Hartrick, Arno Lataster, Frank J.P.M Huygen, Nagy Mekhail, Maarten van Kleef.

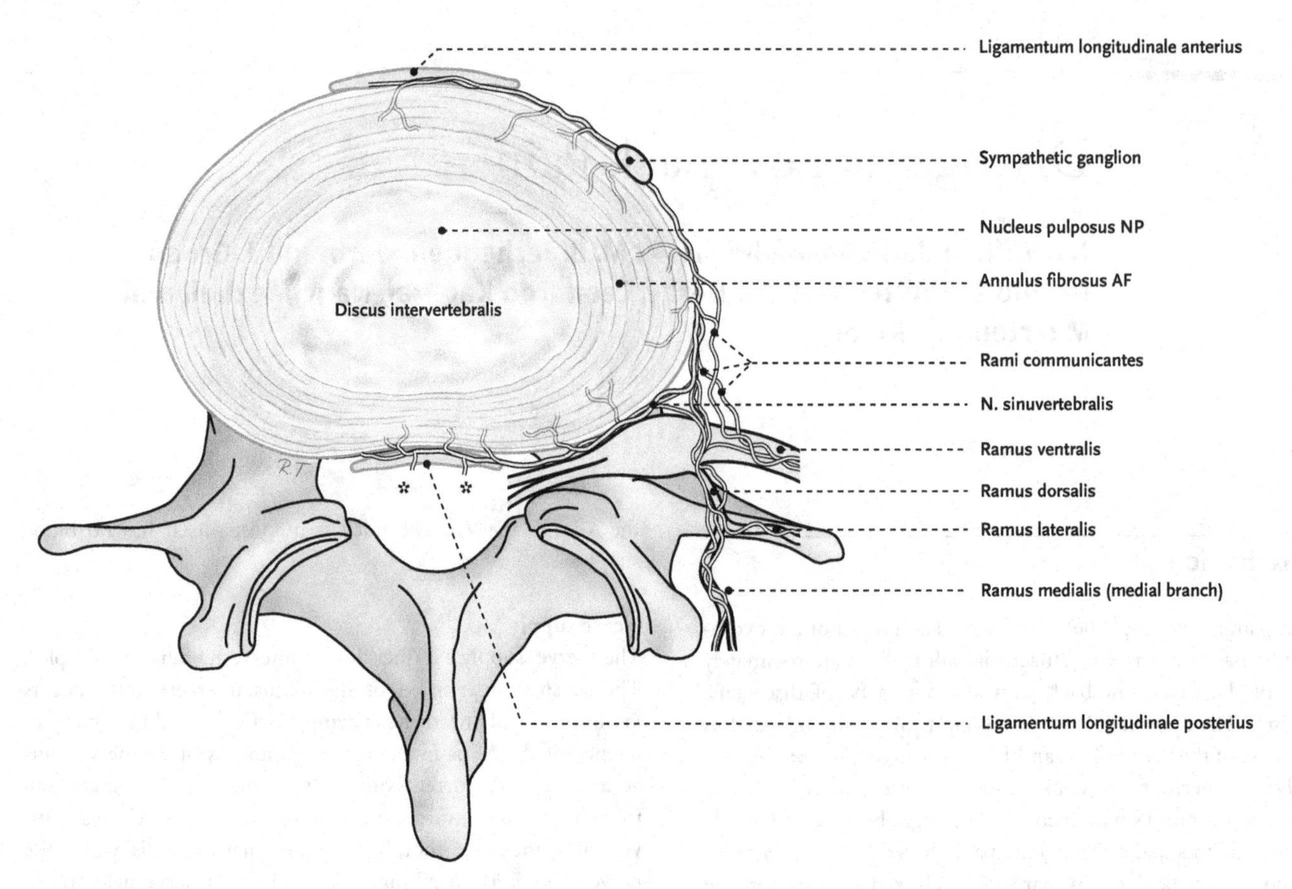

Figure 15.1. Schematic drawing of the lumbosacral innervation.[4] *Connections to the dural nerve plexus. Illustration: Rogier Trompert Medical Art. www.medical-art.nl.

and indirectly supported by a recent RCT showing pain relief following radiofrequency (RF) lesioning of the rami communicantes.[6]

Significance of this innervation pattern

The observation of left-right and cranio-caudal connections in these nerve plexuses further suggest that lateralized disorders, in which nociceptive stimuli reach the spinal cord via nervi sinuvertebrales from the other side, can cause pain at a side that is contralateral to its origin. This could explain why patients complain about pain on the left side at one time and another time about pain on the right. Another implication is that the majority of spinal structures, including the disci intervertebrales are innervated multisegmentally.[4] Via the mechanism of deep somatic referred pain, this innervations pattern leads to an overlap in distribution of referred pain areas from adjacent structures. As a result, the pain projections are not always reliable for determining the source of the pain.

Finally, if the human disci intervertebrales receive significant afferent fibers via sympathetic pathways, their cell bodies may be primarily located in the ganglia spinalia (dorsal root ganglia, DRGs) of C8-L2 nerves, i.e., the levels at which the sympathetic nerve fibers leave the spinal cord.[4] Although it has yet to be proven true, some researchers have utilized this hypothesis to obtain a specific block of the nervus spinalis L2 for low lumbar discogenic pain.[7]

Diagnosis

History

There are no specific characteristics in the patients' history that confirm or disprove the diagnosis of discogenic low back pain.[8] More typical features include persistent, nociceptive low back, groin and/or leg pain that worsens with axial loading and improves with recumbence. Patients may have experienced a prior episode of acute, intense pain caused by an acute tear in the innermost part of the AF (although no scientific proof of this exists).

Discogenic low back pain is often localized medially in the back, and more detailed referral patterns were reported by Ohnmeiss et al. during provocative discography.[9,10] Discogenic pain originating from the L3/L4 level typically radiates to the front (anterior) side of the thigh, L4/L5 to the outside (lateral) of the thigh, and sometimes to the back (posterior) of the thigh, and L5/S1 usually causes pain on the back of the thigh.

Physical examination

There are no typical characteristics of discogenic pain in the physical examination. Biphasic straightening from flexion is considered by some to be an indication of a disk complaint. Pain as a result of pressure on the processus spinosus is considered characteristic of discogenic low back pain ("Federung"). Vanharanta[11] has described pain radiating from the disk due to provocation with a tuning fork pressed on the processus spinosus of the affected segment. Although suggestive, these physical examination characteristics have not been validated, and the current criterion standard for confirming a clinical diagnosis of discogenic pain is a positive discogram and the demonstration of a Grade 3 AF tear.[12,13]

Additional tests

Imaging techniques such as CT and MRI are highly effective means of demonstrating detailed anatomical abnormalities in the vertebral column.[14,15] These imaging techniques are limited in that only an indication can be given for the cause of the pain. Recently, the presence of a high-intensity zone (HIZ) has been correlated with the presence of discogenic pain at that level. The HIZ may be an indication of an AF tear that extends to the outer third of the AF. The HIZ may be caused by the presence of inflammatory cytokines. Conflicting studies can also be found in the literature concerning this subject. On the one hand, a study done by Wolfer and Derby showed an 80% correlation between the HIZ and discogenic pain. Carragee, on the other hand, claims that this HIZ regularly occurs in asymptomatic control patients as well.[12,16] In spite of the regular appearance of conflicting literature, especially between Carragee's and Derby's groups, provocative discography remains the *gold standard* for the diagnosis of discogenic pain. Although MRI images are helpful in visualizing such pathology as disk degeneration and desiccation, HIZs, and loss of disk height, the results commonly correlate poorly with clinical findings, leaving open the critical question of causality. To date, provocation discography is the only available method of linking the morphologic abnormalities seen on MRI with clinically observed pain, and its predictive value has been repeatedly questioned, mainly as a result of reported false positive rates.

Pathophysiology of discogenic pain and discography

In the normal discus intervertebralis, sensory nerves innervate the outermost third of the AF. In the degenerated disk, this innervation is deeper and more widespread; some fibers even penetrate the NP.[17–24] By now, it is also an accepted fact that the discus can be a frequent and significant source of low back pain. Every discus has a NP that is surrounded by a fibrous structure, the AF. As a result of aging, an anomalous posture of the back, or injury, the discus intervertebralis can become weaker, and fissures and tears can arise in the AF (Figure 15.2). These tears can cause chronic pain if the tear in the AF extends to its outermost third.

Based on CT-discography studies, the AF tear is becoming more frequently implicated as the basis for discogenic pain. The emphasis lies more on the extent and the dimensions of the annular tear than on disk degeneration. Sachs et al.[25] developed the "Dallas Discogram Scale," a 4-point scale that specifies the degree of disk degeneration. Grade 0 indicates a disk in which the contrast agent remains entirely in the NP. Grades 1 through 3 indicate tears in which the contrast agent extends to the innermost, middle, and outermost sections, respectively, of the AF. Later, Grade 4 was added; the Grade 4 fissure has expanded into an arcshaped tear outside of or in the innermost ring of the AF (Figure 15.3).

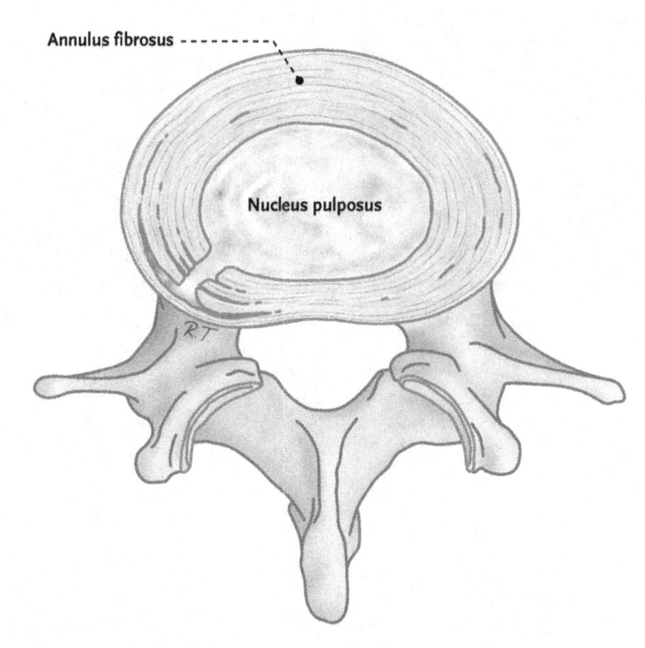

Figure 15.2. Discus intervertebralis with tears and fissures in the annulus fibrosus. Illustration: Rogier Trompert Medical Art. www.medical-art.nl.

Subsequently, Vanharanta[26] demonstrated the relationship between the expansion of the tear in the AF and pain reproduction during discography. Grades 0 and 1 are almost never painful. In Grade 3 annular ruptures, more than 75% of the discographies are accompanied with exact reproduction of concordant pain. On the other hand, it has been shown that in pain reproduction during discography, 77% of the disci intervertebrales have an internal morphology with a Grade 3 rupture. This concordant pain is also present very intermittently in Grade 2 ruptures.

Chemical changes

There are two types of chemical changes that occur in the degenerative disk. First, a fracture in the vertebral endplate can lead to the introduction of inflammatory cytokines in the NP. This inflammation response changes the delicate nutrient balance in the NP, resulting in diminished oxygen diffusion, increase in local lactate concentration, and decrease in pH inside the disk.

In some cases, the cytokines themselves can be the source of pain, and outer annular rupture may facilitate the "leakage" of

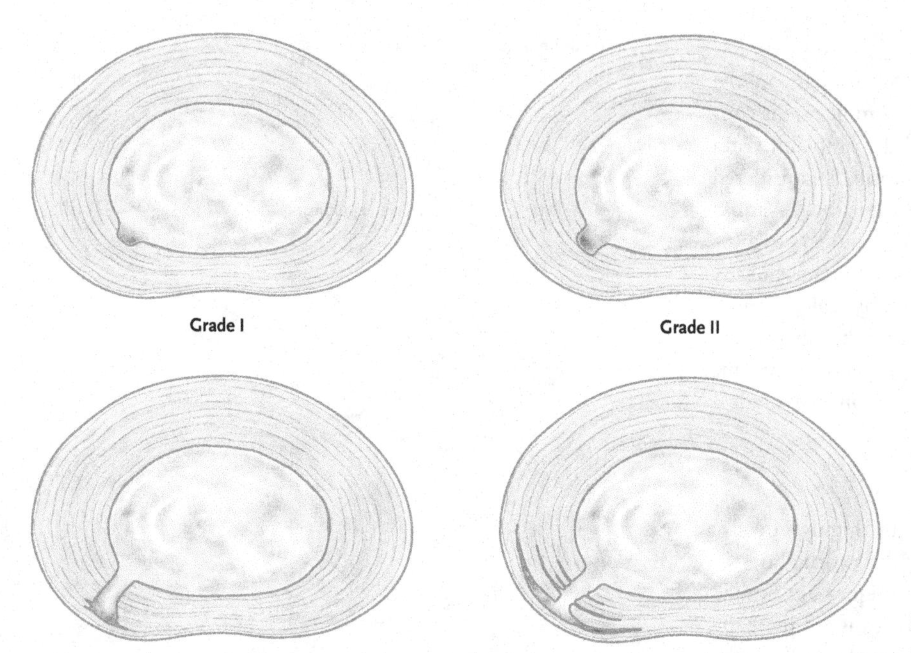

Figure 15.3. Gradation of the radial fissures visible on CT discography. Illustration: Rogier Trompert Medical Art. www.medical-art.nl.

these inflammatory mediators to the adjacent epidural structures such as the ligamentum longitudinale posterius, dura, and ganglion spinale (dorsal root ganglion, DRG). The ingrowth of nociceptors into the deeper layers of the disk may sensitize it to normal mechanical loads. In addition, irritation of the nerve endings in the VE can produce pain. All or some of these mechanisms may cause a "chemically or mechanically" sensitized disk.[26]

Lumbar discography

Definitions

Stimulation of a discus intervertebralis is a procedure that was developed for the purpose of confirming or refuting a clinical hypothesis of discogenic low back pain. The procedure is performed by inserting a needle in the NP of the target disk and injecting contrast agent (or another suitable medium) in order to test the sensitivity of the disk to gradually increasing distending pressures.

Disk stimulation is the more accurate name for a procedure that until now has often been described as (provocative) discography.

Discography is a procedure in which a contrast agent is introduced into the NP of a disk with the goal of describing the morphology of that disk.

Discography thus differs from disk stimulation—a procedure in which attention is focused on the reaction of the patient. Discus stimulation is usually followed by discography in order to verify the correct needle position or to elucidate the internal morphology of the disk. A combination of these definitions could be called provocative discography.

Patient selection

Suitable patients for this procedure are those with chronic low back pain, with or without pseudo-radicular referral, which lasts for longer than 3 months and which does not react to medication, transcutaneous electric nerve stimulation (TENS) and other conservative measures, and for which minimal invasive treatments of the facet joints and the sacroiliac joints do not prove to be effective or are not sufficiently effective. The implementation of the discography procedure is only advisable as a preparation for a possible interventional treatment aimed at reducing discogenic pain. An X-ray and an MRI of the lumbar spinal column must be performed not earlier than 6 months prior to the procedure.

Contraindications

Absolute

- absence of informed consent for discography (or other interventional treatments);
- local infection;
- pregnancy;
- local infection at injection site; and
- systemic infection

Relative

- allergy to contrast agent, local anesthetics, or antibiotics;
- known increased tendency to hemorrhage; and
- use of anticoagulants.

Procedure

Provocative discography is performed in the operating room under strict sterile conditions. Thirty minutes before the intervention, the patient is administered intravenous antibiotics (2 g cephazolin, i.v.). Many interventionalists also mix antibiotics within the intradiscally injected contrast at a concentration between 1 and 10 mg/mL (e.g., 3 mg/mL cephazolin). The administration of antibiotics for the prevention of a discitis is disputed.[27] In their review, Willems et al. indicate that the side effects of antibiotics (allergic reactions) are even greater than the potential benefits and advise against administering antibiotics.[27] Yet currently, international consensus exists to administer periprocedural antibiotics as part of the discography procedure. The most important condition for the prevention of a discitis is observance of strict sterile technique.

Position
In the operation room, the patient lies in the prone position on an X-ray permeable table.

Sterility
The skin of the low back and the gluteal region is thoroughly disinfected. The operator and the assistant must wash their hands according to the local protocol of the hospital, and must wear protective clothing (surgical caps, surgical jackets and sterile gloves). After the injection point has been marked, the patient is covered with a sterile drape. The same must be done with the C-arm. Due to the limited rotation of the C-arm, it must be located on the side of the patient where the needle will be inserted.

Level determination
The levels to be examined are chosen based on a combination of patient history, physical examination, and additional examinations. The symptomatic level and the two adjacent levels are examined. Heretofore, the one or two adjacent disci intervertebrales serve as control levels, although recent evidence[28] showing a ~20% increase in long-term degenerative changes on the side of needle puncture may preclude needle puncture of MRI normal-appearing disks for the sole purpose of a control level. Typically, the least degenerated or more likely asymptomatic levels are studied first. The patient should be blinded to the disk level and should not be aware of the start of the disk stimulation. The patient should preferably be only be lightly sedated during the procedure, but those on copious narcotics should be given a judicious dose so that there pain sensitivity is not exaggerated. The patient must be awake and able to reliably report during the disk stimulation.

The C-arm is first positioned with the direction of the radiation beam parallel to the subchondral plate of the lower vertebral plate of the disk. In the disks above L5-S1, the C-arm is then rotated ipsilaterally until the lateral aspect of the processus articularis overlies the axial middle of the disk to be punctured (Figure 15.4), and the disk height is at its maximum. In this projection, the needle can be inserted parallel to the direction of the radiation beam and brought into position (tunnel view). The target for the puncturing of the AF is the lateral-middle side of the disk, just lateral to the lateral edge of the processus articularis superior (Figure 15.5).

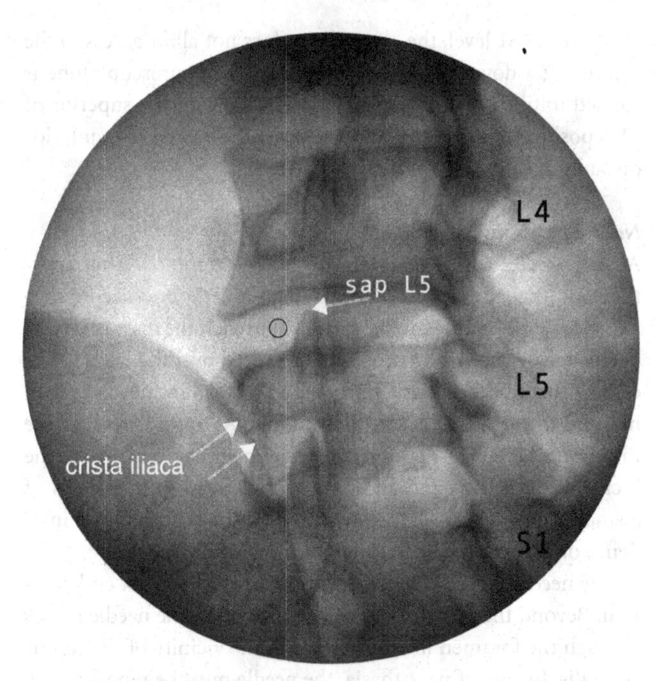

Figure 15.4. Starting point of the needle, assuming a maximal disk height, is such that the C-arm is rotated so that the facet column is between 1/3 and 1/2 of the corpus vertebrae. The injection point is then directly lateral to the processus articularis superior (superior articular process, sap).

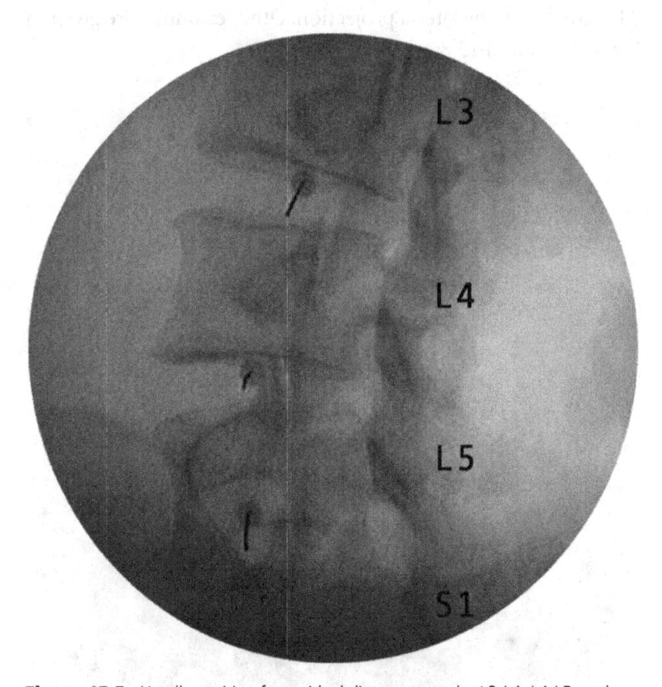

Figure 15.5. Needle position for an ideal discogram at the L3-L4, L4-L5, and L5-S1 levels.

At the L5-S1 level, the crista iliaca does not allow access to the disk using a down-the-beam approach. The fluoroscopy tube is rotated until the lateral edge of processus articularis superior of S1 is positioned approximately 25% over the posterior to anterior distance of the corpus vertebrae.

Needle positioning

A new needle is used for each disk to be examined. After anesthetizing the skin and the underlying tissue, a one-needle or a two-needle technique can be used to approach the disk. In a two-needle technique, a 20-G needle is advanced over the lateral edge of the processus articularis superior. A 25-G hollow needle is then inserted through this needle and into the AF until it reaches the middle of the NP. The two-needle technique may help reduce the incidence of discitis and allow entering the disk with needles of a small diameter (e.g., 27 G) which might help prevent the incidence of iatrogenic disk degeneration.[28]

The needle is carefully advanced to the needle-point end position. Beyond the processus articularis superior, the needle passes through the foramen intervertebrale in the vicinity of the ramus ventralis. In case of paresthesia, the needle must be repositioned. A strong resistance is felt as the needle passes through the AP. The needle is pushed through the AP to the center of the disk. The needle's progress is followed in various projections, first in AP and then in lateral projection (Figure 15.6). Ideally, after placement, the needle is situated in the middle of the disk's NP, as seen in the AP as well as in the lateral projection. Other examples are given in Figures 15.7 and 15.8.

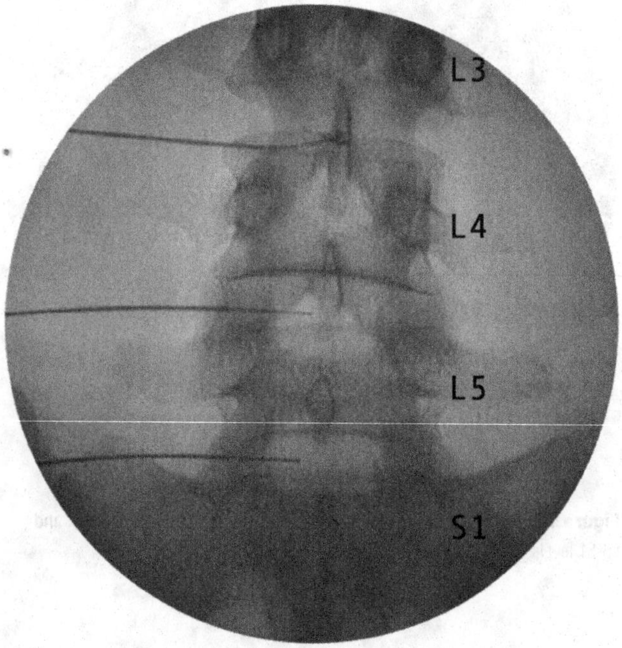

Figure 15.6. AP-position of the needles at discography in which the needles have been positioned in the middle of the nucleus pulposus.

Disk stimulation

After verification of the correct needle position, the stylet is removed from the needle and the needle is connected to a contrast agent delivery system which can measure the intradiscal pressure (manometry). The rate of infusion of the contrast agent should not exceed 0.05 mL/s.[29–31] This rate reflects a static flow that cor-

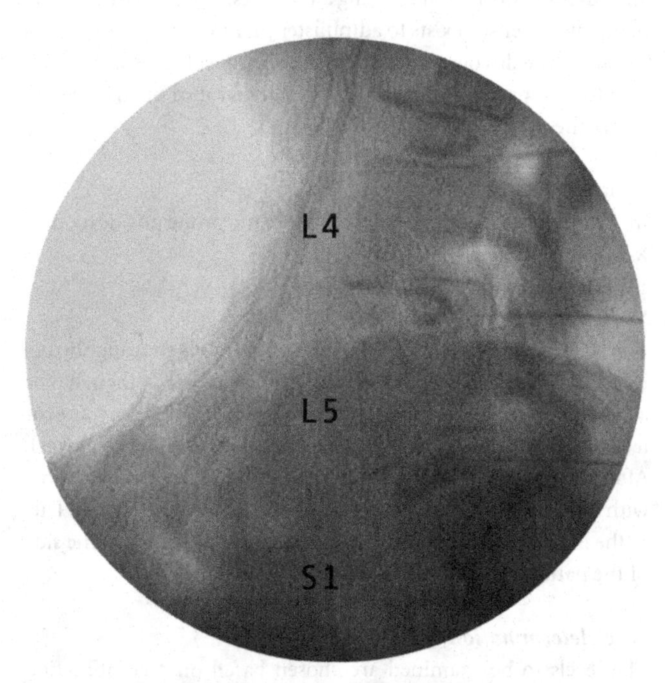

Figure 15.7. Discography at 3 levels where Grades 1 to 2 disks are visible at L3-L4 and L4-L5, and a disk with Grades 3 to 4 rupture is visible at level L5-S1.

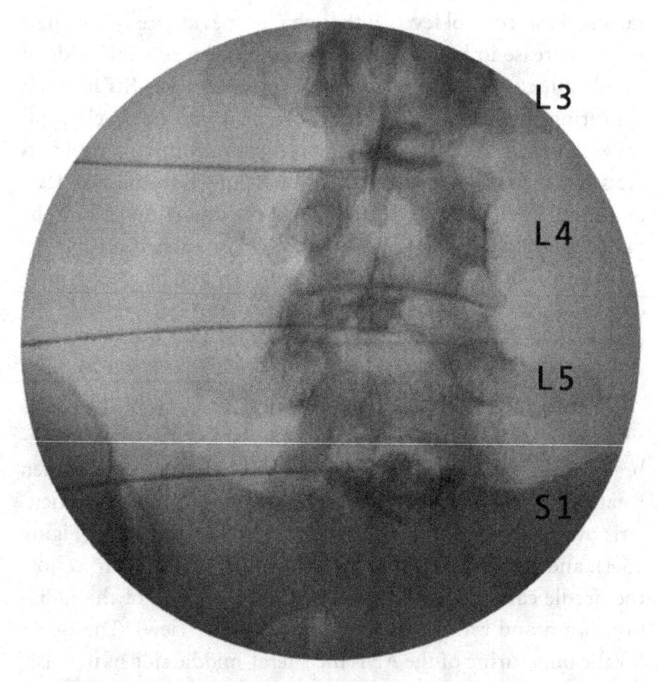

Figure 15.8. Discography at 3 levels: L3-L4, L4-L5 and L5-S1, all in anteroposterior view.

responds to the distension pressure in the discus intervertebralis. If a higher flow is used, false positive discographies can occur due to the resultant pressure peaks. Pain is often provoked by these pressure peaks due to vertebral end-plate compression and distention of the adjacent facet joint. It is important that the disk expected to be most painful is stimulated last; the patient must not be able to see which disk is being stimulated. If the painful disk is stimulated first, it is possible that the echo of that pain lasts long enough to make adequate stimulation at other levels no longer possible. If these conditions have been met, the stimulation can be started.

The following parameters must be carefully monitored during the injection of the contrast solution: the opening pressure (OP), the pressure at which contrast is first visible in the disk; the provocation pressure, the pressure greater than the opening pressure at which complaints of pain arise; and the peak pressure or the final pressure at the end of the procedure. Ideally, pressure, volume, and provocation details are recorded at 0.5 mL increments, with additional notation made for the aforementioned events.

The procedure, per level, is continued until the following events:

- Concordant pain is reproduced at a level of 7 or greater (on a 0 to 10 numeric rating scale; NRS), and subsequent injected volume confirms the response.
- The volume infused reaches the 3.0 mL. (Up to 4 mL may be injected into a very degenerated disk when pressures remain less than 15 psi.).
- The pressure rises to 50 psi above opening pressure in disks with a Grade 3 annular tear.
- If contrast leaks through the outer AF or through the endplates, one may not be able to pressurize the disk to a pressure sufficient to test the disk sensitivity. In these cases, the rapid manual injection may be acceptable, but must be noted and a negative response is a more defendable response.

Assessment criteria

The guidelines of the IASP (International Association for the Study of Pain), as well as those of the ISIS (International Spine Intervention Society), state that two levels must always be tested as controls when performing provocative discography (except if the target disk is that of L5-S1).[32–34] A disk is only considered to be provocative (positive) if concordant pain can be induced at the target level, and if the control levels were negative for provocation of pain.

Manometry: Overestimation of discogenic pain due to a false positive response to provocative discography is also possible. Asymptomatic disks, with overpressurization, may become painful because normally quiescent nociceptors and mechanoreceptors in the endplates and ligamenta longitudinales posteriores, and perhaps capsules of the facet joints, are stimulated. The diagnosis of discogenic pain can only be made if there is reproduction of concordant pain resulting from a pressure that does not produce pain in a normal disk or in an asymptomatic patient.

The concept and definition of a chemically sensitive disk was first described by Derby et al.[35] In 2004, O'Neill further described subgroups: disks with a pain threshold of 0 psi—these disks are described as chemically sensitive disks and[29] disks with a pain threshold of 1 psi or higher—these disks are considered to be pressure sensitive. Pain thresholds ≥50 psi above the opening pressure correlated with a 100% chance of a false positive discography, whereas pain thresholds between 25 and 50 psi above the opening pressure still lead to 50% false positive results. This chance of a false positive disk decreases to 14% in a pain-sensitive disk at 15 psi above opening pressure. The true pressure-sensitive disk probably has a pain threshold of 1–9 psi above opening pressure, or is considered a chemically sensitive disk (0 psi). The latter (chemically sensitive) disk intervertebralis is usually already extremely painful at the time of puncture. The classification of disks based on the pressure at which pain arises is illustrated in Table 15.1.

Morphologically, these disks are Grades 2 to 3 based on the Dallas Discogram Scale (Table 15.2). The international (IASP and ISIS) guidelines are based on these operational criteria:

1 Absolute discogenic pain:
   - Stimulation of target disk reproduces concordant pain.
   - The intensity of this pain has a Numeric Rating Scale (NRS) score of at least 7 on an 11-point scale.
   - The pain is reproduced by a pressure of less than 15 psi above the opening pressure.
   - Stimulation of the two adjacent disks is not painful.

2 Highly probable discogenic pain:
   - Stimulation of target disk reproduces concordant pain.
   - The intensity of this pain has a NRS score of at least 7 on an 11-point scale.
   - The pain is reproduced by a pressure of less than 15 psi above the opening pressure.

Table 15.1. Classification of disks on the basis of the pressure at which pain arises.

- Disks that are painful at a pressure lower than 15 psi above opening pressure
- Disks that are painful between 15 and 50 psi above opening pressure
- Disks that are painful at greater than 50 psi above opening pressure
- Disks that are not painful in spite of the fact that the pressure is higher than 50 psi above opening pressure

Table 15.2. Assessment of the morphology of the discus intervertebralis using discography.

Dallas Discogram Scale:

Grade 0: The contrast remains entirely in the nucleus pulposus.

Grades 1 through 3: Indicate tears in which the contrast agent extends to the innermost, middle, and outermost sections, respectively, of the annulus fibrosus.

Grade 4: Here the Grade 3 fissure has expanded into an arc-shaped tear, outside of or in the innermost ring of the annulus fibrosus.

- Stimulation of *one* of the adjacent disks is not painful.

3 Discogenic pain:
- Stimulation of target disk reproduces concordant pain.
- The intensity of this pain has a NRS score of at least 7 on an 11-point numerical scale.
- The pain is reproduced by a pressure of less than 50 psi above the opening pressure.
- Stimulation of the two adjacent disks is not painful.

4 Possible discogenic pain:
- Stimulation of target disk reproduces concordant pain.
- The intensity of this pain has a NRS score of at least 7 on an 11-point numerical scale.
- The pain is reproduced by a pressure of less than 50 psi above the opening pressure.
- Stimulation of *one* of the adjacent disks is not painful, and stimulation of another disk is painful at a pressure greater than 50 psi above the opening pressure, and the pain is discordant.

Given that a strict selection process will improve the outcome of minimally invasive and surgical treatments, the goal must be to strive toward criteria 1 and 2 for the purpose of concluding that 1 and/or 2 disks are actually positive.

During discography the distribution of the contrast agent is monitored via lateral and AP radiographic examination.

Postoperative care

After the discography, the patient goes to the ward or to the recovery room. The patient may be discharged if the pain is under control and there are no signs of loss of neurological function. The patient may experience worsening of the pain symptoms in the first postoperative days and should be prescribed pain-relieving medication. The patient should be instructed to contact the doctor immediately if she/he experiences an increase in symptoms, loss of neurological function, and/or fever.

Differential diagnosis

The differential diagnosis is first and foremost directed at ruling out *red flags*, such as trauma and fractures, infection, tumors, and neurological complications. Thereafter, one strives to rule out visceral pain. Before making a decision about the interventional treatment plan, it is important to demonstrate that the discus intervertebralis is the cause of the (pseudo-) radicular pain.

Treatment options

Conservative management

There are no known studies that have demonstrated that long-term antinociceptive medication has any significant positive effect in patients with discogenic low back pain. Generally, medication such as NSAIDs and weak opioids are recommended for a limited time (maximum of three months).[36] A systematic review found no evidence for the added value of active exercise therapy in relation to inactive treatment (bed rest) and other conservative treatments such as traction, manipulation, hot packs, or corsets.[37,38]

Interventional management

In the last few years, various minimally invasive treatments have been advanced to treat discogenic pain, such as intradiscal injections, IDET (intradiscal electrothermal therapy), disctrode, biacuplasty, intradiscal radiofrequency (RF) thermocoagulation, and RF treatment of the ramus communicans. Several small-scale prospective and anatomical studies have been published recently concerning the possible role of nucleoplasty in chronic discogenic low back pain. In spite of the fact that these minimally invasive treatments may be an effective alternative to surgical treatments, they remain experimental. The definitive value of these treatments must be determined in the coming years with randomized, controlled studies.

Intradiscal corticosteroid injections

The goal of intradiscal corticosteroid injections is the suppression of the inflammation that is considered to be responsible for discogenic pain. The literature on this topic is limited to case reports that only yield positive results. However, positive and negative results are been found in prospective studies. Butterman published in 2004 a prospective study comparing patients with degenerative disk disease (DDD) and end-plate inflammatory changes on MRI (Modic Type 1) with a patient group having DDD and no end-plate inflammatory changes. The group with Modic Type-1 changes had significantly better results after intradiscal steroid injection compared with the group without Modic Type-1 changes.[39]

In 1992, Simmons published a study in which 25 patients received 80 mg methylprednisolone intradiscally versus a control group to whom 1.5 mL bupivacaine (0.5%) was administered.[40] No significant difference was found between the two groups. Khot et al. published a comparable study of 12 patients in which, after positive discography, the patients were randomly divided into two groups.[41] In one group, intradiscal corticosteroids were administered, and in the control group, physiological saline solution was administered. The authors concluded that intradiscal corticosteroids do not improve clinical outcomes in patients with discogenic low back pain relative to placebo.[42] Intradiscal injections with other chemical substances are being investigated. Klein et al. published a pilot study in which a glucosamine and chondroitin sulfate solution combined with hypertonic dextrose and dimethyl sulfoxide (DMSO) were injected intradiscally.[43] It has been suggested that the injection of these substances synergistically promotes the hypermetabolic response of chondrocytes and retards the enzymatic degradation of cartilage. The authors reported positive results in the VAS score and in the "disability score". Derby et al. performed a comparable study in which he described effects analogous to those of IDET.[44] Given that this was only a pilot study, we must wait for RCTs to be able to make a judgment about the effect of these injections.

Intradiscal electrothermal therapy (IDET)

Saal and Saal published the first use of IDET for discogenic pain. The procedure consists of percutaneous insertion of a thermocoil into the disk under radiographic examination.[45] The catheter must be placed along the internal aspect of the posterior AF. The distal portion of the catheter (5 cm) is heated for 16 min to 90°C. Experimental veterinary studies have demonstrated that this will result in temperatures exceeding 60°C in the posterior AF and to a possible local denervation.

The first results were promising, with 50–70% of the patients experiencing significant pain reduction. Recent controlled studies are fueling much discussion about the actual effectiveness of this treatment.[46,47] Concerning this, it must be said that it is unclear whether the inclusion criteria of the patients was selective enough, and whether the discography was considered the most important method of selection in conformity with what has already been described in this chapter.

Pauza et al. performed a randomized, placebo-controlled prospective study of the effectiveness of IDET in the treatment of chronic discogenic low back pain.[48] His group screened 1,360 patients with low back pain; 64 of these patients were selected for study after positive discography results. Thirty-seven patients were randomized to the IDET group, and 27 patients to the sham group; the IDET catheter was inserted into the sham group, but without application of the RF current. Patients in both groups indicated improvement. In the IDET group, the average improvement in pain score, disability, and depression scale was significantly higher. Approximately 40% of the IDET group patients had an improvement of more than 50% in their pain scores. The NNT (number needed to treat) to reach more than 75% pain reduction was 5. These results suggest that the results of the IDET treatment cannot be completely ascribed to the placebo effect. These results also correspond with the results of various small-scale prospective study populations, which allow one to conclude that IDET can be effective in chronic, discogenic low back pain in a population selected with strict criteria. Pauza used the following inclusion criteria: age between 18 and 65 years, back pain more severe than leg pain, duration of pain symptoms at least 6 months, no improvement after a minimum of 6 weeks of conservative treatment (including medication, physical therapy, rehabilitation), back pain worsens with sitting and standing and is lessened by lying down, a score lower than 20 on the Beck Depression Inventory, no surgical interventions in the last 3 months, and less than 20% loss of disk height in the lumbar spine. In discography, the symptomatic level is indicated by way of negative control levels. A relative contraindication was obesity.

In 2006, Appelby et al. published a systematic review of the literature, and concluded that there was sufficient evidence for the effectiveness and safety of the IDET procedure.[49] Contrary to Appelby's report is that of Freeman et al.[49] This group took a very critical look at the existing literature, and came to the conclusion that the evidence for the effectiveness of the IDET procedure was weak and had a scientifically insufficient foundation. To date, a positive RCT, a negative RCT, various positive prospective studies, and two negative studies have been published. Notably, the fact that no more than two disks are degenerative is important. The outcomes in the cases with more extensive disk degeneration have been shown to be significantly worse. A serious limitation among the available IDET studies is that the selection criteria do not concur: a critical factor for achieving useful results. New studies with internationally defined inclusion criteria are needed in order to arrive at definitive judgments about the clinical effectiveness of the IDET procedure.

The mechanism by which IDET might act is not yet known. Two hypotheses have been proposed. The first hypothesis assumes that electrothermal therapy of the AF produces local pain reduction by way of denervation of the nociceptors. The second mechanism proposed states that changes occur in the structure of the collagen fibers in the AF due to heating; these changes improve the stability of the AF. As of yet, there is little histological proof to support this hypothesis.

The following are described as complications: catheter breakage, nerve injury (cauda equina lesion), post-IDET spinal disk herniation, discitis, local infection, epidural abscess.

Biacuplasty

Intradiscal biacuplasty is the latest in a series of minimally invasive posterior AF heating techniques. This technology works specifically by concentrating RF current between the ends of two straight probes. Relatively even heating over the larger area of the posterior AF is achieved by internally cooling the electrodes.[50,51]

The procedure is completed under fluoroscopy, with the patient lying in the prone position. Two TransDiscal 18 G electrodes via introducers are placed bilaterally in the posterior AF of the discus intervertebralis. The generator controls the delivery of RF energy by monitoring the temperature measured by a thermocouple at the tip of the probe. The temperature increases gradually over a period of 7–8 min to 50°C, with final heating at 50°C for another 7 min. It should be noted that although the temperature is set to 50°C on the RF generator, tissue temperature reaches 65°C due to ionic heating. During this time, the patient should be awake and able to communicate with the physician.

First, two pilot studies involving 8 and 15 patients demonstrated significant pain relief following the disk biacuplasty procedure at 3, 6, and 12 months.[52] In the European case series involving 8 patients, there was an average of about 50% pain reduction at 3 months, with overall good patient satisfaction. In the prospective pilot study involving 15 patients, Kapural et al. reported patient improvements in several pain assessment measures after undergoing disk biacuplasty procedure for discogenic pain.[52] Results from these pain assessment measures included a reduction in the median VAS pain score from 7 to 4 at 1 month, which remained at a level of 3 at 6 and 12 months follow-up, improvement in Oswestry index from 23.3 to 16.5 points at 1 month, which remained similarly improved after 12 months, and an increase in the SF-36 Bodily Pain score from 38 to 54 points.[52] Pilot studies and case series, even when designed as prospective trials, tend to exaggerate the positive outcomes. Therefore, we await results of sham controlled, prospective randomized studies before accepting or refuting this approach to the treatment of discogenic pain. Still, intradiscal biacuplasty may hold several advantages over previous techniques. There is minimal disruption to the native tissue architecture, and thus the biomechanics of the spine are likely unchanged. Additionally, the relative ease of electrode placement eliminates the need to thread a long-heating catheter (e.g., compared with IDET).

Intradiscal radiofrequency (RF) thermocoagulation

Intradiscal RF thermocoagulation is used for the treatment of discogenic pain. Barendse et al. performed a double-blind, randomized prospective study on 28 patients.[53] The discogenic pain diagnosis was made on the basis of the injection of a mixture of 2 mL lidocaine (2%) with contrast agent. Patients who indicated more than a 50% reduction in pain within 30 min were included and randomized into 2 groups. Patients in the RF group ($n = 13$) received an RF treatment of the discus intervertebralis lasting 70 s at 90°C in which the needle was placed in the center of the disk. Patients in the control group underwent the same procedure, except that no RF current was administered. Eight weeks after the treatment, there was no difference between the VAS scores of the two groups for pain and global perceived effect, or in the Oswestry Disability Index. The conclusion was that RF is ineffective for the treatment of discogenic pain. Two important remarks can be made about this study. First of all, the discography was not performed using a method that is currently accepted. It has subsequently become clear that discogenic pain is caused by nociceptors that are found in the outermost layer of the AF. Heating the center of the NP will not necessarily lead to the destruction of nociceptors in the AF.

Ercelen et al. performed another randomized prospective study with RF for discogenic pain using an improved selection and treatment method.[54] Ercelen's group selected 39 patients on the basis of a provocative discography. These patients were randomized into 2 groups. In the first group, the disk was heated for 360 s to 80°C; in the other group, for 120 s to 80°C. In this study, there were also no significant differences in pain reduction and functionality.

Recently a new intradiscal RF method has been introduced—discTRODE™ (Valleylab, Boulder, CO, U.S.A.). The DiscTrode is positioned along the posterior interface between the NP and the AF. In an open trial, Erdine et al.[55] found improvement of symptoms as measured by the SF-36 and the VAS score in 10 of 15 patients (66.6%). Finch et al. reported a case-control study of 46 patients with monodiscopathy with an annular tear confirmed by means of a provocative discography.[56] Thirty-one patients underwent the disk treatment with heat via the DiscTrode, and 15 patients functioned as control group. In the control group, conservative treatment was continued. The VAS score was significantly reduced in the RF group, and this reduction persisted for 12 months. In the control group, the VAS score did not change. The authors concluded that heating the AF, particularly at the level of the annular tear, can potentially be a good alternative for the treatment of discogenic pain. More recently, Kvarstein et al.[57] published a randomized controlled trial comparing intra-annular RF to sham treatment. The authors concluded that there was no beneficial effect of DiscTrode compared with the sham group. Another conclusion was the advice not to use the DiscTrode because of the high number of patients with increased pain in the treatment group.[57] However, the study of Kvarstein et al. was criticized for its lack of power and the fact that the study was terminated early.[58] This technology proved to be ineffective in improving functional capacity and VAS scores when compared with IDET during the study where strict patient selection criteria were employed.[59]

Ramus communicans block

Discogenic low back pain could be considered to be deep somatic pain, if viewed from its neural origin. However, the innervation of the disk shows a multisegmental origin. As described above, the sensory nerve fibers reach the spinal cord via adjacent and more distant rami communicantes and ganglia spinalia (dorsal root ganglia, DRGs) (Figure 15.1). Based on the work of Groen et al., Ohtori's group recently demonstrated that in rats the low lumbar disci intervertebrales are chiefly innervated by L1-L2 ganglia spinalia (DRGs) via the truncus sympathicus and the ramus communicans.[4,60] Fibers from the L3-L6 ganglia spinalia (DRGs) directly innervate the LLP via the nervi sinuvertebrales. Nakamura et al. looked at the afferent pathways that could be responsible for the discogenic low back pain by selectively blocking the L2 root in 33 patients.[7] On the basis of these findings, the authors concluded that the L2 segmental nerve could possibly be the most important afferent pathway for discogenic pain of the low lumbar disks, mainly by way of sympathetic afferent fibers of the nervi sinuvertebrales. Infiltration of the L2 root can then also be useful as a diagnostic procedure and as a therapy.

A block and destruction of the ramus communicans is also described as a treatment for discogenic low back pain or for pain in the vertebra itself.[61] Chandler et al. described the ramus communicans block as being an effective treatment for pain originating from a vertebral compression fracture.[62] Oh and Shim investigated the effectiveness of RF thermocoagulation of the ramus communicans in 49 patients.[5] These patients had chronic discogenic low back pain at 1 level, and had previously received no effect from an IDET treatment. Patients were randomized into an RF group and a control group. The control group received a lidocaine injection near the ramus communicans without RF. After 4 months, there was significant improvement in VAS scores and improvements in the Short Form (36) Health Survey (SF-36) in the RF group relative to the control group. The authors concluded that the RF thermocoagulation of the ramus communicans could be considered as one of the treatments for discogenic low back pain.

In spite of the promising initial results, further randomized studies of the effects of the ramus communicans block on discogenic pain are also needed in this case. A number of questions must still be answered. What is the definitive role of L1-L2 in discogenic low back pain; what is the role of the ramus communicans in this? Which patients react best to a ramus communicans block, and how long is this treatment effective?

Other interventional techniques

Although this overview is not complete, the following techniques have been used frequently in the past. In chemonucleolysis, the enzyme chymopapain is injected into the disk intervertebralis; as a result, the NP is dissolved. This therapy has been almost completely abandoned due to problems related to dosage reliability, difficulties with the supply of chymopapain, and a number of serious complications. Otherwise, the treatment appears to be effective as demonstrated by various RCTs.[63]

Automated percutaneous lumbar nucleotomy (APLD) is a technique in which a section of the NP is mechanically removed percutaneously in order to effect decompression of the NP. However, the technique has been proven to be less effective in comparison with other treatments, and is therefore not advised.[63] A more modern variant of percutaneous nucleotomy using the Dekompressor™ (Stryker Corp., Kalamazoo, MI, U.S.A.) is still being used; it has a smaller diameter than the original APLD apparatus. There is no evidence present in the literature for this technique, and until otherwise shown, it can be considered to be the same as the classic APLD. Percutaneous laser disk-decompression (PLDD) is a treatment method that has been utilized on a large-scale world-wide since the beginning of the 1990s. Laser heat is used to bring about the evaporation of nuclear material. Unfortunately, until now, only case series have been reported.[63] Currently, the following techniques are applied most often worldwide: Nucleoplasty® (Arthrocare, Stockholm, Sweden), Ozone Discolysis, Targeted DISC Decompression, and the aforementioned Dekompressor™.

Percutaneous intradiscal treatments for disk herniation

As previously mentioned in the introduction, there is a clear overlap of the clinical signs of discogenic lumbago and the symptoms of spinal disk herniation. Disk herniation usually leads to a combination of discogenic lumbago and radicular leg pain. There seems to be evidence of a complex interaction between biochemical factors originating from the NP of the discus intervertebralis and mechanical factors (nerve root compression), which together cause the pain. Also, see the chapter on radicular pain.[64]

The goal of epidural injection of steroids in cases of herniated discus is primarily anti-inflammatory and therefore pain lessening. The goal of this treatment is rapid reduction in pain symptoms compared with a conservative treatment. The treatment must be considered conservative during the natural course of the acute lumbosacral radicular syndrome, which is the result of a discus herniation. In the long term, there are no differences in outcome in comparison with conservative treatment without epidural injection of steroids.

The differences between conservative treatment and operative discectomy are also not demonstrated in the long term. Operative discectomy is nonetheless utilized on a large scale. The reason for this is that the intervention can often lead to a more rapid reduction in symptom complaints when compared with a conservative treatment policy.[63] The disadvantages are the operative and anesthesiological risks and the risk of epidural adhesions, which are associated with the so-called postlaminectomy syndrome, or the failed back-surgery syndrome. Otherwise, the indications for operative discectomy are larger discus protrusions and extrusions that show signs of nerve root compression on MRI. Smaller, focal protrusions without nerve root compression appear to be less apt to spontaneously resorb, and have a less favorable natural course; in other words, these small hernias often produce long-term pain symptoms with a slow spontaneous recovery.[65]

Over the years, the aforementioned considerations have led to various percutaneous, minimally invasive intradiscal techniques directed at the mechanical factor of disk herniation with the underlying idea of capitalizing on the advantages of operative therapy with as few of the disadvantages as possible. Most of these techniques—in contrast to the surgical discectomy— have the common goal of decompressing the NP so that there is a change in volume and an accompanying reduction in the pressure on the nerve and/or a lessening of the inflammatory reaction as a result. For these purposes, these techniques are usually only possible in the case of a so-called "contained" hernia.

Nucleoplasty

The decompression method utilizes "coblation," in which a high-energy plasma field is generated with the help of a bipolar RF probe. This plasma field breaks molecular bonds. For this reason, the technique is also called plasma disk decompression (PDD). Tissue can be evaporated in this way at relatively low temperatures (40 to 70°C). However, the plasma field can only arise in conductive surroundings. In practice, this means that the treatment is not effective in a dehydrated disk ("black disk" on MRI). After a 16-G needle has been positioned in the NP, the probe is moved back and forth and rotated intradiscally. In this way, 6 or more tunnels are made in the NP, and the intradiscal pressure drops. Meanwhile, the treatment has been utilized on a large scale, and the complication level appears to be low and acceptable.[66–68]

Percutaneous disk decompression using dekompressor™

The percutaneous disk decompression (Dekompressor™) technology extracts nuclear disk material by an auger within a cannula that ends inside the NP. A significant change in intradiscal pressure should follow the reduction of nuclear volume within the closed hydraulic space. It is imperative that the annular wall should be intact in order to retract the bulging section. Therefore provocative discography may occasionally be needed to confirm the affected level and to rule out any annular disruption. In their case series, Alo and colleagues reported an 80% success rate with this technique.[69] Although there are no controlled studies published on Dekompressor efficacy, a European study reported also pain score improvements in the majority of patients treated with Dekompressor. This seems to suggest that patients with posterolateral foraminal discus protrusions can typically expect more pain relief than those with posteromedian ones.[70] There are no randomized, sham studies on percutaneous discectomy using Dekompressor device.

Ozone discolysis

Ozone discolysis consists of the injection of a mixture of O_3 and O_2, usually both intradiscally, as well as epidurally. As a result, an oxidative dehydration takes place in the NP; this is comparable with chemonucleolysis by means of chymopapain. In addition, upregulation of the intracellular antioxidant scavenger system occurs due to oxidative stress; this results in an increase in the endogenous anti-inflammatory response.[71] In addition to various large case series with remarkably good results, two comparative studies have been published.[72,73] In Gallucci's study, intradiscal and transforaminal epidural corticosteroid injection is compared with intradiscal transforaminal epidural steroid injection with the addition of an O_3/O_2 mixture.[74] Bonnetti et al. had already published a comparative study examining transforaminal epidural injection of an O_3/O_2 mixture versus transforaminal epidural steroid injection.[75] In both studies, ozone resulted in a significantly better effect than corticosteroids. There are no significant complications of the technique described. Ozone discolysis can be utilized for "contained," as well as for "noncontained" spinal disk herniation. The extent to which the degree of disk degeneration has an influence on the clinical result is not yet clear. Although the technique is primarily meant for spinal disk herniation with prominent radicular pain, it is also utilized for discogenic lumbago associated with spinal disk herniation.

Targeted Disk Decompression (TDD)

This technique stems from the IDET technique for discogenic lumbago. In connection with the IDET technique, there have been some reports of unintentional shrinking of the size of disk protrusions as an effect of the technique. TDD makes use of just this property. The catheter used has approximately the same configuration as an IDET catheter; however, the active zone, where coagulation of disk tissue occurs, is markedly shorter. The goal is to position the active zone on the AF-NP boundary at the point of the "contained" protrusion. Given that this technique is a thermocoagulation, the degree of hydration of the NP is, in principle, not important. Although the technique is increasingly utilized and appears to provide good results, no literature has as yet been published about TDD.

Evidence for new developments

The techniques described in new developments above are currently being investigated for effectiveness and complications. At this time, it does not appear to be possible to formulate an evidence rating and recommendations.

Complications of interventional management

Although all these procedures are associated with minimal tissue damage, a short recovery time, and low infection risk, various rare complications have been reported such as catheter breakage, nerve root injuries, post-IDET disk herniation, discitis, radicular pain, severe headache, cauda equina syndrome, and vertebral body osteonecrosis.[57] The most important complication of minimally invasive intradiscal procedures is discitis. The incidence is very low at 0.25% to 0.7%.[27,76] Any patient who complains about increased pain within 1 week after the procedure must be carefully examined. At the very minimum, this examination must include patient history, physical examination, and laboratory examination (infection parameters). If the infection parameters are elevated or abnormal, or in case of doubt, an MRI must be performed in order to rule out discitis.

Staphylococcus aureus is the major cause of discitis. The chance of discitis can be reduced by the routine prophylactic use of intravenous or intradiscal antibiotics. Sharma et al. reviewed the literature and described that the chance of discitis is reduced from 2.7% to 0.7% with the use of the "through the needle technique"; in this technique, the needle is advanced through the skin until the AP is reached, and another thin needle (25 G) is then advanced through the first needle into the disk.[76] Willems published a 0.25% incidence of discitis in a series of 4,981 patients on which the "through the needle" technique was used and to whom no prophylactic antibiotic were administered.[27] They also concluded that the routine use of antibiotics is not necessary for this procedure. However, the international guidelines currently prescribe routine use of periprocedural prophylactic antibiotics.

Evidence for interventional management

A summary of the available evidence is given in Table 15.3.

Recommendations

Intradiscal corticosteroid injections and RF treatment of the disks are not advised for patients with discogenic low back pain. The current body of evidence does not provide sufficient proof to recommend intradiscal treatments, such as IDET and biacuplasty for chronic, nonspecific low back complaints originating from the discus intervertebralis. We are also of the opinion that at this time the only place for intradiscal treatments for chronic low back pain is in a research setting. RF treatment of the ramus communicans is recommended.

Clinical practice algorithm

Figure 15.9 illustrates the practice algorithm for the management of low back pain of discogenic origin.

Table 15.3. Summary of evidence of interventional pain management of discogenic pain.

Technique	Assessment
Intradiscal corticosteroid administration	2 B–
Radiofrequency (RF) treatment of the discus intervertebralis	2 B–
IDET (intradiscal electrothermal therapy)	2 B±
Biacuplasty	0
Disctrode	0
Radiofrequency (RF) of the ramus communicans	2 B+

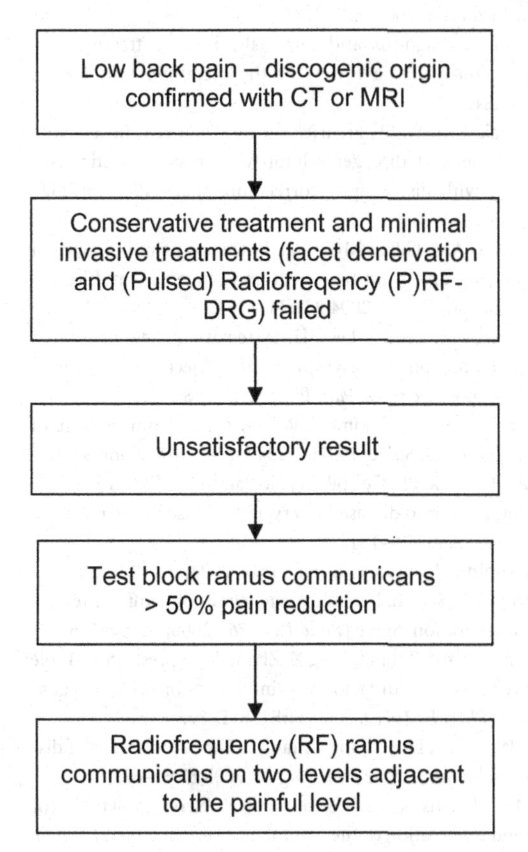

Figure 15.9. Clinical practice algorithm for the interventional management of discogenic pain.

Techniques

IDET

The procedure takes place under sterile OR conditions on a patient lying in the prone position with the aid of radiographic examination. While administering prophylactic antibiotics, a 17 G needle is inserted posterolaterally into the disk, generally on the side with the least complaints. Thereafter, a 30 cm-long catheter with a flexible tip, 5 cm of which can be heated, is advanced through the needle. This tip is advanced circumferentially through the NP until it covers the entire posterior section of the AF. After placement of the tip has been checked radiographically, the tip of the catheter is heated for 18 min to 90°C according to a standard protocol. This temperature is reached after 14 min and is then maintained for 4 min at this level. Then the needle and the catheter are removed, and the patient can be discharged after the recovery period. If during the procedure, the patient complains of leg pain, it is possible that a spinal nerve is being irritated. In this case, the heating process should be immediately terminated. After the procedure, the patient must follow a strict 12-week long rehabilitation protocol. In patients with a large tear in the AF, it may appear to be impossible to maneuver the catheter into the correct position.

Ramus Communicans

Diagnostic block

The C-arm is positioned in such a way that the direction of the radiation beam in the transverse plane is approximately 20° oblique such that the facet joints are projected away and the vertebral column is clearly visible. For the angle in the sagittal plane, the C-arm is rotated on its axis. As a result, the processus transversus changes location relative to the corpus vertebrae. The direction of the radiation beam must be such that the axis of the processus transversus lies slightly above the middle of the corpus vertebrae. Usually, an SMK-C15 cannula (Radionics, Burlington, MA, U.S.A.) is used for this procedure. An injection point is marked just caudally to the processus transversus, and somewhat medially to the lateral edge of the corpus vertebrae. After local anesthetization of the skin, the needle is advanced using a tunnel view, for which the general rules of this technique must be observed; in other words, corrections to the direction of the needle must be made while the needle is in the superficial layers, and the depth of the needle must be checked regularly on the lateral projection. Do not try to make contact with the processus transversus. The needle is advanced until contact is made with the corpus vertebrae. On the lateral projection, the point of the needle lies somewhat ventral to the posterior side of the corpus vertebrae. Contrast agent (0.5 mL) is then injected. On the anteroposterior projection, this usually results in a very compact shadow; on the lateral projection, the contrast agent spreads anteriorly over the corpus vertebrae. In case of intravascular dispersal, a minimal change in position is usually sufficient. Finally, 1 mL lidocaine (2%) is injected.

RF treatment

An SMK-C15 cannula with a 2 mm active point is used. Fluoroscopy and the insertion of the needle conform completely with the technique described for the diagnostic block. When the needle has been correctly positioned, stimulation at 50 Hz causes sensations in the back at a voltage of <1.5 V. Thereafter, 2 Hz stimulation is applied. Contractions of the leg muscles may not be allowed to occur at below twice the value of the sensory threshold. If these conditions are not met, then the needle is moved slightly laterally and anteriorly until a safe position has been achieved. A RF treatment is made for 60 s at 80°C.

The L5 level

This level deserves special mention since the anatomical relationships can require an adapted technique. This can be the result of a high crista iliaca or of a broad processus transversus. In these cases, the L5 segmental nerve exits the foramen intervertebrale more horizontally than the other lumbar nerves do. While adjusting the C-arm axially, it is best to project the processus transversus as high as possible. By doing so, a safe needle position can often be found for this level. Nevertheless, the intervention at this level is not possible in all cases.

Summary

Lumbar discography, provocative discography, and disk manometry are all examinations whose goal is to determine whether a discus intervertebralis is the cause of patients' pain symptoms. In spite of the unceasing stream of contradictory literature, provocative discography remains the gold standard for the determination of the diagnosis of discogenic pain. For the purpose of improving the results of minimally invasive intradiscal treatments, it is important to use a strict selection process to select discography patients' and to perform discography with manometry. It must be noted that the studies performed up to now have not included patients selected in the correct manner generally, and in particular by not adequately performing discography. This has certainly not had a positive influence on the results. For the treatment of discogenic pain, a RF treatment of the ramus communicans can be recommended.

References

1. Kuslich SD, Ulstrom CL, Michael CJ. The tissue origin of low back pain and sciatica: a report of pain response to tissue stimulation during operations on the lumbar spine using local anesthesia. *Orthop Clin North Am.* 1991;22:181–187.
2. Schwarzer AC, Aprill CN, Derby R, Fortin J, Kine G, Bogduk N. The relative contributions of the disc and zygapophyseal joint in chronic low back pain. *Spine.* 1994;19:801–806.
3. Cohen SP, Larkin TM, Barna SA, Palmer WE, Hecht AC, Stojanovic MP. Lumbar discography: a comprehensive review of outcome studies, diagnostic accuracy, and principles. *Reg Anesth Pain Med.* 2005;30:163–183.
4. Groen GJ, Baljet B, Drukker J. Nerves and nerve plexuses of the human vertebral column. *Am J Anat.* 1990;188:282–296.
5. Suseki K, Takahashi Y, Takahashi K, Chiba T, Yamagata M, Moriya H. Sensory nerve fibres from lumbar intervertebral discs pass through rami communicantes. A possible pathway for discogenic low back pain. *J Bone Joint Surg Br.* 1998;80:737–742.
6. Oh WS, Shim JC. A randomized controlled trial of radiofrequency denervation of the ramus communicans nerve for chronic discogenic low back pain. *Clin J Pain.* 2004;20:55–60.
7. Nakamura SI, Takahashi K, Takahashi Y, Yamagata M, Moriya H. The afferent pathways of discogenic low-back pain. Evaluation of L2 spinal nerve infiltration. *J Bone Joint Surg Br.* 1996;78:606–612.
8. Schwarzer AC, Aprill CN, Derby R, Fortin J, Kine G, Bogduk N. The prevalence and clinical features of internal disc disruption in patients with chronic low back pain. *Spine.* 1995;20:1878–1883.
9. Ohnmeiss DD, Vanharanta H, Ekholm J. Relation between pain location and disc pathology: a study of pain drawings and CT/discography. *Clin J Pain.* 1999;15:210–217.
10. Ohnmeiss DD, Vanharanta H, Ekholm J. Relationship of pain drawings to invasive tests assessing intervertebral disc pathology. *Eur Spine J.* 1999;8:126–131.
11. Vanharanta H. The intervertebral disc: a biologically active tissue challenging therapy. *Ann Med.* 1994;26:395–399.
12. Carragee EJ, Hannibal M. Diagnostic evaluation of low back pain. *Orthop Clin North Am.* 2004;35:7–16.
13. Zhou Y, Abdi S. Diagnosis and minimally invasive treatment of lumbar discogenic pain—a review of the literature. *Clin J Pain.* 2006;22:468–481.
14. Ito M, Incorvaia KM, Yu SF, Fredrickson BE, Yuan HA, Rosenbaum AE. Predictive signs of discogenic lumbar pain on magnetic resonance imaging with discography correlation. *Spine.* 1998;23:1252–1258; discussion 9–60.
15. Gilbert FJ, Grant AM, Gillan MG, et al. Low back pain: influence of early MR imaging or CT on treatment and outcome—multicenter randomized trial. *Radiology.* 2004;231:343–351.
16. Wolfer LR, Derby R, Lee JE, Lee SH. Systematic review of lumbar provocation discography in asymptomatic subjects with a meta-analysis of false-positive rates. *Pain Physician.* 2008;11:513–538.
17. Coppes MH, Marani E, Thomeer RT, Groen GJ. Innervation of "painful" lumbar discs. *Spine.* 1997;22:2342–2349; discussion 9–50.
18. Freemont AJ, Peacock TE, Goupille P, Hoyland JA, O'Brien J, Jayson MI. Nerve ingrowth into diseased intervertebral disc in chronic back pain. *Lancet.* 1997;350:178–181.
19. Hurri H, Karppinen J. Discogenic pain. *Pain.* 2004;112:225–228.
20. Peng B, Hao J, Hou S, et al. Possible pathogenesis of painful intervertebral disc degeneration. *Spine (Phila Pa 1976).* 2006;31:560–566.
21. Peng B, Chen J, Kuang Z, Li D, Pang X, Zhang X. Expression and role of connective tissue growth factor in painful disc fibrosis and degeneration. *Spine (Phila Pa 1976).* 2009;34:E178–E182.
22. Peng B, Wu W, Hou S, Li P, Zhang C, Yang Y. The pathogenesis of discogenic low back pain. *J Bone Joint Surg Br.* 2005;87:62–67.
23. Freemont AJ, Watkins A, Le Maitre C, et al. Nerve growth factor expression and innervation of the painful intervertebral disc. *J Pathol.* 2002;197:286–292.
24. Freemont AJ. The cellular pathobiology of the degenerate intervertebral disc and discogenic back pain. *Rheumatology (Oxford).* 2009;48:5–10.
25. Sachs BL, Vanharanta H, Spivey MA, et al. Dallas discogram description. A new classification of CT/discography in low-back disorders. *Spine.* 1987;12:287–294.
26. Vanharanta H, Sachs BL, Spivey MA, et al. The relationship of pain provocation to lumbar disc deterioration as seen by CT/discography. *Spine.* 1987;12:295–298.
27. Willems PC, Jacobs W, Duinkerke ES, De Kleuver M. Lumbar discography: should we use prophylactic antibiotics? A study of 435 consecutive discograms and a systematic review of the literature. *J Spinal Disord Tech.* 2004;17:243–247.
28. Carragee EJ, Don AS, Hurwitz EL, Cuellar JM, Carrino J, Herzog R. Does discography cause accelerated progression of degeneration changes in the lumbar disc: a ten-year matched cohort study. *Spine (Phila Pa 1976).* 2009;34:2338–2345.

29. O'Neill C, Kurgansky M. Subgroups of positive discs on discography. *Spine.* 2004;29:2134–2139.
30. Seo KS, Derby R, Date ES, Lee SH, Kim BJ, Lee CH. In vitro measurement of pressure differences using manometry at various injection speeds during discography. *Spine J.* 2007;7:68–73.
31. Shin DA, Kim SH, Han IB, Rhim SC, Kim HI. Factors influencing manometric pressure during pressure-controlled discography. *Spine (Phila Pa 1976).* 2009;34:E790–E793.
32. Bogduk N. Provocation discography: lumbar disc stimulation. In: ISIS, ed. *Practice Guidelines for Spinal Diagnostic and Treatment Procedures.* Seattle, WA: International Spine Intervention Society; 2004:20–46.
33. Merskey H, Bogduk N. *Classification of Chronic Pain: Descriptions of Chronic Pain Syndromes and Definitions of Pain Terms.* 2nd ed. Seattle, WA: IASP Press; 1994.
34. Saboeiro GR. Lumbar discography. *Radiol Clin North Am.* 2009;47:421–433.
35. Derby R, Howard MW, Grant JM, Lettice JJ, Van Peteghem PK, Ryan DP. The ability of pressure-controlled discography to predict surgical and nonsurgical outcomes. *Spine.* 1999;24:364–371; discussion 71–72.
36. Koes BW, van Tulder MW, Peul WC. Diagnosis and treatment of sciatica. *BMJ.* 2007;334:1313–1317.
37. Luijsterburg PA, Verhagen AP, Ostelo RW, et al. Physical therapy plus general practitioners' care versus general practitioners' care alone for sciatica: a randomised clinical trial with a 12-month follow-up. *Eur Spine J.* 2008;17:509–517.
38. Luijsterburg PA, Verhagen AP, Ostelo RW, van Os TA, Peul WC, Koes BW. Effectiveness of conservative treatments for the lumbosacral radicular syndrome: a systematic review. *Eur Spine J.* 2007;16: 881–899.
39. Buttermann GR. The effect of spinal steroid injections for degenerative disc disease. *Spine J.* 2004;4:495–505.
40. Simmons JW, McMillin JN, Emery SF, Kimmich SJ. Intradiscal steroids. A prospective double-blind clinical trial. *Spine.* 1992;17:S172–S175.
41. Khot A, Bowditch M, Powell J, Sharp D. The use of intradiscal steroid therapy for lumbar spinal discogenic pain: a randomized controlled trial. *Spine.* 2004;29:833–836; discussion 7.
42. Muzin S, Isaac Z, Walker J 3rd. The role of intradiscal steroids in the treatment of discogenic low back pain. *Curr Rev Musculoskelet Med.* 2008;1:103–107.
43. Klein RG, Eek BC, O'Neill CW, Elin C, Mooney V, Derby RR. Biochemical injection treatment for discogenic low back pain: a pilot study. *Spine J.* 2003;3:220–226.
44. Derby R, Eek B, Lee SH, Seo KS, Kim BJ. Comparison of intradiscal restorative injections and intradiscal electrothermal treatment (IDET) in the treatment of low back pain. *Pain Physician.* 2004;7: 63–66.
45. Saal JA, Saal JS. Intradiscal electrothermal treatment for chronic discogenic low back pain: a prospective outcome study with minimum 1-year follow-up. *Spine.* 2000;25:2622–2627.
46. Freeman BJ. IDET: a critical appraisal of the evidence. *Eur Spine J.* 2006;15(suppl 3):S448–S457.
47. Urrutia G, Kovacs F, Nishishinya MB, Olabe J. Percutaneous thermocoagulation intradiscal techniques for discogenic low back pain. *Spine.* 2007;32:1146–1154.
48. Pauza KJ, Howell S, Dreyfuss P, Peloza JH, Dawson K, Bogduk N. A randomized, placebo-controlled trial of intradiscal electrothermal therapy for the treatment of discogenic low back pain. *Spine J.* 2004;4:27–35.
49. Appleby D, Andersson G, Totta M. Meta-analysis of the efficacy and safety of intradiscal electrothermal therapy (IDET). *Pain Med.* 2006;7:308–316.
50. Kapural L, Mekhail N, Hicks D, et al. Histological changes and temperature distribution studies of a novel bipolar radiofrequency heating system in degenerated and nondegenerated human cadaver lumbar discs. *Pain Med.* 2008;9:68–75.
51. Pauza K. Cadaveric intervertebral disc temperature mapping during disc biacuplasty. *Pain Physician.* 2008;11:669–676.
52. Kapural L, Nageeb F, Kapural M, Cata JP, Narouze S, Mekhail N. Cooled radiofrequency system for the treatment of chronic pain from sacroiliitis: the first case-series. *Pain Pract.* 2008;8:348–354.
53. Barendse GA, van Den Berg SG, Kessels AH, Weber WE, van Kleef M. Randomized controlled trial of percutaneous intradiscal radiofrequency thermocoagulation for chronic discogenic back pain: lack of effect from a 90-second 70°C lesion. *Spine.* 2001;26: 287–292.
54. Ercelen O, Bulutcu E, Oktenoglu T, et al. Radiofrequency lesioning using two different time modalities for the treatment of lumbar discogenic pain: a randomized trial. *Spine.* 2003;28:1922–1927.
55. Erdine S, Yucel A, Celik M. Percutaneous annuloplasty in the treatment of discogenic pain: retrospective evaluation of one year follow-up. *Agriculture* 2004;16:41–47.
56. Finch PM, Price LM, Drummond PD. Radiofrequency heating of painful annular disruptions: one-year outcomes. *J Spinal Disord Tech.* 2005;18:6–13.
57. Kvarstein G, Mawe L, Indahl A, et al. A randomized double-blind controlled trial of intra-annular radiofrequency thermal disc therapy—a 12-month follow-up. *Pain.* 2009;145:279–286.
58. van Kleef M, Kessels AG. Underpowered clinical trials: time for a change. *Pain.* 2009;145:265–266.
59. Kapural L, Hayek S, Malak O, Arrigain S, Mekhail N. Intradiscal thermal annuloplasty versus intradiscal radiofrequency ablation for the treatment of discogenic pain: a prospective matched control trial. *Pain Med.* 2005;6:425–431.
60. Ohtori S, Takahashi K, Chiba T, Yamagata M, Sameda H, Moriya H. Sensory innervation of the dorsal portion of the lumbar intervertebral discs in rats. *Spine.* 2001;26:946–950.
61. Sluijter ME. Radiofrequency lesions of the communicating ramus in the treatment of low back pain. In: Raj PP, ed. *Current Management of Pain.* Philadelphia: Kluwer Academic publishers; 1989: 145–159.
62. Chandler G, Dalley G, Hemmer J, Jr, Seely T. Gray ramus communicans nerve block: novel treatment approach for painful osteoporotic vertebral compression fracture. *South Med J.* 2001;94:387–393.
63. Gibson JN, Waddell G. Surgical interventions for lumbar disc prolapse: updated Cochrane Review. *Spine.* 2007;32:1735–1747.
64. Van Boxem K, Cheng J, Patijn J, van Kleef M, Lataster A, Mekhail N, Van Zundert J. 11. Lumbosacral radicular pain. *Pain Pract.* 2010;10:339–358.
65. Jensen TS, Albert HB, Soerensen JS, Manniche C, Leboeuf-Yde C. Natural course of disc morphology in patients with sciatica: an MRI study using a standardized qualitative classification system. *Spine.* 2006;31:1605–1612; discussion 13.
66. Boswell MV, Trescot AM, Datta S, et al. Interventional techniques: evidence-based practice guidelines in the management of chronic spinal pain. *Pain Physician.* 2007;10:7–111.

67. Al-Zain F, Lemcke J, Killeen T, Meier U, Eisenschenk A. Minimally invasive spinal surgery using nucleoplasty: a 1-year follow-up study. *Acta Neurochir (Wien)*. 2008;150:1257–1262.
68. Manchikanti L, Derby R, Benyamin RM, Helm S, Hirsch JA. A systematic review of mechanical lumbar disc decompression with nucleoplasty. *Pain Physician.* 2009;12:561–572.
69. Alo KM, Wright RE, Sutcliffe J, Brandt SA. Percutaneous lumbar discectomy: clinical response in an initial cohort of fifty consecutive patients with chronic radicular pain. *Pain Pract.* 2004; 4:19–29.
70. Amoretti N, David P, Grimaud A, et al. Clinical follow-up of 50 patients treated by percutaneous lumbar discectomy. *Clin Imaging.* 2006;30:242–244.
71. Bocci V. Ozone as a bioregulator. Pharmacology and toxicology of ozonetherapy today. *J Biol Regul Homeost Agents.* 1996;10:31–53.
72. Buric J, Molino Lova R. Ozone chemonucleolysis in non-contained lumbar disc herniations: a pilot study with 12 months follow-up. *Acta Neurochir Suppl.* 2005;92:93–97.
73. Muto M, Andreula C, Leonardi M. Treatment of herniated lumbar disc by intradiscal and intraforaminal oxygen-ozone (O_2-O_3) injection. *J Neuroradiol.* 2004;31:183–189.
74. Gallucci M, Limbucci N, Zugaro L, et al. Sciatica: treatment with intradiscal and intraforaminal injections of steroid and oxygen-ozone versus steroid only. *Radiology.* 2007;242:907–913.
75. Bonetti M, Fontana A, Cotticelli B, Volta GD, Guindani M, Leonardi M. Intraforaminal O(2)-O(3) versus periradicular steroidal infiltrations in lower back pain: randomized controlled study. *AJNR Am J Neuroradiol.* 2005;26:996–1000.
76. Sharma SK, Jones JO, Zeballos PP, Irwin SA, Martin TW. The prevention of discitis during discography. *Spine J.* 2009;9:936–943.

16 Complex Regional Pain Syndrome

Frank van Eijs, Michael Stanton-Hicks, Jan Van Zundert, Catharina G. Faber, Timothy R. Lubenow, Nagy Mekhail, Maarten van Kleef and Frank Huygen

Introduction

Complex Regional Pain Syndrome (CRPS) is a syndrome occurring as a complication of surgery or trauma, most often in 1 extremity, however, CRPS in multiple extremities has also been described. Spontaneous development can occur.[1] The most recent definition from the International Association for the Study of Pain (IASP) is that CRPS is a collection of locally appearing painful conditions following a trauma, which chiefly occur distally and exceed in intensity and duration the expected clinical course of the original trauma, often resulting in considerably restricted motor function. CRPS is characterized by a variable progression over time.

The clinical picture was first described more than 100 years ago by Sudeck and in the 1860s by Mitchell. A review of the literature reveals 72 different names for this syndrome, such as Sudeck's atrophy, algodystrophy, posttraumatic dystrophy, and the most frequently used term, reflex sympathetic dystrophy. Since a consensus meeting of the IASP in Orlando in 1993, "Complex Regional Pain Syndrome" has been the term agreed upon. A distinction is made between Type 1 (without) and Type 2 (with demonstrable nerve damage).[2] More recently, a third type has been added, namely CRPS Not Otherwise Specified (NOS), involving a syndrome that only partially complies with the diagnostic criteria, but where no other diagnosis can be made. Bruehl et al.[3] defined a number of subtypes, namely: a relatively limited syndrome with predominating vasomotor symptoms, a relatively limited syndrome with predominating neuropathic pain/sensory disturbances and a florid CRPS comparable to the classic description of reflex sympathetic dystrophy with the highest levels of motor and trophic signs. The estimated incidence varies from 5.46 to 26.2 per 100,000 person years. CRPS in adults occurs slightly more often in the upper extremities. A fracture is the most common initial event when it occurs in the upper extremity. Women are affected 3.4 to 4 times more often than men. The mean age at diagnosis does not differ between men and women and varies between 47 and 52 years.[4,5]

Pathophysiology

In the literature, there is ongoing debate on the pathophysiology of CRPS.

Current understandings involve peripheral, afferent, efferent and central mechanisms.

Peripheral mechanisms include hypoxia caused by vasoconstriction induced by endothelial dysfunction, leading to a decreased level of nitric oxide (NO) and increased level of endothelin-1 (ET-1) in the affected extremity. Sterile inflammation has been demonstrated by increased levels of pro-inflammatory cytokines, such as interleukin 6 (IL-6) and tumor necrosis factor alpha (TNF-alpha).[6] Neurogenic inflammation is caused by excretion of neuropeptides from nociceptive C-fibers, which was demonstrated by elevated levels of substance P, bradykinin, and calcitonin gene-related peptide (CGRP).[7] Denervation hypersensitivity can be caused by peripheral degeneration of small fiber neurons in the skin of affected limbs, leading to inappropriate firing.[8] Nociceptive afferent input may be caused by an increase in the number of alpha 1 receptors in the affected extremity, increased peripheral alpha adrenergic receptor hypersensitivity, and chemical coupling between sympathetic and nociceptive neurons in the skin of CRPS affected limbs.[9] Possible efferent mechanisms are sympathetic dysfunction leading to variable vasoconstriction, hypoxia, and sweating abnormalities. Dysfunctional efferent motor pathways may lead to involuntary movements, dystonia, and decreased range of motion. Central mechanisms, such as (supra)

Evidence-Based Interventional Pain Medicine: According to Clinical Diagnoses, First Edition. Edited by Jan Van Zundert, Jacob Patijn, Craig T. Hartrick, Arno Lataster, Frank J.P.M Huygen, Nagy Mekhail, Maarten van Kleef.

spinal sensitization through N-methyl-D-aspartate (NMDA) and neurokinin-1 (NK-1) receptor interaction, have also been described, as well as (secondary) psychological factors like pain-related fear and movement anxiety.[10]

Diagnosis

History

CRPS is usually preceded by trauma or surgery, the affected area usually extends beyond the original injury. The disease arises mostly glove-like in an arm or sock-like in a leg. The symptoms consist of a combination of continuous pain, sensory dysfunction, vasomotor and sudomotor dysfunction, and motor and trophic signs. Case reports of CRPS-like symptoms without pain are mentioned, yet these are rare.

Physical examination

Sensory dysfunction of the skin may include hyperalgesia and mechanical allodynia, but also hypoalgesia and mechanical hypoesthesia. Asymmetry of skin temperature and changes in skin color occur, as well as edema and hyper- or hypohidrosis. Signs of motor dysfunction include a reduction in the "range of motion" of affected joints and/or weakness, tremor, involuntary movements, bradykinesia, and dystonia. Abnormal skin hair growth and changes in nail growth may be observed. Symptoms may vary over time, and pain and other symptoms are often exacerbated with exertion of the affected extremity.[2]

Additional tests

There is no specific diagnostic test available, but various additional tests can be important in excluding other diagnoses. Laboratory tests such as full blood count, erythrocyte sedimentation rate, and C-reactive protein are normal in CRPS, but may help to exclude infection or rheumatologic disease. Duplex scanning and ultrasound may exclude peripheral vascular disease. Nerve conduction studies are helpful in excluding peripheral neuropathic disease or confirming nerve involvement in CRPS-2. Plain radiographs of the skeleton and contrastenhanced magnetic resonance imaging (MRI) may demonstrate osteoporosis in the affected limb, but are of no diagnostic value.[11] Three-phase bone scanning may demonstrate increased uptake of technetium Tc 99m biphosphonates due to increased bone metabolism.[12] Skin temperature measurements by infrared thermometry may reveal long-term changes in skin temperature and skin temperature dynamics between the affected and non-affected side.[13] Other tests may only be of value to quantify or substantiate the clinical symptoms and are predominantly of use in scientific research. These include: quantitative sensory testing; resting sweat output; provocative sweat output test by the quantitative sudomotor axon reflex test; sympathetic skin response; volumetry in edema of the extremities; visual analogue scales for pain; impairment level sumscore; skills questionnaires; walking, rising and sitting down skills questionnaires, and upper limb activity monitoring.[14]

Differential diagnosis

Diagnosis is based upon criteria obtained from medical history and physical examination. The most commonly used criteria are the original IASP-criteria and the modified diagnostic criteria according to Harden and Bruehl.[15–17] The criteria as described by Veldman are often used in the Netherlands.[1] All criteria have essentially been determined empirically and overlap partially, whereby the IASP criteria are the most sensitive, and the modified criteria according to Harden and Bruehl the most specific (Tables 16.1 to 16.3).[16,17]

CRPS requires an extensive differential diagnosis, because many of the symptoms can also be caused by other diseases. Distinction should be made with vascular and myofascial pain syndromes, inflammation, vascular diseases, and psychological problems. (Table 16.4)

Table 16.1. IASP criteria (Merskey, 1994).

1. Develops after tissue damage (CRPS type-1) or nerve damage (CRPS type-2)
2. Continuous pain, allodynia or hyperalgesia disproportional to the inciting event.
3. Evidence at some time of edema, abnormal skin blood flow and sudomotor abnormalities in the region of pain.
4. Other causes of pain or dysfunction are excluded.

Criteria 2, 3, and 4 must be fulfilled.

Table 16.2. Modified diagnostic criteria (Harden, 2007).

1. Continuous pain, disproportionate to the inciting event.
2. Patients should have at least 1 symptom in each of the following categories and 1 sign in 2 or more categories.

Categories:

1. Sensory (allodynia, hyperalgesia, hypoesthesia)
2. Vasomotor (temperature or skin color abnormalities)
3. Sudomotor (edema or sweating abnormalities)
4. Motor/trophic (muscle weakness, tremor, hair, nail, skin abnormalities)

Table 16.3. Dutch criteria (Veldman 1993).

A. 4 or 5 of the following symptoms:
1. Inexplicable diffuse pain
2. Difference in skin color between affected and contralateral extremity
3. Diffuse edema
4. Difference in skin temperature between affected and contralateral extremity
5. Limited "active range of motion"

B. The occurrence or increase of above-mentioned symptoms with use of the involved extremity.

C. Above-mentioned symptoms are present in an area that is greater than the area of original trauma or surgery and distal to this area.

Table 16.4. Differential diagnosis of complex regional pain syndrome.

Neuropathic pain syndromes	*Inflammation*
• Peripheral (poly)neuropathy	• Erysipelas
• Nerve entrapment	• Inflammation NOS
• Radiculopathy	• Bursitis
• Postherpetic neuralgia	• Seronegative arthritis
• Deafferentation pain after CVA	• Rheumatologic diseases
• Plexopathy	*Myofascial pain*
• Motor neuron disease	• Overuse
Vascular diseases	• Disuse
• Thrombosis	• Tennis elbow
• Acrocyanosis	• Repetitive strain injury
• Atherosclerosis	• Fibromyalgia
• Raynaud's disease	*Psychiatric problems*
• Erythromelalgia	• Somatoform pain disorders
	• Münchhausen syndrome

Treatment options

Conservative management

The primary treatment of CRPS consists of early active mobilization physical therapy combined with pharmacological pain treatment.

Physical therapy

Physical therapy proved superior to occupational therapy and superior to a control group in a randomized controlled trial (RCT) of 135 CRPS-1 patients.[18] More recently, good results with a high level of evidence have been described with graded motor imagery therapy with imagined hand movements and mirror therapy for upper extremity CRPS.[19–21] The use of pharmacological agents is guided by the involved mechanism (symptom oriented treatment, see algorithm in (Figure 16.1). Psychological support may be initiated if there is no improvement with the above mentioned regime.

Anti-inflammatory therapy

Nonsteroidal anti-inflammatory drugs (NSAIDs) for the treatment of CRPS were only studied in a small trial comparing scintigraphic outcome of calcitonin with NSAIDs. NSAIDs were inferior to calcitonin.[22]

A number of RCTs studied the effect of oxygen radical scavengers. Topical application of dimethyl sulfoxide 50% (DMSO-50%) has been found superior to placebo and oral N-acetylcysteine was generally equally effective as DMSO in the treatment of CRPS-1.[23,24]

Intravenous mannitol, however—another free radical scavenger—has proven to be ineffective.[25] Biphosphonates, which reduce the increased bone turnover, such as oral alendronate or intravenous pamidronate, were studied in 2 RCTs showing effect in favor of the biphosphonates.[26,27] Calcitonin, a polypeptide hormone with a similar mode of action as the biphosphonates, can be administered subcutaneously or by intranasal spray. The different studies on these preparations for the management of CRPS show mixed results. A critical review concluded that in well-designed trials, the effectiveness cannot be demonstrated.[28]

In a placebo-controlled RCT with 23 CRPS patients, the use of prednisone maximum 10 mg thrice daily for 3 weeks and then taper the dose during the next weeks until a maximum treatment period of 12 weeks, led to 75% improvement in all 13 treated patients as compared to only 2 out of 10 patients who received placebo.[29] Another RCT compared the use of 40 mg prednisolone per day with piroxicam in CRPS following stroke and found significant improvement after 1 month of prednisolone treatment.[30] However, since the use of corticosteroids may lead to potential serious complications, long-term use of corticosteroids is not recommended.

Analgesic therapies

There are no studies on the analgesic action of acetaminophen (paracetamol) in CRPS. As such, the usefulness of acetaminophen and NSAIDs is questionable. Slow release morphine (90 mg/d) was not effective in a double-blind placebo-controlled trial, so opioids are not likely to be of any benefit. The pain in CRPS is of neuropathic nature. First-line therapy of neuropathic pain consists of tricyclic antidepressants (TCA) like amitriptyline, the most frequently investigated drug for neuropathic pain. It improves pain and sleep impairment and can be given in CRPS although there are no trials that evaluate TCAs in CRPS.[31] Carbamazepine in a dose of 600 mg/d significantly reduced pain in a placebocontrolled RCT.[32] Gabapentin has a mild effect on pain in a subpopulation of CRPS patients and is therefore worth trying.[33] The NMDA blocker, ketamine, administered intravenously in subanesthetic dosages of maximal 20 to 25 mg/h/70 kg, has been shown to be effective in relieving CRPS-associated pain in 1 retrospective case series report and 2 randomized double-blind placebo-controlled trials.[34–36]

Vasodilatory therapy

Patients with hyperactive vasomotor symptoms leading to (intermittent) cold extremity CRPS may respond to alpha 1 adrenergic blockers like phenoxybenzamine and terazosin, or calcium channel blockers like nifedipine.[37,38]

Spasmolytic therapy

Oral spasmolytic therapy with oral benzodiazepines or oral baclofen may be used in CRPS related dystonia, tremor or myoclonus.[14]

In conclusion: Physical therapy with active mobilization and graded motor imagery treatment, together with a symptom-oriented pharmacological treatment, is the best initial approach of CRPS.

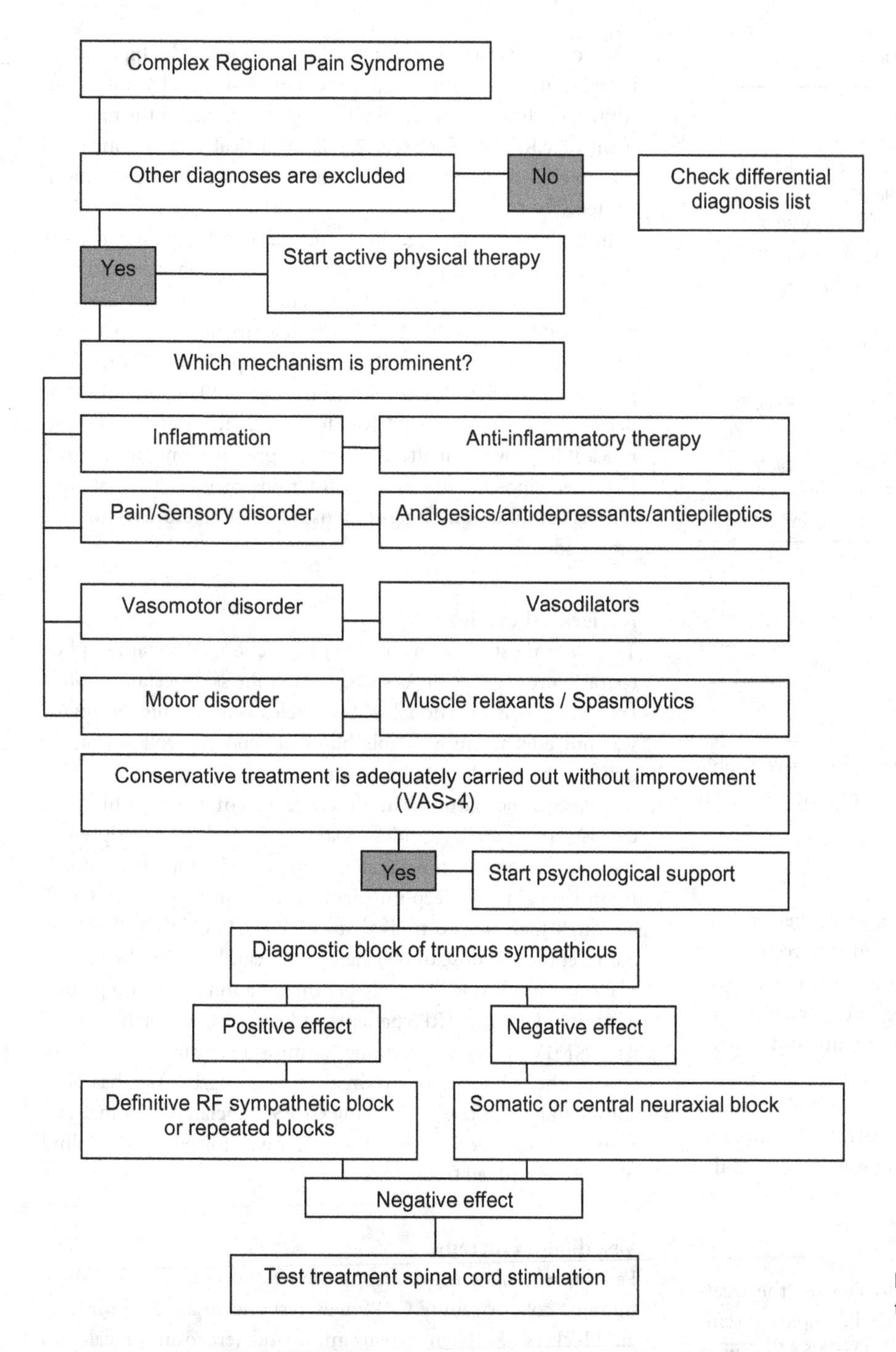

Figure 16.1. Clinical practice algorithm for the treatment of CRPS.

Interventional management

If conventional therapy fails to give adequate relief of symptoms (eg, pain score more than 4), interventional pain management techniques may be considered. These techniques are: intravenous regional blocks, sympathetic blocks of the ganglion stellatum for CRPS in the arm, and of the lumbar truncus sympathicus for CRPS in the leg. Peripheral and spinal cord stimulation and epidural or intrathecal drug administration may also be considered. Somatic and central neuraxial blocks for the management of CRPS have also been described.

Intravenous regional blocks

Intravenous regional blocks (IVRBs) with guanethidine for the treatment of CRPS-1 were first described by Hannington–Kiff.[39] The technique consists of the intravenous administration of 10 mg to 20 mg of guanethidine in a heparinized, isotonic saline solution of 25 mL, after elevating the arm for 1 minute and inflating a tourniquet at 50 mm Hg above the patient's systolic blood pressure. The tourniquet is maintained for 15 minutes to 30 minutes, after which it is let down slowly. This technique causes displacement of noradrenalin (NA) from presynaptic vesicles and prevents the re-uptake of NA leading to an increase in skin blood flow for several days.

Intravenous regional blocks with guanethidine

The effect of IVRB with guanethidine for CRPS was studied in several the case series,[40–42] prospective trials[43] and 3 RCTs.[44–46] The outcome of case series is variable.

One study of 17 patients treated with a series of IVRB guanethidine and lidocaine resulted in successful outcome in all patients. The high success rate in this series in attributed to the fact that 25 blocks were given over a period of 11 weeks compared to the usual 1 block to 6 blocks.[41] This high frequency of IVRB is not common practice and cannot be supported.

In a prospective case-controlled study of 26 patients with CRPS of the hand significantly better pain reduction and improvement of function was observed after treatment with DMSO-50% ointment 4 times daily during 3 weeks when compared to treatment with IVRB guanethidine twice a week during 3 weeks.[43] In a double-blind crossover study with saline, high-dose guanethidine, and low-dose guanethidine, no significant difference between groups was found. All groups reported less than 30% pain reduction; there was no evidence of a dose-response for guanethidine. The trial was stopped prematurely after serious adverse events in 2 patients with the high dose of guanethidine.[44] A double-blind controlled multicenter RCT comparing IVRB with guanethidine or placebo in a group of 60 CRPS patients found no differences in long-term outcome.[45] In another RCT, in a group of 57 CRPS patients, comparing IVRB with guanethidine to saline, again, no significant long-term differences were found.[46]

Intravenous regional blocks with other medications

IVRB with lidocaine and methylprednisolone was not effective when compared to saline in a RCT in 22 CRPS-1 patients.[47] In a retrospective case series of 61 patients treated with IVRB containing lidocaine and ketorolac, 26% of patients had complete resolution of pain, 43% had partial response, and 31% had no response to this therapy.[48] In 1 double-blind placebo-controlled study, the use of intravenous regional ketanserin, a potent vasodilator, had a pain relieving effect.[49]

In conclusion, there is evidence that IVRB with guanethidine is not effective for the management of CRPS. The use of ketanserin was only studied in an earlier small trial.

Sympathetic blocks: ganglion stellatum (stellate ganglion) and lumbar block

The sympathetic nervous system has been implicated in numerous pain syndromes ranging from neuropathic pain to vascular pain to visceral pain. A role for sympathetic block (SB) is presumed. Recently, this was extensively reviewed by Day.[50] He concluded that despite frequent use of minimally invasive sympathetic blocks and neurolysis, their efficacy for providing analgesia has been sparsely reported in the literature. Focusing on sympathetic block for CRPS, we could identify 13 articles: 2 on SB (Ganglion stellatum, stellate ganglion block [SGB] and lumbar sympathetic block [LSB]), 6 on SGB, and 5 on LSB.

Ganglion stellatum (stellate ganglion) block

Ganglion stellatum (stellate ganglion) block (SGB) is commonly performed for CRPS of the upper extremity. This cervicothoracic ganglion sends sympathetic efferents to the truncus cervicalis and the plexus brachialis, and is located anterolaterally to the head of the first rib, lateral to the musculus longus colli, and posteromedial to the arteria vertebralis[51] (Figure 16.2).

Linson et al.[52] described the use of SGB for patients with CRPS in the upper arm. Twenty-eight patients were all treated with indwelling-catheter injections of bupivacaine 0.5%, 4 times a day during a mean of 7 days (range 1 day to 14 days). Short-term outcomes were good: 90% of patients improved during treatment. In the long-term, at 6 months to 6 years, 2 patients were lost to follow-up. Of the remaining 26 patients, 19 felt that their pain had remained improved. Seven patients however, judged the pain improvement in the long term as minimal. Another study also found prolonged SGB with bupivacaine useful if intermittent SGBs plus conservative treatment with analgesics, tranquilizers and physical therapy failed. After an average of 3 years follow-up, there was 25% relapse rate and 75% marked to complete improvement in a group of 26 posttraumatic CRPS patients.[53] The combination therapy of daily SGB with up to 10 to 15 injections, together with oral amitriptyline up to 100 mg per day, was found to give significant improvements in both VAS pain ratings and grip force strength.[54] In another study, SGB performed within 16 weeks after onset of symptoms gave significantly better pain relief than if performed later than 16 weeks after symptom onset. Moreover, it was found that a decrease in skin perfusion of the CRPS extremity as compared to the normal side, adversely affected the efficacy of the SGB.[55]

In a small case series of 6 patients, the effect of opioid infiltration for CRPS-1 was examined; the data showed no efficacy of morphine when injected around the ganglion stellatum.[56]

Radiofrequency (RF) denervation of the ganglion stellatum was found comparably effective to other methods of SGB blockade with 40.7% of patients having more than 50% pain relief, in a selected group of patients who responded positively to a diagnostic block with 4 mL to 6 mL lidocaine 1%.[57]

Lumbar sympathetic block

LSB is frequently performed at the L2 to L4 lumbar levels for complex regional pain syndrome of the lower extremity. Pre- and post ganglionic fibers form a synapse in the sympathetic ganglia. These ganglia are located at the anterolateral side of the lumbar vertebrae (Figure 16.3). Unlike the SGBs, imageguided techniques are mandatory. Under fluoroscopic guidance, the technique has been demonstrated to be easy to perform.[58] Computerized tomography (CT),[59] MRI,[60] and ultrasound based techniques have also been described and their reliability demonstrated.[61] However, since CT and MRI are time-consuming and less suitable for daily practice, fluoroscopy remains the method of choice. Ultrasound-based techniques, however, may become more important in the near future.

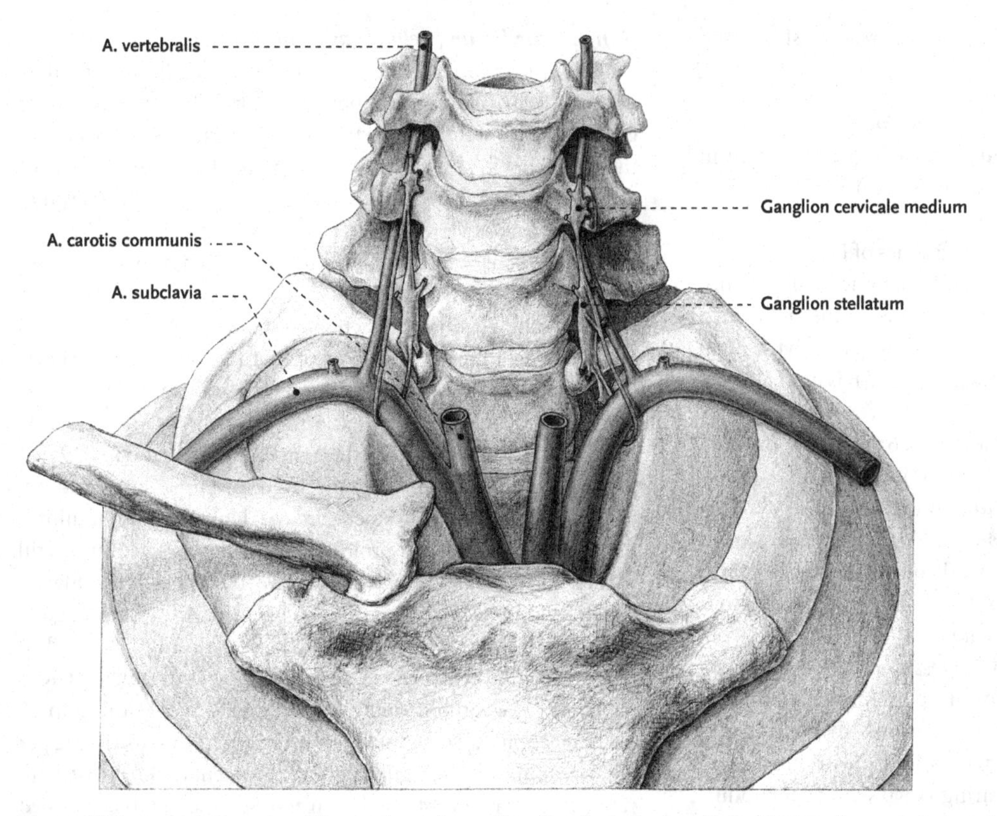

Figure 16.2. Anatomic illustration of the ganglion stellatum; Illustration: Rogier Trompert Medical Art. http://www.medical-art.nl

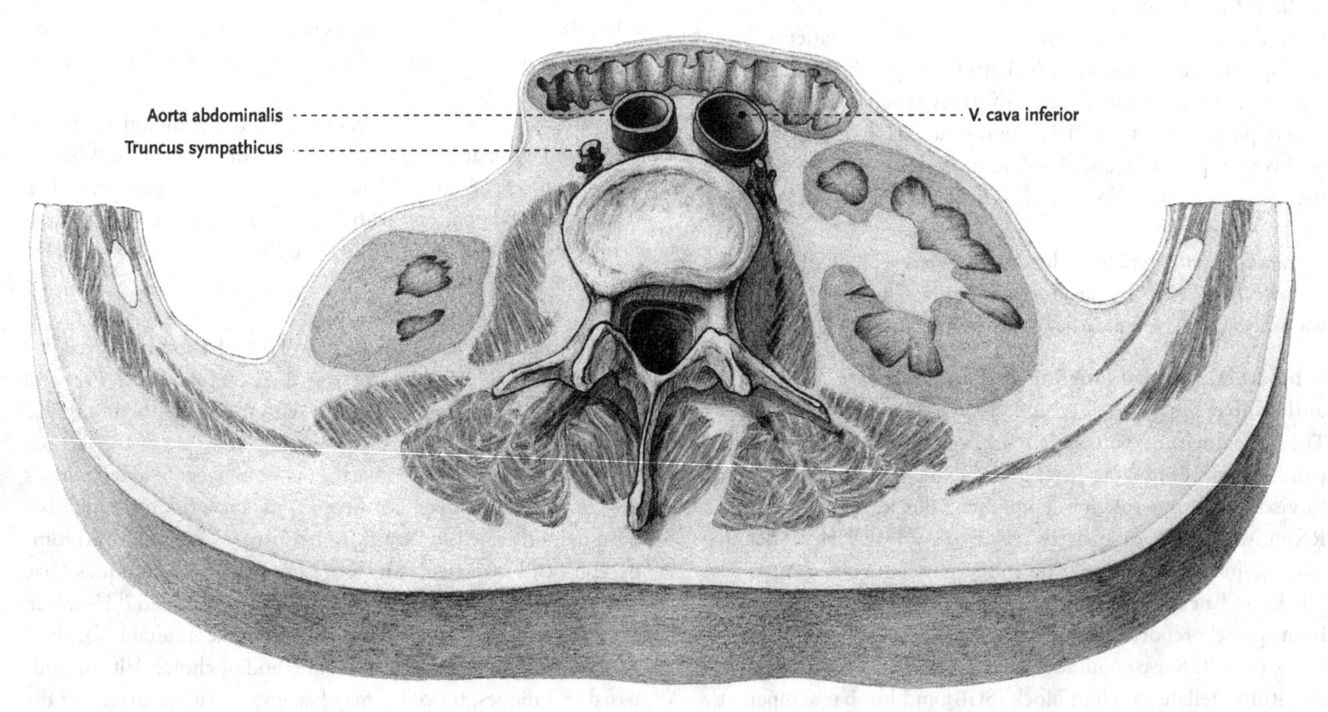

Figure 16.3. Anatomic illustration of the lumbar truncus sympathicus; Illustration: Rogier Trompert Medical Art. http://www.medical-art.nl

LSBs can be performed by repeated injections of local anesthetic. In order to achieve longer-lasting results, neurolysis with, for example, phenol, has been used. Radiofrequency treatment of the lumbar truncus sympathicus is a third method for performing LSB.

In 29 patients with CRPS of the lower limb following total knee replacement, LSB was performed with intermittent injections of 20 mL bupivacaine 0.375%. Complete pain relief was found in 13 (45%) patients, partial pain relief in 12 (41%) patients and no pain relief in 3 (10%) patients. One patient dropped out due to technical failure.[62] Iohexol, a regularly used water-soluble contrast dye, was found not to alter the effect of LSB and even improved pain relief. In a subset of 11 patients, who agreed to report some aspects of pain in more detail, it was noted that the increase in skin temperature correlated significantly with the relief of allodynia.[63]

RF LSB at the L2–L4 sympathetic ganglia was documented in a case series of 20 patients with CRPS; 5 (25%) became pain free and 9 (45%) had temporary pain relief.[64] RF LSB was compared with phenol neurolysis. It was found that phenol retained sympatholytic effects in 89% of patients after 8 weeks, as compared to only 12% in the RF group.[65] In a RCT performed in 20 CRPS-1 patients, it was found that RF treatment at 80°C for 90 seconds at the L2–L4 sympathetic ganglia was as effective as phenol neurolysis at the same ganglia (3 mL phenol 7% at each lumbar level). All patients had statistically significant reduction from baseline of various pain scores at 4 months follow-up; however, phenol caused neuropathic pain symptoms in 1 patient (10%).[66]

Sympathetic blocks

In a double-blind, placebo-controlled crossover study, it was found that the duration of pain relief by SB with local anesthetics was reliably longer (90 hours) as compared to saline (20 hours).[67] Sympathetic blocks were examined (SGB and LSB) with weekly injections of 14 mL to 16 mL bupivacaine 0.25%, or continuous bupivacaine 0.25% infusions of 5 mL per hour for 5 days (if pain relief was limited to the duration of the local anesthetic). Significant long-term improvement of pain (47% reduction in VAS pain score) and functionality was found in all patients at a mean follow-up of 9.4 months. A 50% or greater relief from pain after diagnostic block was highly correlated with improvement at long-term follow-up. Mechanical and thermal allodynia predicted a positive response to initial sympathetic block. Anxiety negatively influenced pain relief and functional outcome.[68]

A recent trial in 9 patients with CRPS-1 of more than 6 months duration compared the analgesic action of LSB with bupivacaine to LSB with bupivacaine mixed with botulinum toxin A (BTA); it was found that BTA significantly increased the analgesic action of the LSB. Analgesia duration was prolonged from fewer than 10 days (95% CI: 0 to 12) to 71 days (95% CI: 12 to 253). The mechanism of action being explained by the BTA preventing the release of acetylcholine from the preganglionic sympathetic nerves and thus inducing long-lasting but not permanent sympathetic block.[69]

In conclusion: SGB by means of intermittent injections of local anesthetic for the management of CRPS of the upper limb was documented in retrospective and prospective studies. RF SGB was evaluated in a retrospective study. LSB with local anesthetic was demonstrated to be superior to placebo injection. RF LSB yields comparable results to phenol neurolysis. The latter may produce a longer effect but the risk for deafferentation pain is higher; therefore, RF treatment is preferred.

Neurostimulation

Transcutaneous electrical stimulation

Transcutaneous electrical nerve stimulation (TENS) may give pain relief in a subgroup of patients with CRPS.[70] Although there is no conclusive evidence for the use and effectiveness of TENS, this therapy is noninvasive with only minimal adverse events, the most common being a contact allergy for the skin electrodes.[71] This makes TENS suitable as a preliminary or adjunctive therapy.[72]

Spinal cord stimulation

For patients with chronic CRPS who do not respond to conservative medical and rehabilitation therapy or sympathetic blocks, Spinal Cord Stimulation (SCS) may be considered. The short-term effect of this therapy in patients with CRPS has been demonstrated in a randomized study.[73] In this study, 54 patients with CRPS were included and randomized 2:1 to receive SCS and physical therapy or a standard regimen of physical therapy alone. Thirty-six patients were assigned to and treated with a test SCS. Twenty-four of those reported a reduction in pain and in these patients a definitive system was implanted. Eighteen patients only received physical therapy. Six months posttreatment, the intention to treat (ITT) analysis showed a clear reduction in pain intensity in the group with stimulated patients despite the fact that only 24 of the 36 patients were actually treated with SCS. The positive effects on pain and global perceived effect remained in an ITT analysis 2 years after implantation.[74] Pain reduction was identical in patients treated with a cervical lead compared to a lumbar lead.[75] Five years after the start of treatment the differences were smaller, but the patients who were treated with SCS were still doing better than the patients who had a negative test SCS or those who were in the control group. At the end of the follow-up period, despite the diminishing effect, 95% of the patients treated with the SCS indicated that they would have been willing to undergo the treatment again to achieve the same result.[76] A recent review on the clinical and cost-effectiveness of SCS in the management of chronic neuropathic or ischemic pain suggests that this treatment is effective in reducing the chronic neuropathic pain of CRPS type 1.[77]

Peripheral nerve stimulation

In a prospective case series, peripheral nerve stimulation (PNS) with surgically placed plate type electrodes connected with an implantable pulse generator reduced allodynic and spontaneous pain in 19 (63%) out of 30 implanted patients with CRPS and symptoms in the distribution of 1 major peripheral nerve.[78] In a retrospective study with 52 patients (48 CRPS-2 patients and 4 phantom limb patients), 47 patients were implanted after a positive trial stimulation. Of these patients, 43 (91%) had lasting excellent to good success with marked pain reduction and reduction of pain related disability.[79] In another retrospective study 41 PNS devices were implanted in 38 patients with pain in a peripheral nerve distribution. Over 60% of patients had significant improvement of their pain of more than 50% following implantation of the peripheral nerve stimulator.[80] The technique can only be applied if the pain is in the distribution of a peripheral nerve and is thus less suitable for most CRPS-1 patients.

Somatic and central neuraxial blocks

Plexus brachialis block

Somatic nerve block of the plexus brachialis also blocks the efferent sympathetic nerves around it. Theoretically somatic blockade increases the ability to tolerate physical therapy, especially if the shoulder is also affected. In a retrospective case series in 25 patients, of which 17 CRPS patients, improvement in pain and range of motion was found after interscalcne block with 30 mL to 40 mL bupivacaine 0.125% injected every other day up to a total of 10 injections. This approach was suggested if sympathetic blockade failed.[81]

In a small case series of 6 CRPS patients treated with continuous or daily axillary injections with bupivacaine together with physical and occupational therapy, 3 out of 6 patients responded well to this therapy; another patient also responded well initially, but the catheter had to be removed due to infection at the insertion site. The 2 poor responders were chronic CRPS patients.[82]

Epidural administration of drugs

The epidural administration of opioids and other drugs is increasingly being offered for non-malignant pain. Epidural bupivacaine in high anesthetic doses for 2 to 3 days followed by epidural infusion of opioids for up to 7 days together with continuous passive motion allowed for recovery of the knee function in patients with CRPS of the knee.[83] Epidural clonidine has been demonstrated to give short-term pain relief in chronic CRPS and to be possibly effective in the long term with small VAS reductions from 7.0 ± 0.4 to 5.1 ± 0.6 ($P < 0.05$).[84]

Unilateral cervical epidural analgesia with low dose bupivacaine and clonidine by continuous infusion for CRPS may be an interesting approach. The low bupivacaine dose gives only minimal limb muscle weakness and allows for active rehabilitation therapy.[85] In a retrospective study, 37 CRPS-1 patients were treated with this unilateral epidural catheter technique with continuous bupivacaine and fentanyl infusions. Of these patients almost 90% improved significantly when treated within 1 year after onset of symptoms. If treatment was initiated more than 1 year after onset and if more than 1 limb was involved, the success rate decreased dramatically.[86]

Intrathecal administration of drugs

The intrathecal administration of drugs has been utilized increasingly in the last 30 years. Intrathecal administration of morphine with a totally implantable drug delivery system gave >50% pain relief in a case series of 5 patients with chronic CRPS.[87] Intrathecal treatment of CRPS pain with bupivacaine in high anesthetic doses up to 90 mg per day was studied in a small series of 3 patients. The infusion improved pain but did not prevent the syndrome from becoming chronic and was therefore not recommended.[88]

Intrathecal baclofen improves dystonia, pain, disability, and quality of life in patients with CRPS-1 associated dystonia but is associated with a high complication rate as described below.[89]

Intrathecal ziconotide (a nonopioid analgesic) may be a promising drug for the treatment of refractory CRPS pain but requires more research.[90]

Complications of interventional management

Complications of the intravenous regional blocks

The IVRB technique is a relatively safe procedure to perform but with frequent minor side effects like dizziness (41% of patients) after release of the tourniquet.[48] Serious orthostatic hypotension may occur.[44]

Complications of the ganglion stellatum (stellate ganglion) block

The incidence of severe complications is 1.7 in 1,000 patients. Potentially life-threatening complications usually arise from inadvertent subarachnoid injection or injection in the arteria vertebralis. This makes ECG monitoring and placement of an intravenous line prior to performing the procedure mandatory.[91] Actually the autonomic innervation of the arm occurs via Th1. However puncture at this level gives a small chance of injecting into the thoracic pleural cavity. To prevent this it is possible to first inject towards C7 and then adjust the needle in the direction of Th1. One potential side effect is the occurrence of Horner's syndrome caused by the local anesthetic spreading to the cervical truncus sympathicus. Hoarseness can also occur via spread to the nervus laryngeus recurrens.

Complications of the lumbar sympathetic block

Blocking the sympathetic nervous system causes vasodilatation in the extremity which may lead to (orthostatic) hypotension. Therefore patients should receive intravenous fluid infusion prior to treatment. During recovery blood pressure should be measured intermittently over a period of 45 minutes. After the recovery period sufficient fluid intake during the first 24 hours is advised. Patients can sometimes develop a warm and edematous leg that can possibly be interpreted as overshoot. These symptoms usually disappear spontaneously after about 6 weeks. Another possible complication is damage to the nervus ilioinguinalis or more frequently (5% to 10%) the nervus genitofemoralis. This can give a neuropathic deafferentation pain. An alternative approach, the transdiscal technique, has been demonstrated to lower the risk of nervus genitofemoralis neuritis.[92] Similarly, this risk is reduced if RF denervation of the lumbar truncus sympathicus is used instead of injecting a neurolytic agent.[65] With bilateral chemical LSB men can become impotent.

Complications of spinal cord stimulation

Possible complications that require reoperation include electrode dislocation or pain from the implanted pulse generator pocket.[74] Life-threatening complications like meningitis are rare but other adverse events like infection, dural puncture, pain in the region of a stimulator component, equipment failure, revision procedures other than battery change and removal operations occur in 34% of the patients.[93]

Complications of peripheral nerve stimulation

Possible complications requiring reoperation are related to the surgical technique or PNS equipment design and include migration of the electrode in 33%, infection in 15% and the need for placement in an alternative location in 11% of patients.[94]

Complications of plexus brachialis block

Plexus brachialis block is a relatively safe procedure with the most common complication being infection of the catheter skin insertion site.

Complications of epidural and intrathecal drug administration

Frequent complications of epidural drug administration include infections and catheter or pump failure.[95] Adverse effects of intrathecal drug administration include infections, catheter and pump system failures, post dural puncture headache, and the formation of intrathecal granulomas, carrying the potential to produce spinal cord compression.

Evidence for interventional management

A summary of the available evidence is given in Table 16.5.

Recommendations

Based upon the available evidence with regard to effect and complications, we recommend the following interventional techniques for the treatment of CRPS.

Table 16.5. Summary of evidence for interventional pain management of CRPS.

Technique	Score
Intravenous regional block guanethidine	2 A–
Ganglion stellatum (stellate ganglion) block	2 B+
Lumbar sympathetic block	2 B+
Plexus brachialis block	2 C+
Epidural infusion analgesia	2 C+
Spinal cord stimulation	2 B+
Peripheral nerve stimulation	2 C+

For CRPS patients with severe pain, allodynia, or with a clear skin temperature difference as compared to the nonaffected extremity that do not respond to medication and physical therapy, a diagnostic block of the ganglion stellatum or the lumbar sympathetic nervous system may be performed. If this block provides at least 50% pain reduction, this procedure can be repeated a few times with local anesthetic. Radiofrequency therapy of the ganglion stellatum or the lumbar sympathetic ganglia is a suitable alternative. In the case of persistent symptoms, SCS can be recommended after multidisciplinary evaluation. Somatic plexus brachialis block, epidural analgesia and PNS can be considered, preferentially within the context of a clinical study.

Clinical practice algorithm

The practice algorithm is illustrated in Figure 16.1.

Technique(s)

Ganglion stellatum (stellate ganglion) block

Injections have traditionally been guided by palpable anatomical landmarks.[96] Supportive technology such as fluoroscopy,[97] computed tomography[98] and ultrasound[99] have been demonstrated to make the procedure technically more reliable. SGB's may be performed by injection of local anesthetics or by RF denervation.

The patient is placed in a supine position with the head slightly hyperextended. The level of C6–C7 is determined by fluoroscopy with the C-arm in anteroposterior position. The C-arm is adjusted until the vertebral end plates are aligned. After local disinfection, the skin is anesthetized using 1% lidocaine and a needle is inserted at the junction of the processus transversus and the corresponding C6 or C7 corpus vertebralis. After contact with the bone, oblique projection is used to check if the needle is anterior to the foramen intervertebrale. If the needle is past this level and no contact has been made with the base of the processus transversus, the needle needs to be repositioned. Once the needle is in the correct position a small amount (0.5 mL to 1 mL) of contrast dye is injected in order to prevent intravascular injection. The contrast dye must spread craniocaudally. (Figures 16.4 and 16.5)

For a test block, the injection is given using a 60 mm, 20 gauge radiocontrast needle. After C-arm fluoroscopy confirmation of the correct position 5 mL 1% lidocaine or 0.25% bupivacaine is injected depending on the spread of the contrast dye.

For a definitive block using RF, a 60 mm, 20 gauge RF needle is combined with a thermocouple probe for thermometry and thermal lesioning. After confirmation of the correct needle position with fluoroscopy, electrical stimulation is performed at 50 Hz (sensory stimulation) and 2 Hz (motor stimulation) to 1 mA, to ensure that there is no contact with a segmental nerve root (the patient should not feel anything apart from a faint feeling in the shoulder and/or arm). Then 0.7 mL 1% lidocaine in injected, after which a thermal lesion is carried out for 1 minute at 80°C. This procedure may be repeated if necessary.

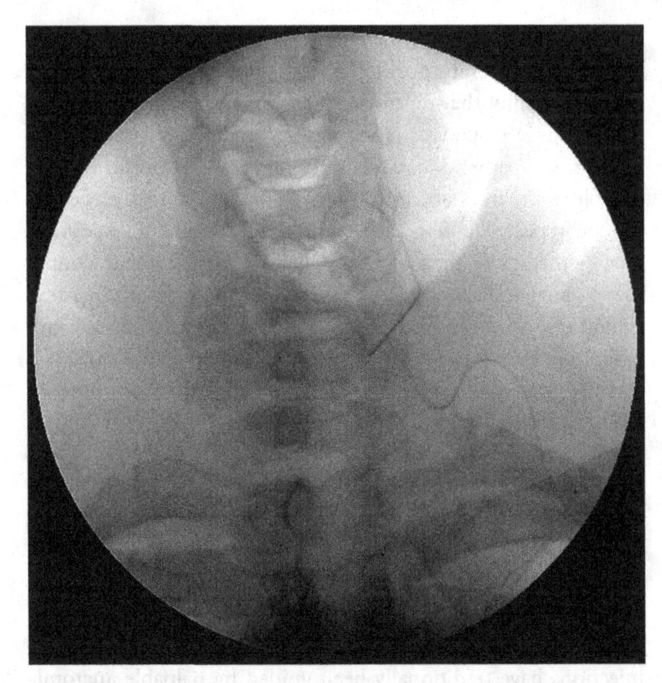

Figure 16.4. Ganglion stellatum (stellate ganglion) block: anteroposterior view of the needle position.

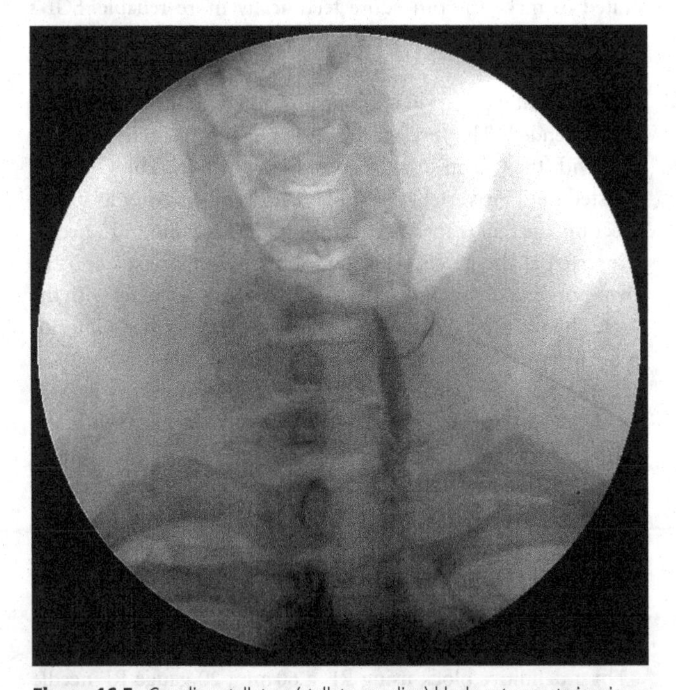

Figure 16.5. Ganglion stellatum (stellate ganglion) block: anteroposterior view with contrast solution.

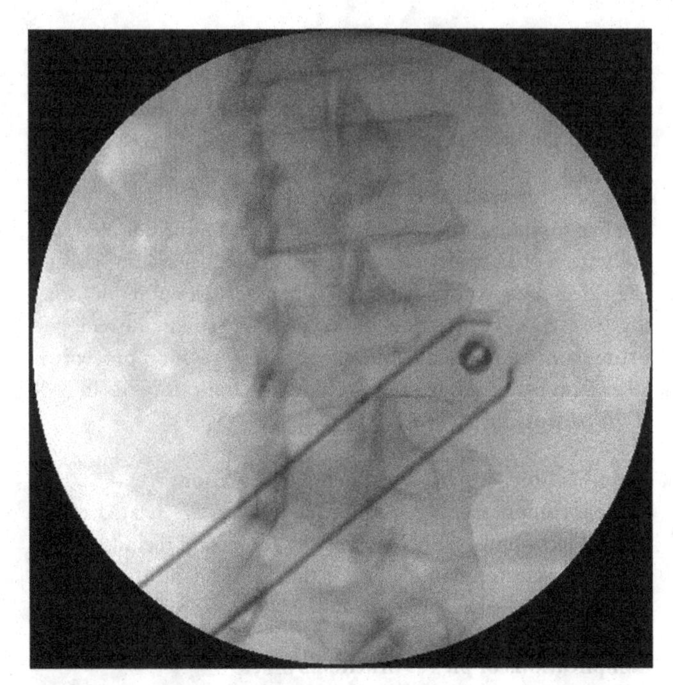

Figure 16.6. Lumbar sympathetic diagnostic block injection point: oblique projection.

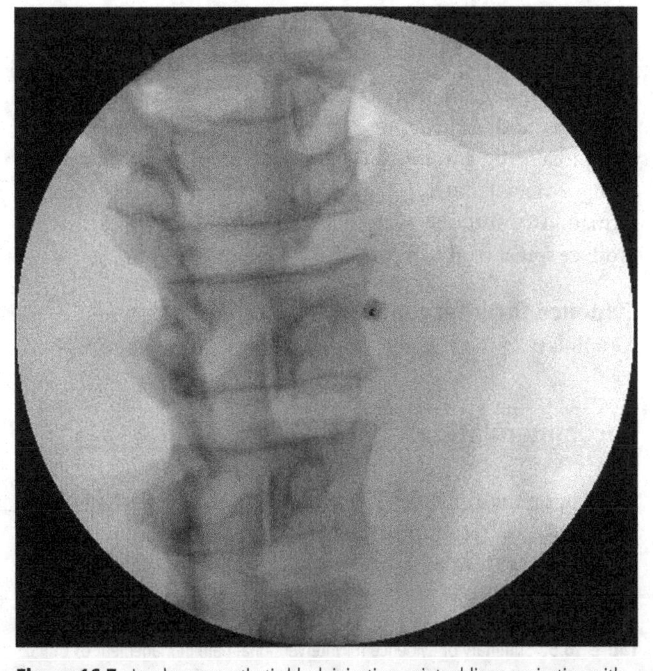

Figure 16.7. Lumbar sympathetic block injection point: oblique projection with needle using a tunnel view.

Lumbar sympathetic block

The patient is placed in the prone position on the treatment table, a cushion can be placed under the abdomen in order to reduce the lumbar lordosis. The C-arm fluoroscope is used to identify the L2–L4 levels. The C-arm is adjusted in the cranio-caudal direction until the vertebral end plates are aligned. Then the C-arm, is turned laterally until the distal end of the processus transversus projects inline with the lateral edge of the corresponding L2–L4 corpora vertebrae. After local disinfection, the skin is anesthetized using 1% lidocaine and a needle is inserted using a tunnel view until the front of the vertebra has been reached (Figures 16.6 and 16.7). The lateral projection is used to assure that the needle does not pass the anterior border of the corpus vertebrae. Also an AP projection is used to assure that the needle point projects over the facet joint of the spinal column. The truncus sympathicus can be reached by a single needle approach at the L3 corpus vertebrae[100] or by a multiple needle approach at the L2–L4 corpora vertebrae. If there is a good contrast outline of the dye when starting with the single needle approach at L3 there is no need for the multiple needle approach. In either case, a small amount (0.5 mL to 1 mL) of contrast dye should be injected (injection of too much contrast dye makes repositioning of the needle more difficult). In the AP projection, the contrast dye should be visible as a cloud in front of the corpus vertebrae, but not laterally. In the case of a streaky lateral spread the needle could be in the musculus psoas compartment and the needle needs to be inserted more deeply. Using lateral projection, a string will be seen running along the anterolateral aspect of the corpus vertebrae (Figure 16.8).

A 20 gauge, 150 mm needle at the level of L3 is used for a test block. After confirmation of the correct needle positioning by radiocontrast dye, 5 mL to 10 mL of 1% lidocaine or 0.25% bupivacaine is injected.

For a definitive block using RF a 20 gauge, 150 mm long RF needle with a 10 mm non-insulated tip is used combined with a thermocouple probe for thermometry and thermal lesioning. Consideration can be given to only blocking at 2 levels, L3 and L4. After confirmation of the correct position with the fluoroscope, electrical stimulation is carried out, using consecutively 50 Hz (sensory stimulation) and 2 Hz (motor stimulation) to 1 mA, to ensure that there is no contact with a segmental nerve root (patient should not feel anything apart from a faint feeling in the abdomen). At each level 0.7 mL 1% lidocaine is injected after which a thermal lesion is carried out for 1 minute at 80°C. This procedure may be repeated if necessary.

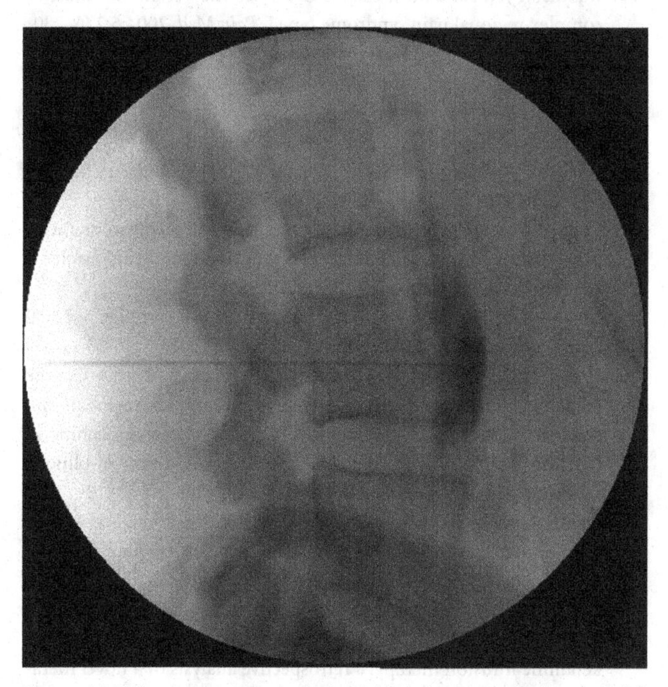

Figure 16.8. Lumbar sympathetic diagnostic block: lateral view with spread of contrast solution.

Spinal cord stimulation

All patients in the discussed studies received trial SCS with a temporary electrode after the prophylactic administration of 1,500 mg of cefuroxime (a cephalosporin) intravenously. With the patient in prone position, under direct fluoroscopy a Tuohy needle was introduced in the epidural space. The electrode was advanced until the tip was at C4 in the case of upper extremity CRPS and at T10 in the case of lower extremity CRPS. The electrode was positioned so that there was adequate stimulation as reported by the patient as paresthesias covering the area of pain. The needle was then withdrawn and the electrode connected to an external stimulator. The trial SCS was carried out at home for at least 1 week. Meanwhile, patients were encouraged to perform their normal daily activities. A permanent implant was performed if there was a 50% pain reduction score or if there was a score of at least 6 (meaning much improvement) on a 7 point scale for global perceived effect of treatment.

The permanent implantation technique used consisted of the introduction of an epidural stimulation electrode via a 5-cm midline incision with the patient in prone position after prophylactic administration of 1,500 mg of cefuroxime intravenously. The electrode was fixed with special clips. After placing the patient in a lateral position the electrode was connected with an internal pulse generator in the left lower anterior abdominal wall by a tunneled extension lead. The patient remained in the hospital for 24 hours after implantation and was given 2 additional doses of 750 mg cefuroxime. Stimulation parameters used consisted of high frequency stimulation (rate 85 Hz) with a pulse width of 210 ms. The pulse intensity was controlled by means of a patient programmer that allowed the patient to adjust the amplitude of stimulation from 0 V to 10 V.

Summary

There is no gold standard for diagnosis of CRPS. Clinical history and physical examination form the cornerstones of the diagnostic process.

When conservative treatment with physical and medical treatment fails, multidisciplinary evaluation should follow. If there is no improvement in pain and dysfunction, sympathetic blockade may be performed. If this block is effective, it may be followed by repeated injections or RF treatment. If symptoms persist, a continuous epidural infusion, intermittent or continuous plexus brachialis block in combination with exercise therapy may be useful. If symptoms persist SCS after a successful trial stimulation period may yield positive results.

References

1. Veldman PH, Reynen HM, Arntz IE, Goris RJ. Signs and symptoms of reflex sympathetic dystrophy: prospective study of 829 patients. *Lancet.* 1993;342:1012–1016.
2. Stanton-Hicks M, Janig W, Hassenbusch S, Haddox JD, Boas R, Wilson P. Reflex sympathetic dystrophy: changing concepts and taxonomy. *Pain.* 1995;63:127–133.
3. Bruehl S, Harden RN, Galer BS, Saltz S, Backonja M, Stanton-Hicks M. Complex regional pain syndrome: are there distinct subtypes and sequential stages of the syndrome? *Pain.* 2002;95:119–124.
4. de Mos M, de Bruijn AG, Huygen FJ, Dieleman JP, Stricker BH, Sturkenboom MC. The incidence of complex regional pain syndrome: a population-based study. *Pain.* 2007;129:12–20.
5. Sandroni P, Benrud-Larson LM, McClelland RL, Low PA. Complex regional pain syndrome type I: incidence and prevalence in Olmsted county, a population-based study. *Pain.* 2003;103:199–207.
6. Groeneweg JG, Huygen FJ, Heijmans-Antonissen C, Niehof S, Zijlstra FJ. Increased endothelin-1 and diminished nitric oxide levels in blister fluids of patients with intermediate cold type complex regional pain syndrome type 1. *BMC Musculoskelet Disord.* 2006;7:91.
7. Birklein F, Schmelz M. Neuropeptides, neurogenic inflammation and complex regional pain syndrome (CRPS). *Neurosci Lett.* 2008;437:199–202.
8. Oaklander AL, Fields HL. Is reflex sympathetic dystrophy/complex regional pain syndrome typeIa small-fiber neuropathy? *Ann Neurol.* 2009;65:629–638.
9. Gibbs GF, Drummond PD, Finch PM, Phillips JK. Unravelling the pathophysiology of complex regional pain syndrome: focus on sympathetically maintained pain. *Clin Exp Pharmacol Physiol.* 2008;35:717–724.
10. de Mos M, Sturkenboom MC, Huygen FJ. Current understandings on complex regional pain syndrome. *Pain Pract.* 2009;9:86–99.
11. Schurmann M, Zaspel J, Lohr P, et al. Imaging in early posttraumatic complex regional pain syndrome: a comparison of diagnostic methods. *Clin J Pain.* 2007;23:449–457.
12. Zyluk A. The usefulness of quantitative evaluation of three-phase scintigraphy in the diagnosis of post-traumatic reflex sympathetic dystrophy. *J Hand Surg Br.* 1999;24:16–21.
13. Krumova EK, Frettloh J, Klauenberg S, Richter H, Wasner G, Maier C. Long-term skin temperature measurements—a practical diagnostic tool in complex regional pain syndrome. *Pain.* 2008; 140:8–22.
14. Perez RS, Zollinger PE, Dijkstra PU, et al. [Clinical practice guideline "Complex regional pain syndrome type I"]. *Ned Tijdschr Geneeskd.* 2007;151:1674–1679.
15. Merskey H, Bogduk N. *Radicular Pain—Radicular Pain and Radiculopathy, Classification of Chronic Pain.* 2nd ed. Seattle, Washington: IASP Press; 1994:13–16.
16. Harden RN, Bruehl S, Stanton-Hicks M, Wilson PR. Proposed new diagnostic criteria for complex regional pain syndrome. *Pain Med.* 2007;8:326–331.
17. Bruehl S, Harden RN, Galer BS, et al. External validation of IASP diagnostic criteria for Complex Regional Pain Syndrome and proposed research diagnostic criteria. International Association for the Study of Pain. *Pain.* 1999;81:147–154.
18. Oerlemans HM, Oostendorp RA, de Boo T, Goris RJ. Pain and reduced mobility in complex regional pain syndrome I: outcome of a prospective randomised controlled clinical trial of adjuvant physical therapy versus occupational therapy. *Pain.* 1999;83: 77–83.
19. Moseley GL. Graded motor imagery is effective for long-standing complex regional pain syndrome: a randomised controlled trial. *Pain.* 2004;108:192–198.
20. Daly AE, Bialocerkowski AE. Does evidence support physiotherapy management of adult Complex Regional Pain Syndrome Type One? A systematic review. *Eur J Pain.* 2009;13:339–353.
21. Ezendam D, Bongers RM, Jannink MJ. Systematic review of the effectiveness of mirror therapy in upper extremity function. *Disabil Rehabil.* 20091–20015.
22. Rico H, Merono E, Gomez-Castresana F, Torrubiano J, Espinos D, Diaz P. Scintigraphic evaluation of reflex sympathetic dystrophy: comparative study of the course of the disease under two therapeutic regimens. *Clin Rheumatol.* 1987;6:233–237.
23. Zuurmond WW, Langendijk PN, Bezemer PD, Brink HE, de Lange JJ, van Loenen AC. Treatment of acute reflex sympathetic dystrophy with DMSO 50% in a fatty cream. *Acta Anaesthesiol Scand.* 1996;40:364–367.
24. Perez RS, Zuurmond WW, Bezemer PD, et al. The treatment of complex regional pain syndrome type I with free radical scavengers: a randomized controlled study. *Pain.* 2003;102:297–307.
25. Perez RS, Pragt E, Geurts J, Zuurmond WW, Patijn J, van Kleef M. Treatment of patients with complex regional pain syndrome type I with mannitol: a prospective, randomized, placebo-controlled, double-blinded study. *J Pain.* 2008;9:678–686.
26. Manicourt DH, Brasseur JP, Boutsen Y, Depreseux G, Devogelaer JP. Role of alendronate in therapy for posttraumatic complex regional pain syndrome type I of the lower extremity. *Arthritis Rheum.* 2004;50:3690–3697.
27. Robinson JN, Sandom J, Chapman PT. Efficacy of pamidronate in complex regional pain syndrome type I. *Pain Med.* 2004;5:276–280.
28. Kingery WS. A critical review of controlled clinical trials for peripheral neuropathic pain and complex regional pain syndromes. *Pain.* 1997;73:123–139.
29. Christensen K, Jensen EM, Noer I. The reflex dystrophy syndrome response to treatment with systemic corticosteroids. *Acta Chir Scand.* 1982;148:653–655.
30. Kalita J, Vajpayee A, Misra UK. Comparison of prednisolone with piroxicam in complex regional pain syndrome following stroke: a randomized controlled trial. *QJM.* 2006;99:89–95.
31. Rowbotham MC. Pharmacologic management of complex regional pain syndrome. *Clin J Pain.* 2006;22:425–429.
32. Harke H, Gretenkort P, Ladleif HU, Rahman S, Harke O. The response of neuropathic pain and pain in complex regional pain syndrome I to carbamazepine and sustained-release morphine in patients pretreated with spinal cord stimulation: a double-blinded randomized study. *Anesth Analg.* 2001;92:488–495.
33. van de Vusse AC, Stomp-van den Berg SG, Kessels AH, Weber WE. Randomised controlled trial of gabapentin in Complex Regional Pain Syndrome type 1 [ISRCTN84121379]. *BMC Neurol.* 2004; 4:13.
34. Correll GE, Maleki J, Gracely EJ, Muir JJ, Harbut RE. Subanesthetic ketamine infusion therapy: a retrospective analysis of a novel therapeutic approach to complex regional pain syndrome. *Pain Med.* 2004;5:263–275.

35. Sigtermans MJ, van Hilten JJ, Bauer MC, et al. Ketamine produces effective and long-term pain relief in patients with Complex Regional Pain Syndrome Type 1. *Pain.* 2009;145:304–311.
36. Schwartzman RJ, Alexander GM, Grothusen JR, Paylor T, Reichenberger E, Perreault M. Outpatient intravenous ketamine for the treatment of complex regional pain syndrome: a double-blind placebo controlled study. *Pain.* 2009;147:107–115.
37. Muizelaar JP, Kleyer M, Hertogs IA, DeLange DC. Complex regional pain syndrome (reflex sympathetic dystrophy and causalgia): management with the calcium channel blocker nifedipine and/or the alpha-sympathetic blocker phenoxybenzamine in 59 patients. *Clin Neurol Neurosurg.* 1997;99:26–30.
38. Inchiosa MA Jr, Kizelshteyn G. Treatment of complex regional pain syndrome type I with oral phenoxybenzamine: rationale and case reports. *Pain Pract.* 2008;8:125–132.
39. Hannington-Kiff JG. Intravenous regional sympathetic block with guanethidine. *Lancet.* 1974;1:1019–1020.
40. Field J, Monk C, Atkins RM. Objective improvements in algodystrophy following regional intravenous guanethidine. *J Hand Surg Br.* 1993;18:339–342.
41. Paraskevas KI, Michaloglou AA, Briana DD, Samara M. Treatment of complex regional pain syndrome type I of the hand with a series of intravenous regional sympathetic blocks with guanethidine and lidocaine. *Clin Rheumatol.* 2006;25:687–693.
42. Kaplan R, Claudio M, Kepes E, Gu XF. Intravenous guanethidine in patients with reflex sympathetic dystrophy. *Acta Anaesthesiol Scand.* 1996;40:1216–1222.
43. Geertzen JH, de Bruijn H, de Bruijn-Kofman AT, Arendzen JH. Reflex sympathetic dystrophy: early treatment and psychological aspects. *Arch Phys Med Rehabil.* 1994;75:442–446.
44. Jadad AR, Carroll D, Glynn CJ, McQuay HJ. Intravenous regional sympathetic blockade for pain relief in reflex sympathetic dystrophy: a systematic review and a randomized, double-blind crossover study. *J Pain Symptom Manage.* 1995;10:13–20.
45. Ramamurthy S, Hoffman J. Intravenous regional guanethidine in the treatment of reflex sympathetic dystrophy/causalgia: a randomized, double-blind study. Guanethidine Study Group. *Anesth Analg.* 1995;81:718–723.
46. Livingstone JA, Atkins RM. Intravenous regional guanethidine blockade in the treatment of post-traumatic complex regional pain syndrome type 1 (algodystrophy) of the hand. *J Bone Joint Surg Br.* 2002;84:380–386.
47. Taskaynatan MA, Ozgul A, Tan AK, Dincer K, Kalyon TA. Bier block with methylprednisolone and lidocaine in CRPS type I: a randomized, double-blinded, placebocontrolled study. *Reg Anesth Pain Med.* 2004;29:408–412.
48. Connelly NR, Reuben S, Brull SJ. Intravenous regional anesthesia with ketorolac-lidocaine for the management of sympathetically-mediated pain. *Yale J Biol Med.* 1995;68:95–99.
49. Hanna MH, Peat SJ. Ketanserin in reflex sympathetic dystrophy. A double-blind placebo controlled cross-over trial. *Pain.* 1989;38:145–150.
50. Day M. Sympathetic blocks: the evidence. *Pain Pract.* 2008;8:98–109.
51. Hogan QH, Erickson SJ. MR imaging of the stellate ganglion: normal appearance. *AJR Am J Roentgenol.* 1992;158:655–659.
52. Linson MA, Leffert R, Todd DP. The treatment of upper extremity reflex sympathetic dystrophy with prolonged continuous stellate ganglion blockade. *J Hand Surg Am.* 1983;8:153–159.
53. Todd DP. Prolonged stellate block in treatment of reflex sympathetic dystrophy. *Agressologie.* 1991;32:5 Spec No:281–282.
54. Karakurum G, Pirbudak L, Oner U, Gulec A, Karadasli H, Satana T. Sympathetic blockade and amitriptyline in the treatment of reflex sympathetic dystrophy. *Int J Clin Pract.* 2003;57:585–587.
55. Ackerman WE, Zhang JM. Efficacy of stellate ganglion blockade for the management of type 1 complex regional pain syndrome. *South Med J.* 2006;99:1084–1088.
56. Glynn C, Casale R. Morphine injected around the stellate ganglion does not modulate the sympathetic nervous system nor does it provide pain relief. *Pain.* 1993;53:33–37.
57. Forouzanfar T, van Kleef M, Weber WE. Radiofrequency lesions of the stellate ganglion in chronic pain syndromes: retrospective analysis of clinical efficacy in 86 patients. *Clin J Pain.* 2000;16:164–168.
58. Sprague RS, Ramamurthy S. Identification of the anterior psoas sheath as a landmark for lumbar sympathetic block. *Reg Anesth.* 1990;15:253–255.
59. Redman DR, Robinson PN, Al-Kutoubi MA. Computerised tomography guided lumbar sympathectomy. *Anaesthesia.* 1986;41:39–41.
60. Konig CW, Schott UG, Pereira PL, et al. MR-guided lumbar sympathicolysis. *Eur Radiol.* 2002;12:1388–1393.
61. Kirvela O, Svedstrom E, Lundbom N. Ultrasonic guidance of lumbar sympathetic and celiac plexus block: a new technique. *Reg Anesth.* 1992;17:43–46.
62. Cameron HU, Park YS, Krestow M. Reflex sympathetic dystrophy following total knee replacement. *Contemp Orthop.* 1994;29:279–281.
63. Tran KM, Frank SM, Raja SN, El-Rahmany HK, Kim LJ, Vu B. Lumbar sympathetic block for sympathetically maintained pain: changes in cutaneous temperatures and pain perception. *Anesth Analg.* 2000;90:1396–1401.
64. Rocco AG. Radiofrequency lumbar sympatholysis. The evolution of a technique for managing sympathetically maintained pain. *Reg Anesth.* 1995;20:3–12.
65. Haynsworth RF Jr, Noe CE. Percutaneous lumbar sympathectomy: a comparison of radiofrequency denervation versus phenol neurolysis. *Anesthesiology.* 1991;74:459–463.
66. Manjunath PS, Jayalakshmi TS, Dureja GP, Prevost AT. Management of lower limb complex regional pain syndrome type 1: an evaluation of percutaneous radiofrequency thermal lumbar sympathectomy versus phenol lumbar sympathetic neurolysis—a pilot study. *Anesth Analg.* 2008;106:647–649, table of contents.
67. Price DD, Long S, Wilsey B, Rafii A. Analysis of peak magnitude and duration of analgesia produced by local anesthetics injected into sympathetic ganglia of complex regional pain syndrome patients. *Clin J Pain.* 1998;14:216–226.
68. Hartrick CT, Kovan JP, Naismith P. Outcome prediction following sympathetic block for complex regional pain syndrome. *Pain Pract.* 2004;4:222–228.
69. Carroll I, Clark JD, Mackey S. Sympathetic block with botulinum toxin to treat complex regional pain syndrome. *Ann Neurol.* 2009;65:348–351.
70. Robaina FJ, Rodriguez JL, de Vera JA, Martin MA. Transcutaneous electrical nerve stimulation and spinal cord stimulation for pain relief in reflex sympathetic dystrophy. *Stereotact Funct Neurosurg.* 1989;52:53–62.

71. Nnoaham KE, Kumbang J. Transcutaneous electrical nerve stimulation (TENS) for chronic pain. *Cochrane Database Syst Rev.* 2008;(3):CD003222.
72. Cruccu G, Aziz TZ, Garcia-Larrea L, et al. EFNS guidelines on neurostimulation therapy for neuropathic pain. *Eur J Neurol.* 2007;14:952–970.
73. KemLer MA, Barendse GA, van Kleef M, et al. Spinal cord stimulation in patients with chronic reflex sympathetic dystrophy. *N Engl J Med.* 2000;343:618–624.
74. KemLer MA, De Vet HC, Barendse GA, Van Den Wildenberg FA, Van Kleef M. The effect of spinal cord stimulation in patients with chronic reflex sympathetic dystrophy: two years' follow-up of the randomized controlled trial. *Ann Neurol.* 2004;55:13–18.
75. Forouzanfar T, KemLer MA, Weber WE, Kessels AG, van Kleef M. Spinal cord stimulation in complex regional pain syndrome: cervical and lumbar devices are comparably effective. *Br J Anaesth.* 2004;92:348–353.
76. KemLer MA, de Vet HC, Barendse GA, van den Wildenberg FA, van Kleef M. Effect of spinal cord stimulation for chronic complex regional pain syndrome Type I: five-year final follow-up of patients in a randomized controlled trial. *J Neurosurg.* 2008;108:292–298.
77. Simpson EL, Duenas A, Holmes MW, Papaioannou D, Chilcott J. Spinal cord stimulation for chronic pain of neuropathic or ischaemic origin: systematic review and economic evaluation. *Health Technol Assess.* 2009;13:iii, ix–iix, 1–154.
78. Hassenbusch SJ, Stanton-Hicks M, Schoppa D, Walsh JG, Covington EC. Long-term results of peripheral nerve stimulation for reflex sympathetic dystrophy. *J Neurosurg.* 1996;84:415–423.
79. Buschmann D, Oppel F. [Peripheral nerve stimulation for pain relief in CRPS II and phantom-limb pain]. *Schmerz.* 1999;13:113–120.
80. Mobbs RJ, Nair S, Blum P. Peripheral nerve stimulation for the treatment of chronic pain. *J Clin Neurosci.* 2007;14:216–221.
81. Gibbons JJ, Wilson PR, Lamer TJ, Elliott BA. Interscalene blocks for chronic upper extremity pain. *Clin J Pain.* 1992;8:264–269.
82. Ribbers GM, Geurts AC, Rijken RA, Kerkkamp HE. Axillary brachial plexus blockade for the reflex sympathetic dystrophy syndrome. *Int J Rehabil Res.* 1997;20:371–380.
83. Cooper DE, DeLee JC, Ramamurthy S. Reflex sympathetic dystrophy of the knee. Treatment using continuous epidural anesthesia. *J Bone Joint Surg Am.* 1989;71:365–369.
84. Rauck RL, Eisenach JC, Jackson K, Young LD, Southern J. Epidural clonidine treatment for refractory reflex sympathetic dystrophy. *Anesthesiology.* 1993;79:1163–1169, discussion 27A.
85. Buchheit T, Crews JC. Lateral cervical epidural catheter placement for continuous unilateral upper extremity analgesia and sympathetic block. *Reg Anesth Pain Med.* 2000;25:313–317.
86. Moufawad S, Malak O, Mekhail NA. Epidural infusion of opiates and local anesthetics for Complex Regional Pain Syndrome. *Pain Pract.* 2002;2:81–86.
87. Kanoff RB. Intraspinal delivery of opiates by an implantable, programmable pump in patients with chronic, intractable pain of nonmalignant origin. *J Am Osteopath Assoc.* 1994;94:487–493.
88. Lundborg C, Dahm P, Nitescu P, Appelgren L, Curelaru I. Clinical experience using intrathecal (IT) bupivacaine infusion in three patients with complex regional pain syndrome type I (CRPS-I). *Acta Anaesthesiol Scand.* 1999;43:667–678.
89. van Rijn MA, Munts AG, Marinus J, et al. Intrathecal baclofen for dystonia of complex regional pain syndrome. *Pain.* 2009;143:41–47.
90. Kapural L, Lokey K, Leong MS, et al. Intrathecal ziconotide for complex regional pain syndrome: seven case reports. *Pain Pract.* 2009;9:296–303.
91. Wulf H, Maier C. [Complications and side effects of stellate ganglion blockade. Results of a questionnaire survey]. *Anaesthesist.* 1992;41:146–151.
92. Ohno K, Oshita S. Transdiscal lumbar sympathetic block: a new technique for a chemical sympathectomy. *Anesth Analg.* 1997;85:1312–1316.
93. Turner JA, Loeser JD, Deyo RA, Sanders SB. Spinal cord stimulation for patients with failed back surgery syndrome or complex regional pain syndrome: a systematic review of effectiveness and complications. *Pain.* 2004;108:137–147.
94. Ishizuka K, Oaklander AL, Chiocca EA. A retrospective analysis of reasons for reoperation following initially successful peripheral nerve stimulation. *J Neurosurg.* 2007;106:388–390.
95. Hassenbusch SJ. Epidural and subarachnoid administration of opioids for nonmalignant pain: technical issues, current approaches and novel treatments. *J Pain Symptom Manage.* 1996;11: 357–362.
96. Carron H, Litwiller R. Stellate ganglion block. *Anesth Analg.* 1975;54:567–570.
97. Abdi S, Zhou Y, Patel N, Saini B, Nelson J. A new and easy technique to block the stellate ganglion. *Pain Physician.* 2004;7:327–331.
98. Erickson SJ, Hogan QH. CT-guided injection of the stellate ganglion: description of technique and efficacy of sympathetic blockade. *Radiology.* 1993;188:707–709.
99. Narouze S, Vydyanathan A, Patel N. Ultrasound-guided stellate ganglion block successfully prevented esophageal puncture. *Pain Physician.* 2007;10:747–752.
100. Hatangdi VS, Boas RA. Lumbar sympathectomy: a single needle technique. *Br J Anaesth.* 1985;57:285–289.

17 Herpes Zoster and Post-Herpetic Neuralgia

Albert J. M. van Wijck, Mark Wallace, Nagy Mekhail and Maarten van Kleef

Introduction

Herpes zoster is a viral condition that appears mainly in older people. The incidence in the Dutch population is 3.4 per 1,000 people per year; in a population above 75 years, this amounts to 9.1 per 1,000 people per year.[1] Approximately 20% of all people are affected by herpes zoster in their lifetime. In contrast to other herpes infections, herpes zoster relatively rarely relapses. Only a small percentage of patients are referred to the hospital by their family doctor, this mainly for the management of severe pain.

There is no consensus about the definition of PHN. It is usually defined as a zoster-related pain, which is still present 1 month after the development of the vesicles. Sometimes, however, this persists for a period of 3 to 6 months. In clinical trials, a cutoff pain intensity of 30 on a 100-point scale is used. Obviously, the definition used influences the reported incidence of PHN. This can vary from 10% to more than 50%. The risk for PHN increases with age. Figure 17.1 represents an estimated natural course of pain from herpes zoster and PHN.[2] Even though persistent serious pain occurs in a small percentage of herpes zoster patients, in those affected, it can have great consequences. Their quality of life is largely affected, not only directly by the pain, but also indirectly by fatigue, and diminished mobility and social contacts.

Pathophysiology

Herpes zoster develops through reactivation of the varicella zoster virus (VZV), which infects people during childhood and leads to chicken pox (varicella). After recovery from chicken pox, the virus becomes latent in the sensory ganglia. The specific immunity to the virus gradually reduces with age, and the virus can overcome this defense. The virus disperses from the ganglia via the axon to the epidermis where it causes the characteristic unilateral rash of herpes zoster in one or, sometimes, a few dermatomes. The vesicles contain a virus and are therefore infectious to people who have not yet built up a natural defense. It is possible for grandparents with herpes zoster to be the source of chicken pox for one of their grandchildren. The reverse, however, is impossible. To the contrary, contact with chicken pox can reinforce the resistance against VZV, which reduces the risk for herpes zoster.

The pain from herpes zoster primarily develops because of inflammation of the sensory nerves.

The pathophysiology of PHN is not fully understood yet. In any case, two processes play a role: sensitization and deafferentation. Peripheral sensitization develops because inflammatory mediators, such as substance P, histamines, and cytokines reduce the stimulus threshold of nociceptors. Central sensitization is related to an increasingly stronger response from nerve cells in the occipital horn to continuous stimulation by nociceptive C fibers. Deafferentation can develop through the replication of the virus in the cell and/or the subsequent inflammatory reaction. The swelling accompanying the inflammation can compress the sensory ganglion in the foramen intervertebrale, resulting in ischemia and nerve tissue damage. In addition, Schwann cell activation may play a role.[3]

Diagnosis

History

Patients with *herpes zoster* report unilateral symptoms in the dermatome that corresponds with the affected ganglion spinale (dorsal root ganglion, DRG). In addition to pain, there are paresthesias, dysesthesias, and pruritus. Likewise, general malaise, fever, and headache may occur. These symptoms usually begin as a prodrome a few days before the rash occurs.

Evidence-Based Interventional Pain Medicine: According to Clinical Diagnoses, First Edition. Edited by Jan Van Zundert, Jacob Patijn, Craig T. Hartrick, Arno Lataster, Frank J.P.M Huygen, Nagy Mekhail, Maarten van Kleef.

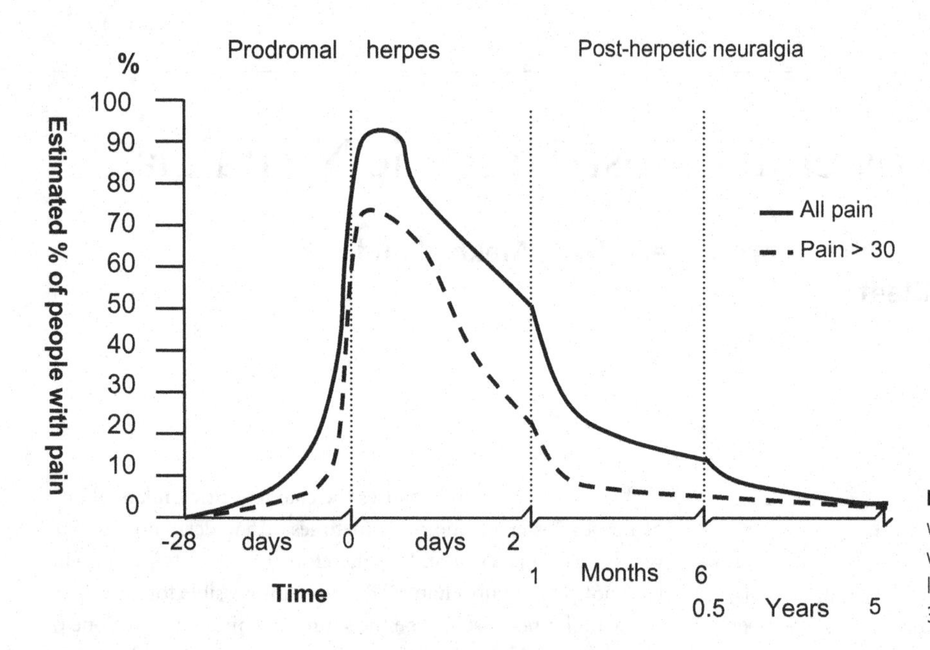

Figure 17.1. Estimate of the number of people with pain at different times after the development of vesicles. The solid line represents all pain; the dotted line represents all pain with an intensity of more than 30 on a scale from 0 to 100.

The dermatome-related pain is described as burning, throbbing, numbing, and itching.

Patients with *post-herpetic neuralgia* describe the pain as being sharp, burning, aching, or shooting that is constantly present in the dermatome that corresponds with the earlier rash. Stimulation-induced pain, allodynia, and hyperalgesia are often present. Wearing clothes can be very unpleasant or even painful for these patients.[4]

Physical examination

During the acute phase, the patient shows the typical rash with redness, papules, and vesicles in the painful dermatome. Healing vesicles show crust formation. The rash is generally unilateral and does not cross the midline of the body. Concomitant sensory defects such as hypesthesia, hyperalgesia, or allodynia frequently occur.[4] Motor defects are rare. The painful area can increase in size and exceed the limits of the affected dermatome with PHN.

Additional tests

Additional laboratory testing, such as polymerase chain reaction (PCR), can establish or rule out the presence of herpes simplex virus when there is an atypical presentation of epidermal rash and relapsing rash in the same area.

A strong increase of antibody titer can establish the so-called *zoster sine herpete* if dermatome-related pain is present without vesicles.

Differential diagnosis

During the prodromal phase and depending on the dermatome involved, there is a long list of possible differential diagnoses, such as coronary artery disease, pleurodynia, costochondritis (Tietze's syndrome), pericarditis, cholecystitis, acute abdominal diseases, disk diseases, nerve diseases, and myofascial pain. The diagnosis of herpes zoster is usually easy to establish as soon as the rash is visible. However, in 10% to 20% of the cases, it turns out that the clinical diagnosis of herpes zoster cannot be confirmed with serology or PCR.[5,6] The distinction from herpes simplex is somewhat difficult in young people. In contrast to herpes zoster, with herpes simplex, the rash can cross the midline of the body, and the symptoms can relapse. Contact dermatitis and epidermal rash resulting from food poisoning also must be ruled out.[4] The diagnosis of PHN is established based on medical history and physical examination. Scarring or vitiligo is often visible. If no vesicles are seen or documented, the distinction between PHN and other neuropathic pain syndromes cannot be established. The therapeutic consequences of this are, however, minimal.

Treatment options

The objectives of treating herpes zoster are: (1) the reduction of severity and duration of the pain; (2) the promotion of recovery of epidermal defects and prevention of secondary infections; and (3) the reduction or prevention of PHN.

The objective of the treatment of PHN is primarily pain alleviation and—directly related to that—an improvement of the quality of life.

Conservative management

Pharmacological treatment of herpes zoster

Antiviral medicines

Antiviral medicines, such as acyclovir, famcyclovir, or valacyclovir, should be started as quickly as possible after the onset of clinical signs. A review regarding the efficacy of this treatment showed that antiviral treatment, provided it starts within 72 hours after the development of the vesicles, accelerates the healing of the vesicles by approximately 1 to 2 days.[7] It is, however, doubtful if antiviral treatment can prevent PHN. There were four systematic reviews published with different conclusions.[8–11] Antiviral medicines reduce, at most to a slight degree, the incidence and duration of PHN.

Corticosteroids

A large randomized study compared the effect of acyclovir with that of a combination of acyclovir and prednisolone.[12] A significantly better pain reduction was gained in the first 2 weeks for the group that was treated with prednisolone.

Another study compared the effect of acyclovir– prednisolone, acyclovir–placebo, prednisolone–placebo, and placebo–placebo. The patients who received prednisolone alone or in combination with acyclovir had 2.3 times more chance of being free of pain after a month in comparison with the patients who did not receive prednisolone. The corticosteroid treatment, however, had no influence on the healing of the rash.[7]

A Cochrane review studied the effect of oral, intramuscular, or intravenous corticosteroid administration during the acute phase of herpes zoster for the prevention of PHN 6 months after the acute infection. Inadequate evidence was found to determine if corticosteroids are safe and effective in the prevention of PHN.[13]

Analgesics

There are no studies that evaluate the effect nonsteroidal anti-inflammatory drugs (NSAIDs) and/or paracetamol. Clinical experience has shown that these analgesics reduce acute pain. Opioids are effective in reducing acute herpes zoster pain.[14]

Local anesthetics

Clinical evidence and a single randomized controlled trial (RCT) show that topical lidocaine was effective without significant side effects.[15]

Adjuvant analgesics

A small placebo-controlled study showed that amitriptyline (25 mg a day taken for 90 days in the evening) during the acute phase of herpes zoster reduced the risk of PHN by 50%.[16] Another study showed that gabapentin reduced acute herpes zoster pain.[17]

Pharmacological treatment of PHN

To a great extent, the pharmacological treatment of PHN is the same as that for other neuropathic pain syndromes. However, a number of randomized controlled studies, meta-analyses, and systematic reviews mainly concentrate on PHN. The key findings are summarized below, although in the U.S.A., formally only lidocaine patch, pregabalin, gabapentin, and 8% capsaicin patch are approved by the Food and Drug Administration (FDA) for this indication.[18]

Tricyclic antidepressants

The most frequently used and investigated tricyclic antidepressant is amitriptyline. The collective data from different RCTs show a number needed to treat (NNT) of 2.6 in order to obtain significant pain relief. The most important products in the group of tricyclic antidepressants in addition to amitriptyline are nortriptyline and desipramine. All of these medicines provide comparable results.[19]

Antiepileptics

The effect of gabapentin with PHN was extensively investigated. A meta-analysis of two RCTs estimated a collective NNT of 4.4. In these studies, the average daily doses ranged from 1,800 mg to 2,400 mg.[19] An RCT compared gabapentin in doses up to 3,600 mg a day with placebo and found a significant pain reduction in the active group.[20]

Pregabalin is assumed to have a mechanism of action comparable to gabapentin. The only difference is that pregabalin is better absorbed with linear kinetics, making it easier to titrate. There are no meta-analyses regarding the effect of pregabalin, but different RCTs show that pregabalin, in daily doses of 150 to 600 mg, relieve pain better than placebo.[21]

Tramadol

A placebo-controlled study, in which 127 patients with PHN were treated with long-acting tramadol with a mean dose of 275 mg per day for 6 weeks, showed significant pain reduction and improvement of quality of life.[22]

Opioids

The role of opioids in the treatment of neuropathic pain was controversial for a long time. It has now been shown that oral and intravenous administration of opioids provide significant alleviation of neuropathic pain.[23–25] The analgesic effect of oxycodone for the treatment of PHN was evaluated in a double-blind randomized crossover study. The oxycodone treatment resulted in a significantly better reduction of pain (allodynia, steady state pain, and paroxysmal spontaneous pain).[24]

An NNT of 2.7 was found for the opioid treatment in an RCT. These data imply that opioids can be useful in the treatment of PHN.[26]

Local treatments

Local anesthetics

The 5% lidocaine patch was investigated for the treatment of PHN. An RCT and two open-label studies suggest a positive effect when the patch is applied to the most painful area.[18] A Cochrane review concluded that there is inadequate evidence to recommend topical lidocaine as first-line treatment for PHN, although some clinicians prefer lidocaine patch as first-line treatment.[27]

Capsaicin

A 6-week study with parallel groups followed by a 2-year open follow-up study showed that 0.075% capsaicin cream provides pain alleviation in 64% of the patients after 6 weeks in comparison with 25% of the patients who received placebo.[28] The application must take place three to four times a day and is often accompanied by local irritation and an unpleasant burning sensation, which can be a threat to treatment compliance. A single administration of a patch with 8% capsaicin on a lidocaine-pretreated skin proved effective in a large RCT.[29]

Other treatments

A number of other treatments are used, such as NMDA receptor antagonists, ketamine, topical NSAIDs and tricyclic antidepressants, Botox, vincristine iontophoresis, homeopathy, and acupuncture. There is, however, little evidence that justifies evaluation of the efficacy of these therapeutic options.[18]

Combination treatments

The different medicinal treatments are typically investigated and addressed individually. However, there is a tendency to implement more than one therapeutic class simultaneously in order to achieve an additive or synergistic effect. In a crossover trial with 41 patients, there was better analgesia with a combination of gabapentin and morphine in lower dosages than with monotherapy using either of these products alone.[30]

Interventional management

Epidural and paravertebral injection

Several studies have shown that epidural injections of corticosteroids with or without local anesthetics reduce the pain during the acute phase. The question is, however, if this treatment prevents PHN. An Italian study with 600 herpes zoster patients older than 55 years with a visual analog scale greater than 70 compared repeated injections of bupivacaine and methylprednisolone by way of an epidural catheter with intravenous prednisolone and acyclovir. The epidural injections were repeated every 3 to 4 days (for a maximum of 3 weeks) until the patient was free of pain. Analysis after 1 year of the 485 patients who completed the study showed an incidence of 22% of PHN in the group that received intravenous acyclovir and prednisolone, and 1.6% of PHN in the group that received epidural bupivacaine and methylprednisolone.[31] However, in view of the risk of major endocrinological adverse effects, this is not regular practice.

In many countries, it is more common to administer an epidural injection without a catheter.[32] In a multicenter study in the Netherlands, 598 patients age 50 or over with herpes zoster below dermatome C6 were studied to see if a single interlaminar epidural injection of bupivacaine (10 mg) and methylprednisolone (80 mg) had any supplemental value over the standard treatment with antiviral medicines and painkillers.[33] The epidural injection provided a reduction in pain for 1 month after the development of vesicles, but there was no long-term effect, such as the prevention of PHN. Interlaminar epidural injection was used in this randomized study. The transforaminal technique with radiography is an alternative approach to the epidural space where dispersion of the medication to the affected ganglion spinale (dorsal root ganglion, DRG) would possibly be better. A difficulty with this technique, especially in the thorax, is that the affected dermatome cannot be determined with certainty, which causes one to easily treat at a level too high or too low. There is no research of the efficacy of this technique for herpes zoster. Theoretically, a technique, which requires the needle position and the dispersion of the medication to be monitored, should preferably be executed under radiographic control. The value of epidural injections for the treatment of existing PHN has also not been investigated.

A recent single-center study randomized 132 herpes zoster patients to either standard therapy of oral antivirals and analgesics, or a series of 4 paravertebral injections of bupivacaine and methylprednisolone in addition to standard therapy. After 12 months, the incidence of PHN after paravertebral injections was 2% compared with 16% after standard therapy alone. The authors of the latter study concluded that a series of paravertebral blocks seemed to be effective in preventing PHN but that a larger multicenter trial was needed.

Intrathecal injection

A Japanese study of 277 patients with PHN reported a clearly positive effect from 4 weekly intrathecal injections of 60 mg of methylprednisolone dissolved in lidocaine 3%.[34] Complications such as hypotension, symptoms of nerve root irritation, and arachnoiditis were not reported. The authors received much criticism, and the treatment is scarcely applied. Confirmation of the results in an independent second study is necessary.[35]

Sympathetic nerve block

The value of a sympathetic nerve block for the treatment of acute herpes zoster is described mainly in retrospective studies. A small, randomized study compared bupivacaine administration with physiological saline solution. A review concluded that based on the retrospective data, there was evidence that sympathetic nerve block reduced the duration of acute herpes zoster pain.[36]

The influence of sympathetic nerve block on the risk for the development of PHN can be somewhat derived from the retrospective studies that investigated the acute phase. The results are difficult to interpret, because the time of the initial sympathetic nerve block and the evaluation criteria differ.[36]

Sympathetic nerve block for the treatment of PHN was evaluated mainly in retrospective studies as well. In a few studies, a reduction in pain was noted initially, but this effect was not maintained for the longer term. There is inadequate evidence for a long-term effect from sympathetic nerve block for PHN.

Spinal cord stimulation

Twenty-eight consecutive patients suffering PHN refractory to pharmacological treatment received spinal cord stimulation.[37] The majority of these patients had serious underlying pathology such as cardiovascular, respiratory, endocrine conditions, or cancer. A long-lasting alleviation of pain, the duration of which was not reported in the publication, was obtained in 23 patients, and the pain medication could be reduced or even completely terminated (inclusion criterion was a positive response to a sympathetic nerve block). This study has various weak points including the absence of a comparative treatment group, which is certainly most important. The type of patient suggests, however, that randomization was difficult for ethical and practical reasons.

Other interventional treatments

The effect on herpes zoster and PHN from subcutaneous injections, transcutaneous nerve stimulation, percutaneous nerve stimulation, and pulsed and conventional radiofrequency has not been established. There is minor anecdotal evidence for the efficacy of these techniques, and the risk for complications, such as exacerbation of the pain, is unknown. There are no controlled studies.

Complications of interventional management

Complications of epidural and paravetebral injections

Complications of injections include hematoma or abscess, but the risk is low. Corticosteroids can cause a temporary depression of the adrenal cortex. At the time of injection, cellular immunity has already reached its peak because the intervention takes place at least a few days after the onset of the condition. Therefore, an increased risk for the dissemination or spread of the infection because of the immunosuppressive activity of corticosteroids is not expected. The risk for infarction of the spinal cord by accidental intra-arterial injection exists with the transforaminal epidural method. It is known that application of methylprednisolone at cervical levels is associated with increased risk.[38,39] Steroid particles may cause an embolic process in the spinal cord. Pneumothorax is a risk with paravertebral injection.

Sympathetic nerve block complications

Vasodilatation occurs in extremities when sympathetic nerves are blocked. This can be accompanied by hypotension. The establishment of an intravenous access before treatment is recommended. Intermittent blood pressure should be measured in the recovery room. Intravenous crystalloids can potentially be administered depending on the blood pressure.

Orthostatic hypotension may occur when standing up quickly. After the recovery period, it is recommended that the patient take additional oral fluids during the first 24 hours. Another infrequent complication is damage to the nervus ilioinguinalis; more frequently (5% to 10%), the nervus genitofemoralis is injured. This can cause neuropathic deafferentation pain.

Complications of spinal cord stimulation

Spinal cord stimulation and the potential complications have been described in the chapter on complex regional pain syndrome (CRPS).[40]

Evidence for interventional management

The available evidence for interventional pain management techniques is summarized in Table 17.1

Table 17.1. Summary of evidence for interventional management of pain due to herpes zoster infection.

Technique	Evaluation
Interventional pain treatment of acute herpes zoster	
Epidural injections	2 B+
Sympathetic nerve block	2 C+
Prevention of PHN	
One-time epidural injection	2 B–
Repeated paravertebral injections	2 C+
Sympathetic nerve block	2 C+
Treatment of PHN	
Epidural injections	0
Sympathetic nerve block	2 C+
Intrathecal injection	?
Spinal cord stimulation	2 C+

PHN, post-herpetic neuralgia.

Recommendations

An epidural injection of corticosteroids with local anesthesia can be used in patients with pain caused by herpes zoster that has been inadequately reduced by pharmacological treatment. Monitoring of the correct needle position with radiography has a theoretical benefit compared with a "blind" technique. Effectiveness and safety of transforaminal epidural corticosteroid injections for patients with herpes zoster have not been investigated and should subsequently only be performed as part of a study. A series of paravertebral injections of corticosteroids with local anesthetics every second day for a week can be an alternative. A sympathetic nerve block can also be considered, particularly during the acute stage, but has no advantage over epidural corticosteroid with or without local anesthetic.

Sympathetic nerve block can be considered for patients suffering from PHN refractory to conservative treatment. For patients who have inadequate pain control with sympathetic nerve block, spinal cord stimulation can be considered. Considering the degree of invasiveness and the costs of this treatment, it should preferentially be performed in a study context.

Vaccination

The observation that herpes zoster mainly appears in older patients (>50 years) and that the reduced immunity is accompanied by an increased risk for herpes zoster stimulated research into a common factor in this risk population: This proved to be a reduced VZV-specific immune response. In addition, it was also observed that contact with children with varicella increased the immunity for varicella zoster. Theoretically, the immunity of adults for VZV is increased by a booster vaccination. With this method, the incidence of herpes zoster infections and, consequently, PHN is reduced.

The shingles prevention study included 38,456 adults who, *at random*, received a zoster vaccine or placebo. The participants in

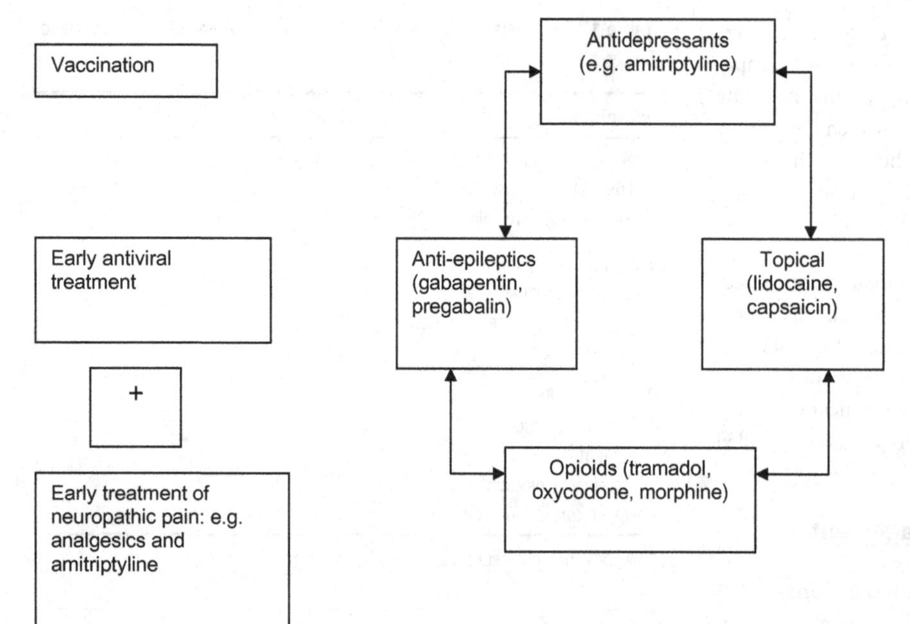

Figure 17.2. Algorithm for pharmacological prevention and treatment of post-herpetic neuralgia (from: Baron and Wasner,[35] with the publisher's permission).

the study were followed for an average duration of 3.13 years after vaccination.[5] The vaccination reduced the burden of illness in a significant way, which is a composite end point consisting of the incidence of herpes zoster, duration, and intensity of the pain. The burden of illness was 61.1% lower in the vaccination group compared with placebo. The incidence of PHN in the active group was 66.5% lower than in the placebo group. These findings certainly provide hope and place the prevention plan first in the treatment algorithm.

In an editorial on the prevention by epidural injection of post-herpetic neuralgia in the elderly study that was described above, Baron and Wasner[35] proposed the algorithm (Figure 17.2).

Clinical practice algorithm

Figure 17.3 illustrates the clinical practice algorithm for the management of PHN.

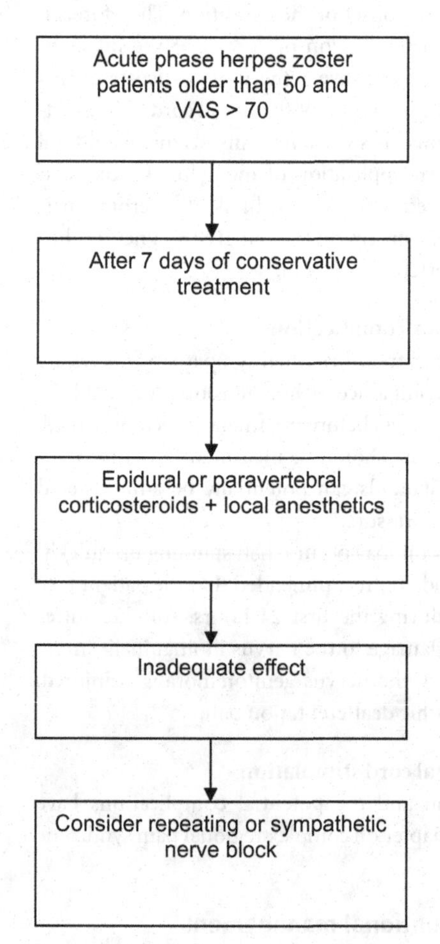

Figure 17.3. Clinical practice algorithm for anesthesiological treatment of post-herpetic neuralgia. VAS, visual analog scale.

Technique(s)

For the description of epidural injection, the reader is referred to the following chapters: cervical radicular,[41] thoracic pain,[42] and lumbosacral radicular pain.[43] Sympathetic nerve block is described in the chapter on CRPS.[40]

Summary

Herpes zoster is a condition that mainly affects older people. Its course is usually favorable, and the symptoms disappear spontaneously within a few weeks. Some patients, however, have prolonged pain: PHN. This persistent pain syndrome is difficult to treat. Interventional treatments, such as epidural injections of corticosteroids and local anesthetic drugs, have an effect on the acute pain but are of limited use in preventing PHN.

References

1. Opstelten W, Mauritz JW, de Wit NJ, van Wijck AJ, Stalman WA, van Essen GA. Herpes zoster and postherpetic neuralgia: incidence and risk indicators using a general practice research database. *Fam Pract.* 2002;19:471–475.
2. Van Wijck A. Postherpetic neuralgia. Phd Thesis, University Utrecht, Dept. Anesthesiology and Pain Management, Utrecht, 2006.
3. Bartley J. Post herpetic neuralgia, Schwann cell activation and vitamin D. *Med Hypotheses.* 2009;73:927–929.
4. Dworkin RH, Gnann JW Jr, Oaklander AL, Raja SN, Schmader KE, Whitley RJ. Diagnosis and assessment of pain associated with herpes zoster and postherpetic neuralgia. *J Pain.* 2008;9:S37–S44.
5. Oxman MN, Levin MJ, Johnson GR, et al. A vaccine to prevent herpes zoster and postherpetic neuralgia in older adults. *N Engl J Med.* 2005;352:2271–2284.
6. Opstelten W, van Loon AM, Schuller M, et al. Clinical diagnosis of herpes zoster in family practice. *Ann Fam Med.* 2007;5:305–309.
7. Opstelten W, Eekhof J, Neven AK, Verheij T. Treatment of herpes zoster. *Can Fam Physician.* 2008;54:373–377.
8. Lancaster T, Silagy C, Gray S. Primary care management of acute herpes zoster: systematic review of evidence from randomized controlled trials. *Br J Gen Pract.* 1995;45:39–45.
9. Jackson JL, Gibbons R, Meyer G, Inouye L. The effect of treating herpes zoster with oral acyclovir in preventing postherpetic neuralgia. A meta-analysis. *Arch Intern Med.* 1997;157:909–912.
10. Wood MJ, Kay R, Dworkin RH, Soong SJ, Whitley RJ. Oral acyclovir therapy accelerates pain resolution in patients with herpes zoster: a meta-analysis of placebo-controlled trials. *Clin Infect Dis.* 1996;22:341–347.
11. Alper BS, Lewis PR. Does treatment of acute herpes zoster prevent or shorten postherpetic neuralgia? *J Fam Pract.* 2000;49: 255–264.
12. Wood MJ, Johnson RW, McKendrick MW, Taylor J, Mandal BK, Crooks J. A randomized trial of acyclovir for 7 days or 21 days with and without prednisolone for treatment of acute herpes zoster. *N Engl J Med.* 1994;330:896–900.
13. He L, Zhang D, Zhou M, Zhu C. Corticosteroids for preventing postherpetic neuralgia. *Cochrane Database Syst Rev.* 2008;1: CD005582.
14. Dworkin RH, Barbano RL, Tyring SK, et al. A randomized, placebo-controlled trial of oxycodone and of gabapentin for acute pain in herpes zoster. *Pain.* 2009;142:209–217.
15. Lin PL, Fan SZ, Huang CH, et al. Analgesic effect of lidocaine patch 5% in the treatment of acute herpes zoster: a double-blind and vehicle-controlled study. *Reg Anesth Pain Med.* 2008;33:320–325.
16. Bowsher D. The effects of pre-emptive treatment of postherpetic neuralgia with amitriptyline: a randomized, double-blind, placebo-controlled trial. *J Pain Symptom Manage.* 1997;13:327–331.
17. Berry JD, Petersen KL. A single dose of gabapentin reduces acute pain and allodynia in patients with herpes zoster. *Neurology.* 2005;65:444–447.
18. Wu CL, Raja SN. An update on the treatment of postherpetic neuralgia. *J Pain.* 2008;9:S19–S30.
19. Hempenstall K, Nurmikko TJ, Johnson RW, A'Hern RP, Rice AS. Analgesic therapy in postherpetic neuralgia: a quantitative systematic review. *PLoS Med.* 2005;2:e164.
20. Rowbotham M, Harden N, Stacey B, Bernstein P, Magnus-Miller L. Gabapentin for the treatment of postherpetic neuralgia: a randomized controlled trial. *JAMA.* 1998;280:1837–1842.
21. Frampton JE, Foster RH. Pregabalin: in the treatment of postherpetic neuralgia. *Drugs.* 2005;65:111–118, discussion 119–120.
22. Boureau F, Legallicier P, Kabir-Ahmadi M. Tramadol in post-herpetic neuralgia: a randomized, double-blind, placebo-controlled trial. *Pain.* 2003;104:323–331.
23. Rowbotham MC, Reisner-Keller LA, Fields HL. Both intravenous lidocaine and morphine reduce the pain of postherpetic neuralgia. *Neurology.* 1991;41:1024–1028.
24. Watson CP, Babul N. Efficacy of oxycodone in neuropathic pain: a randomized trial in postherpetic neuralgia. *Neurology.* 1998;50: 1837–1841.
25. Watson CP, Moulin D, Watt-Watson J, Gordon A, Eisenhoffer J. Controlled-release oxycodone relieves neuropathic pain: a randomized controlled trial in painful diabetic neuropathy. *Pain.* 2003;105:71–78.
26. Raja SN, Haythornthwaite JA, Pappagallo M, et al. Opioids versus antidepressants in postherpetic neuralgia: a randomized, placebo-controlled trial. *Neurology.* 2002;59:1015–1021.
27. Khaliq W, Alam S, Puri N. Topical lidocaine for the treatment of postherpetic neuralgia. *Cochrane Database Syst Rev.* 2007;2: CD004846.
28. Watson CP, Tyler KL, Bickers DR, Millikan LE, Smith S, Coleman E. A randomized vehicle-controlled trial of topical capsaicin in the treatment of postherpetic neuralgia. *Clin Ther.* 1993;15:510–526.
29. Backonja M, Wallace MS, Blonsky ER, et al. NGX-4010, a high-concentration capsaicin patch, for the treatment of postherpetic neuralgia: a randomised, double-blind study. *Lancet Neurol.* 2008;7:1106–1112.
30. Gilron I, Bailey JM, Tu D, Holden RR, Weaver DF, Houlden RL. Morphine, gabapentin, or their combination for neuropathic pain. *N Engl J Med.* 2005;352:1324–1334.
31. Pasqualucci A, Pasqualucci V, Galla F, et al. Prevention of post-herpetic neuralgia: acyclovir and prednisolone versus epidural local anesthetic and methylprednisolone. *Acta Anaesthesiol Scand.* 2000; 44:910–918.
32. van Wijck A, Opstelten W, Van Essen GA. Herpes zoster en post-herpetische neualgie: beleid in eerste en tweede lijn. *NTTP.* 2003;22:18–21.
33. van Wijck AJ, Opstelten W, Moons KG, et al. The PINE study of epidural steroids and local anaesthetics to prevent postherpetic neuralgia: a randomised controlled trial. *Lancet.* 2006;367: 219–224.
34. Kotani N, Kushikata T, Hashimoto H, et al. Intrathecal methylprednisolone for intractable postherpetic neuralgia. *N Engl J Med.* 2000;343:1514–1519.
35. Baron R, Wasner G. Prevention and treatment of postherpetic neuralgia. *Lancet.* 2006;367:186–188.
36. Wu CL, Marsh A, Dworkin RH. The role of sympathetic nerve blocks in herpes zoster and postherpetic neuralgia. *Pain.* 2000;87: 121–129.
37. Harke H, Gretenkort P, Ladleif HU, Koester P, Rahman S. Spinal cord stimulation in postherpetic neuralgia and in acute herpes zoster pain. *Anesth Analg.* 2002;94:694–700, table of contents.

38. Scanlon GC, Moeller-Bertram T, Romanowsky SM, Wallace MS. Cervical transforaminal epidural steroid injections: more dangerous than we think? *Spine.* 2007;32:1249–1256.
39. Dawley JD, Moeller-Bertram T, Wallace MS, Patel PM. Intra-arterial injection in the rat brain: evaluation of steroids used for transforaminal epidurals. *Spine.* 2009;34:1638–1643.
40. van Eijs F, Stanton-Hicks M, Van Zundert J, et al. 16. Complex regional pain syndrome. *Pain Pract.* 2010 Aug 26. [Epub ahead of print].
41. Van Zundert J, Huntoon M, Patijn J, Lataster A, Mekhail N, van Kleef M. 4. Cervical radicular pain. *Pain Pract.* 2009;10:1–17.
42. van Kleef M, Stolker RJ, Lataster A, Geurts J, Benzon HT, Mekhail N. 10. Thoracic pain. *Pain Pract.* 2010;10:327–338.
43. Van Boxem K, Cheng J, Patijn J, et al. 11. Lumbosacral radicular pain. *Pain Pract.* 2010;10:339–358.

18 Painful Diabetic Polyneuropathy

Wouter Pluijms, Frank Huygen, Jianguo Cheng, Nagy Mekhail, Maarten van Kleef, Jan Van Zundert and Robert van Dongen

Introduction

In the industrialized world, polyneuropathy induced by diabetes mellitus (DM) is one of the most prevalent forms of neuropathy. An estimated 246 million people worldwide have DM, between 20 and 30 million of them are at risk for polyneuropathy. Diabetic neuropathy is related to the chronicity of diabetes and to the glycemic control. As the duration of diabetes is beyond our control, every effort should be directed toward tight control of the blood sugar level in order to provide any success to control or prevent painful diabetic neuropathy. The incidence of DM will probably continue to escalate because of increased risks for obesity. Inadequate treatment of DM in young people can lead to diabetic polyneuropathy within only a few months.[1] Polyneuropathy occurs to a lesser degree also with the non-insulin dependent form of DM, and proper monitoring and control of the glucose level is essential for prevention and intervention.[2]

Although diabetic polyneuropathy has been known since the second half of the 19th century, the pathophysiological mechanisms were only recently elucidated. Diabetic neuropathy can result from a direct toxic effect of glucose on nerve cells. Additionally, the damage of the nerve structures (central and peripheral) is accompanied by a microvascular dysfunction, which damages the vasa nervorum. The latter is secondary to the oxidative stress caused by hyperglycemia and other metabolic/homeostatic disorders. This is undoubtedly the reason why neuropathy and neuropathic pain occur more often in patients whose diabetes is chronically poorly controlled and who also have other cardiovascular risk factors such as hypertension and—more importantly—hyperlipidemia and especially dyslipidemia (high triglycerides and low high-density lipoprotein cholesterol). Actually, the same type of microvascular ischemia is responsible for diabetic retinopathy and nephropathy. Thus, the microvascular dysfunction, secondary to chronic hyperglycemia and dyslipidemia, is a common pathophysiological basis of microvascular complications with diabetes.

There are various types of diabetic neuropathy (Figure 18.1).[3] A *distal and symmetric peripheral neuropathy* is the most frequent form, which can be subdivided depending on the damaged fibers. These can be small and unmyelinated (C fibers) or thicker fibers that are more or less myelinated (Aδ, Aβ). Small fiber damage is thought to result in painful symptoms, leading to painful diabetic polyneuropathy (PDP). A *motor neuropathy*, caused by damage to the Aα fibers of motorneurons that innervate skeletal muscles, can lead to disorders in the ocular, facial, extremity, and trunk motor functions (i.e., mononeuropathy and multiplex neuropathy). An *autonomic neuropathy*, consequent to C fiber damage, causes dysfunction of the digestive and urogenital tracts, cardiac conduction system, and the cutaneous structures. Finally, an *inflammatory neuropathy*, caused by lymphoplasmacytic infiltration with damage to the vasa nervorum and to myelin, can result in a severe deterioration of the general condition.[3]

Diagnosis

History

More than 80% of the patients with DM-induced polyneuropathy have a distal, symmetric type of this condition. The symptoms usually present initially in the feet and gradually work their way up. This can be explained by the pathophysiological mechanism that the longest nerves are damaged first. This is also termed length dependent diabetic polyneuropathy (LDDP). The shorter fibers then follow, and in extreme situations, the trunk can also be affected. Sensory defects can usually be observed in the hands when the sensation around the knee is affected. Although there is an interval of a few years between the appearance of DM and the manifestation of LDDP, these symptoms can be the first symptoms of type 2 DM. The initial symptoms are: signs of diminished

Evidence-Based Interventional Pain Medicine: According to Clinical Diagnoses, First Edition. Edited by Jan Van Zundert, Jacob Patijn, Craig T. Hartrick, Arno Lataster, Frank J.P.M Huygen, Nagy Mekhail, Maarten van Kleef.

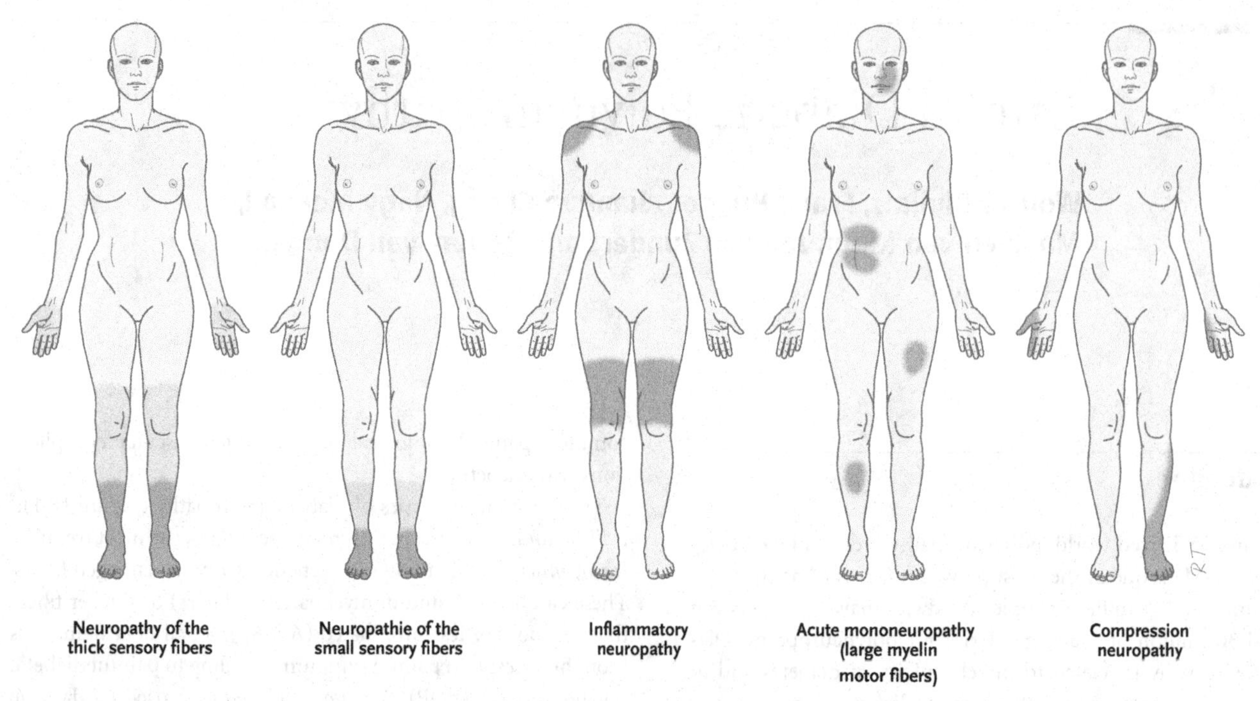

Figure 18.1. Various types of diabetic polyneuropathy (from: Vinik and Mehrabyan.[3] With the publisher's permission).

sensation; burning feet, which may occur particularly during the night and worsen when touched; and the sensation of tingling in the feet. Attacks of shooting pain also occur. If the pain is tolerable, variation in sensitivity can often already be established, which makes the diagnosis of diabetic polyneuropathy probable especially when this is accompanied by trophic disorders and poor wound healing. Generally speaking, recovery of sensory disturbances cannot be expected when LDDP has occurred. The polyneuropathy guideline of the Dutch Institute for Healthcare Improvement (*CBO*)[4] recommends the use of standardized questionnaires when taking the medical history. Two studies showed that the specificity of the medical history for patients with diabetic neuropathy is high (87%) and the sensitivity is 60% when these questionnaires are used.[5,6]

Physical examination

Medical history and a specific physical examination determine the diagnosis. A proper neurological evaluation is important as part of the additional clinical examination. The neurological examination should include at least the following: (1) examination of all qualities of somatosensory function, which should take symmetry and a distal-proximal gradient into account; (2) reflexes; and (3) muscle strength.[4] One of the signs is diminished sensitivity to a pinprick along with reduced temperature sensitivity (i.e., sensory examination of the tractus spinothalamicus). A decrease in proprioception may be manifested as, for example, abnormal sensation of position of the joints (toes, increased risk of falling), reduced pressure sensation, blunted two-point discrimination, or a reduced sense of vibration. Allodynia and hyperpathia can also occur.

Additional tests

Microscopic examination of nerves with diabetic polyneuropathy showed axonal degeneration and demyelination because of the dysfunction of the Schwann cells. Disturbances in the "repair process" of these defects lead to a disrupted function of the different cells and changes in their shape. This explains the occurrence of a reduction of the axonal conduction velocity and a conduction delay in the electromyogram (EMG), as a result of demyelination and degeneration of the thicker fibers. A "normal" EMG, however, does not rule out LDDP because this examination mainly measures the larger fibers and should therefore be combined with a proper clinical evaluation.[2] A reduction of the measured action potentials is also an indication for axonal degeneration which, however, might incidentally only occur later in the disease process. Motor disturbances because of diabetes are very rare. It is not a standard practice to stimulate the thinner, unmyelinated nociceptive fibers at much higher stimulation intensities during these types of examinations. Laser-evoked potentials[7] could possibly have an additional value. Because abnormal vascularization occurs, a so-called micro-angiopathy might also be detected at a microscopic level. This may further damage the already compromised nerve fibers. Finally, inflammatory processes may also play a role in the development of neurological defects. This is then called multifocal diabetic polyneuropathy.

The autonomic manifestations in DM may include orthostasis, rhythm disorders, gastroparesis, gastric function disorders, renal function disorders, and pupillary defects. *Autonomic neuropathy* may lead to a severe interaction with the pharmacological therapy of neuropathic pain. Finally, defects in the diameter of the spinal cord in DM could be a contributing factor for the occurrence of generalized neurological defects.[8]

Differential diagnosis

The presence of DM makes the diagnosis of polyneuropathy resulting from diabetes likely. Further examination for another possible cause of polyneuropathy is required if there are reports of the following alarm symptoms: acute onset, asymmetry, much pain, a particularly proximal condition, considerable motor symptoms, or rapid progression of motor symptoms.[4] Specific examinations can distinguish other forms of polyneuropathy. Specifically, toxic forms are of importance because of the possible reversibility.

Treatment options

Conservative management

Pharmacological treatment

Proper treatment of the underlying DM is essential to prevent the onset of painful symptoms. Spontaneous recovery is rare once the painful symptoms have developed. There are now several guidelines regarding pharmacological treatment of neuropathic pain, including PDP.[9–11] However, the result of pharmacological treatment has been disappointing so far, despite the fact that various new medications have been developed in recent years.

Aldose reductase inhibitors

The effects of drugs that specifically interfere with the causative mechanisms of DM, such as aldose reductase inhibitors, for example, have also been disappointing so far, specifically because of systemic toxicity and lack of potency.[12–16]

Neuropathic pain medications

To a large extent, the treatment of PDP is based on the drugs that are commonly used for neuropathic pain, such as anticonvulsants, antidepressants, and opioids. An international panel of experts recently established a guideline of drug treatment.[11] The objectives of the treatment of PDP are to (1) reduce peripheral sensitization, (2) reduce ectopic activity, (3) reduce central sensitization, (4) reduce central facilitation, and (5) increase central inhibition.

The effects of tricyclic antidepressants (TCAs) on PDP were demonstrated in a few, relatively small-sized studies.[10,17] Comparison of several pharmacological treatments for PDP indicates that TCAs are the most effective drugs. Their use in a sufficiently high dosage, however, is often limited because of a high frequency of adverse effects. Also, specific contraindications often prevent their use.

On the basis of published results, it seems that the selective serotonin and noradrenaline reuptake inhibitors (SNRIs) duloxetine and venlafaxine have a favorable effect on the pain complaints caused by PDP.[18,19] The effect of duloxetine was investigated in three studies. The pooled data showed that between 45% and 55% of the patients experienced more than 50% reduction of pain intensity, which was a higher percentage in comparison with the placebo group (25% to 28%). This yields a number needed to treat of 4.9 and 5.2, with a dosage of 120 mg and 60 mg per day, respectively. The SNRIs, however, also have many adverse effects, which frequently cause patients to discontinue the medication prematurely.

Several anticonvulsants were studied in PDP. Gabapentin was investigated in a number of large studies, in which only a small difference between treatments with gabapentin, amitriptyline, and placebo was found.[20,21] Data from six larger studies with pregabalin showed a pain reduction of more than 50% in 39% and 46% of the patients, with 300 mg and 600 mg per day, respectively, compared with an improvement of 22% in the placebo group.[22] Carbamazepine is less effective than pregabalin. Duloxetine, pregabalin, and gabapentin seem to have a similar effect on pain in PDP.

A limited number of studies have tested the application of local anesthetics in painful diabetic neuropathy. The efficacy of 5% lidocaine-medicated plaster treatment was compared with pregabalin in patients with diabetic peripheral neuropathy (DPN) in a two-stage, adaptive, randomized, controlled, open-label, multicenter trial.[23] In the interim analysis of the first stage of the two-stage adaptive trial, 91 patients with DPN were available for analysis. Overall, 65.3% of patients treated with the 5% lidocaine-medicated plaster and 62.0% receiving pregabalin responded to treatment with a reduction from baseline of ≥2 points or an absolute value of ≤4 points on the 11-item numerical rating scale of recalled average pain intensity over the last 3 days (NRS-3), after 4 weeks of treatment. Both treatments improved secondary endpoints: ≥30% and ≥50% reduction in NRS-3 scores, changes in neuropathic pain symptom inventory scores, and allodynia severity. Patients administering lidocaine plaster experienced fewer drug-related adverse events (3.9% vs. 39.2%) and there were substantially fewer discontinuations because of drug-related adverse events (1.3% vs. 20.3%). After 4 weeks, 5% lidocaine-medicated plaster treatment was associated with similar levels of analgesia in PDP patients but substantially fewer adverse events than with pregabalin.

The effectiveness of intravenous lidocaine in patients with intractable painful diabetic neuropathy was studied in a small double-blind, placebo-controlled crossover trial of two doses of intravenous lidocaine (5 and 7.5 mg/kg) vs. saline.[24] Infusions were administered in random order over 4 hours at four weekly intervals in 15 patients with painful DPN. Both doses of lidocaine significantly ($P < 0.05$ to $P < 0.001$ for the different measures) reduced the severity of pain compared with placebo. This reduction was present at both 14 and 28 days after the infusion. The qualitative nature of the pain was also significantly ($P < 0.05$ to $P < 0.01$) modified by lidocaine compared with placebo for up to 28 days. This study shows that intravenous lidocaine ameliorates pain in some diabetic participants with intractable neuropathic pain, who have failed to respond to, or are intolerant of, available conventional therapy.

A favorable effect of opioid agonists on PDP was demonstrated in three studies.[25–27] Opioids are frequently used as supplementary therapy together with another pharmacological approach. The algorithm for pharmacological treatment of diabetic polyneuropathy is represented in Figure 18.2.

Based on a recently published National Institute for Health and Clinical Excellence guidelines,[28] duloxetine is the first-line agent of choice. If duloxetine is contraindicated, treatment should be initiated with amitriptyline. If first-line therapy does not result in sufficient pain relief, treatment should be continued with amitriptyline, pregabalin, or a combination of both. Third-line treatment options include tramadol and topical lidocaine. In refractory cases, intravenous lidocaine infusion may be considered as part of an investigational trial.

Interventional management

Neurostimulation can be considered if an adequate pharmacological treatment does not lead to sufficient pain reduction or it is accompanied by serious adverse effects. So far, there are four studies that specifically investigate the treatment of diabetic polyneuropathy by means of spinal cord stimulation. The first is a retrospective analysis of 30 patients who were treated for peripheral neuropathy. In four of these patients, the etiology of the pain was diabetic neuropathy.[29] They all had good pain relief in the short term. The pain relief was maintained in the long term for three of the four patients. Despite that, the follow-up period was not described separately for this subgroup; the entire patient group was followed for a mean duration of 87 months.

The second and third studies described diabetes patients who had inadequate pain relief with conventional treatments.[30,31] The trial period for spinal cord stimulation consisted of a crossover between a placebo and active stimulator. The standardized measurement instruments were used in different evaluation points in time with the stimulator "on" or "off." A significant improvement was reported with the generator "on" whereas no significant differences were found with the generator "off," in comparison with the baseline evaluations. A long-term effect was reported.[31] The fourth study reported the results of spinal cord stimulation in diabetic neuropathy patients suffering from PDP that was unresponsive to conventional treatment.[32] Trial stimulation resulted in ≥50% pain relief in 82% of patients. In long-term follow-up, clinically relevant pain relief was achieved in 64% of patients at 1 year and 60% of patients at 2.5 years. These studies show that spinal

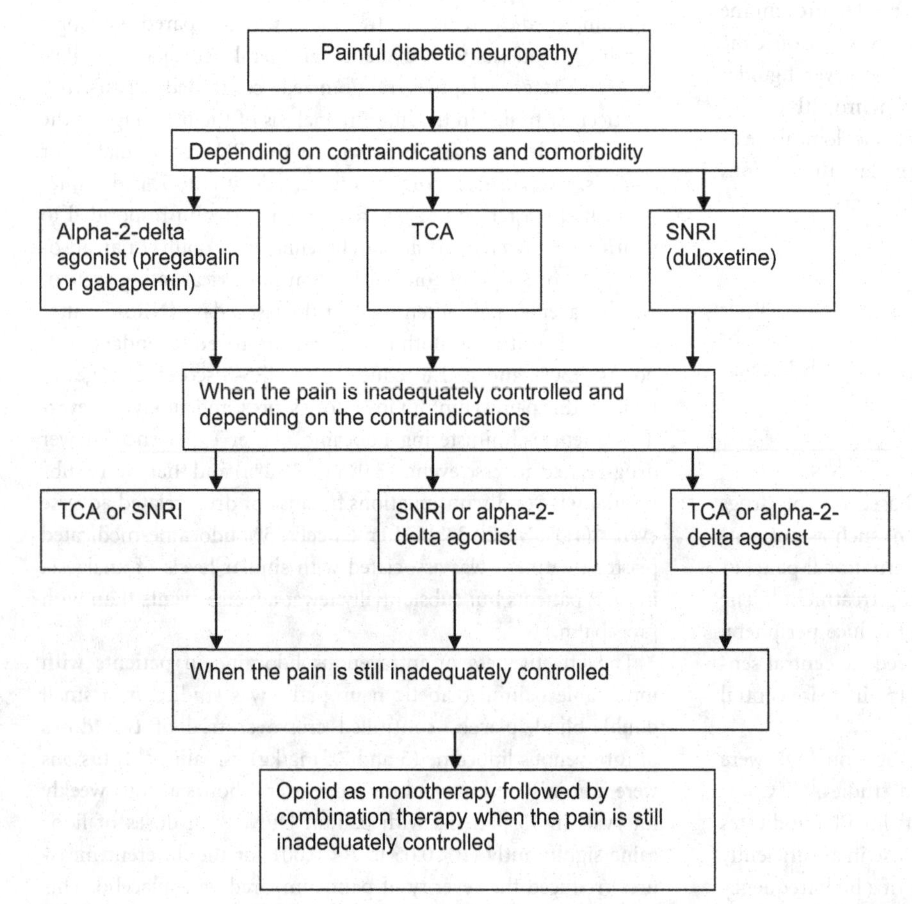

Figure 18.2. Algorithm for the pharmacological treatment of diabetic polyneuropathy (from: Jensen et al.[11] With the publisher's permission). SNRI, serotonin and noradrenaline reuptake inhibitor; TCA, tricyclic antidepressants.

Table 18.1. Summary of the evidence for interventional management of painful diabetic polyneuropathy.

Technique	Evaluation
Spinal cord stimulation	2 C+

cord stimulation can potentially provide pain alleviation for a longer term in patients with PDP. However, vigorously designed, controlled studied are needed to demonstrate a long-term efficacy in pain reduction, functional improvement, and medication sparing. It is also important to be able to predict in which patient groups or at what stage of the disease process spinal cord stimulation is most beneficial.

Complications of interventional management

Complications associated with the device of spinal cord stimulation include lead migration (14%), lead breakage (7%), implanted pulse generator migration (1%), and loss of therapeutic effect/paresthesias.[33] Technical adverse events can be solved by lead replacement, repositioning of the pulse generator, or reprogramming of stimulation parameters. Medical adverse events of spinal cord stimulation include infection or wound breakdown (10%), pain at pulse generator implantation site (12%), and fluid collection at pulse generator implantation site (5%).[33] Infection can be treated with antibiotics and removal of the implant.

Evidence for interventional management

The summary of the evidence for the interventional management of PDP is given in Table 18.1.

Recommendations

Proper monitoring and control of the glucose levels is the essential treatment for PDP. If drug treatment fails, spinal cord stimulation can be considered as part of a study, because of its invasiveness and the costs.

Clinical practice algorithm

Figure 18.3 represents the treatment algorithm for PDP based on the available evidence.

Technique(s)

We refer to the article in this series on "Complex Regional Pain Syndrome" for the technique.[34]

Summary

DM type 1 and type 2 can lead to a painful polyneuropathy.

The first line of treatment consists of pharmacological management with well-studied neuropathic pain medications.

If pharmacological treatment fails, spinal cord stimulation as part of a study can be considered.

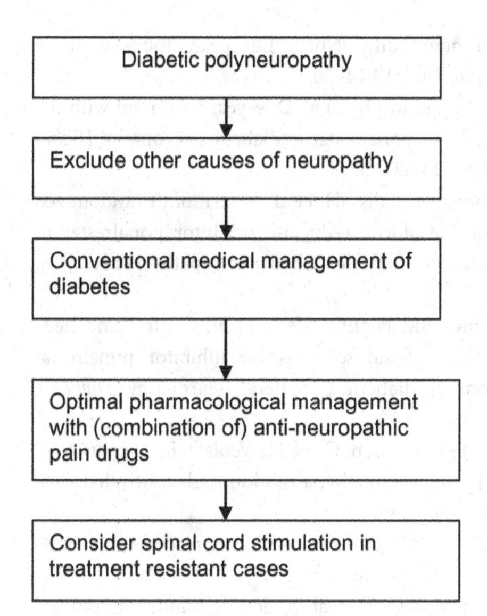

Figure 18.3. Clinical practice algorithm for the treatment of diabetic polyneuropathy.

References

1. Said G. Diabetic neuropathy—a review. *Nat Clin Pract Neurol.* 2007;3:331–340.
2. Partanen J, Niskanen L, Lehtinen J, et al. Natural history of peripheral neuropathy in patients with non-insulindependent diabetes mellitus. *N Engl J Med.* 1995;333:89–94.
3. Vinik AI, Mehrabyan A. Diabetic neuropathies. *Med Clin North Am.* 2004;88:947–999.
4. van Doorn P, van Engelen B. *Richtlijn Polyneuropatie.* Alphen aan den Rijn: Van Zuiden Communications BV; 2005.
5. Franse LV, Valk GD, Dekker JH, et al. "Numbness of the feet" is a poor indicator for polyneuropathy in type 2 diabetic patients. *Diabet Med.* 2000;17:105–110.
6. Gentile S, Turco S, Corigliano G, et al. Simplified diagnostic criteria for diabetic distal polyneuropathy. Preliminary data of a multicentre study in the Campania region. S.I.M.S.D.N. Group. *Acta Diabetol.* 1995;32:7–12.
7. Cruccu G, Anand P, Attal N, et al. EFNS guidelines on neuropathic pain assessment. *Eur J Neurol.* 2004;11:153–162.
8. Eaton SE, Harris ND, Rajbhandari SM, et al. Spinalcord involvement in diabetic peripheral neuropathy. *Lancet.* 2001;358:35–36.
9. Attal N, Cruccu G, Haanpaa M, et al. EFNS guidelines on pharmacological treatment of neuropathic pain. *Eur J Neurol.* 2006;13:1153–1169.
10. Finnerup NB, Otto M, McQuay HJ, et al. Algorithm for neuropathic pain treatment: an evidence based proposal. *Pain.* 2005;118:289–305.
11. Jensen TS, Backonja MM, Hernandez Jimenez S, et al. New perspectives on the management of diabetic peripheral neuropathic pain. *Diab Vasc Dis Res.* 2006;3:108–119.
12. Boulton AJ, Levin S, Comstock J. A multicentre trial of the aldose-reductase inhibitor, tolrestat, in patients with symptomatic diabetic neuropathy. *Diabetologia.* 1990;33:431–437.
13. Macleod AF, Boulton AJ, Owens DR, et al. A multicentre trial of the aldose-reductase inhibitor tolrestat, in patients with symptomatic

diabetic peripheral neuropathy. North European Tolrestat Study Group. *Diabete Metab.* 1992;18:14–20.

14. Ziegler D, Mayer P, Rathmann W, et al. One-year treatment with the aldose reductase inhibitor, ponalrestat, in diabetic neuropathy. *Diabetes Res Clin Pract.* 1991;14:63–73.
15. Krentz AJ, Honigsberger L, Ellis SH, et al. A 12-month randomized controlled study of the aldose reductase inhibitor ponalrestat in patients with chronic symptomatic diabetic neuropathy. *Diabet Med.* 1992;9:463–468.
16. Florkowski CM, Rowe BR, Nightingale S, et al. Clinical and neurophysiological studies of aldose reductase inhibitor ponalrestat in chronic symptomatic diabetic peripheral neuropathy. *Diabetes.* 1991;40:129–133.
17. Sindrup SH, Bach FW, Madsen C, et al. Venlafaxine versus imipramine in painful polyneuropathy: a randomized, controlled trial. *Neurology.* 2003;60:1284–1289.
18. Goldstein DJ, Lu Y, Detke MJ, et al. Duloxetine vs. placebo in patients with painful diabetic neuropathy. *Pain.* 2005;116:109–118.
19. Raskin J, Pritchett YL,Wang F, et al. A double-blind, randomized multicenter trial comparing duloxetine with placebo in the management of diabetic peripheral neuropathic pain. *Pain Med.* 2005;6: 346–356.
20. Backonja M, Beydoun A, Edwards KR, et al. Gabapentin for the symptomatic treatment of painful neuropathy in patients with diabetes mellitus: a randomized controlled trial. *JAMA.* 1998;280: 1831–1836.
21. Morello CM, Leckband SG, Stoner CP, et al. Randomized double-blind study comparing the efficacy of gabapentin with amitriptyline on diabetic peripheral neuropathy pain. *Arch Intern Med.* 1999;159:1931–1937.
22. Griesing T, Freeman R, Rosenstock J. Efficacy, safety, and tolerability of pregabalin treatment for diabetic peripheral neuropathy: findings from 6 randomized controlled trials. *Diabetologia.* 2005; 48:A351.
23. Baron R, Mayoral V, Leijon G, et al. Efficacy and safety of 5% lidocaine (lignocaine) medicated plaster in comparison with pregabalin in patients with postherpetic neuralgia and diabetic polyneuropathy: interim analysis from an open-label, two-stage adaptive, randomized, controlled trial. *Clin Drug Investig.* 2009;29:231–241.
24. Viola V, Newnham HH, Simpson RW. Treatment of intractable painful diabetic neuropathy with intravenous lignocaine. *J Diabetes Complications.* 2006;20:34–39.
25. Eisenberg E, McNicol ED, Carr DB. Efficacy and safety of opioid agonists in the treatment of neuropathic pain of nonmalignant origin: systematic review and meta-analysis of randomized controlled trials. *JAMA.* 2005;293:3043–3052.
26. Gimbel JS, Richards P, Portenoy RK. Controlledrelease oxycodone for pain in diabetic neuropathy: a randomized controlled trial. *Neurology.* 2003;60:927–934.
27. Harati Y, Gooch C, Swenson M, et al. Double-blind randomized trial of tramadol for the treatment of the pain of diabetic neuropathy. *Neurology.* 1998;50:1842–1846.
28. NICE. Neuropathic pain: the pharmacological management of neuropathic pain in adults in non-specialist settings. *NICE Guidelines* 2010;96:1–155.
29. Kumar K, Toth C, Nath RK. Spinal cord stimulation for chronic pain in peripheral neuropathy. *Surg Neurol.* 1996;46:363–369.
30. Tesfaye S, Watt J, Benbow SJ, et al. Electrical spinalcord stimulation for painful diabetic peripheral neuropathy. *Lancet.* 1996;348:1698–1701.
31. Daousi C, Benbow SJ, MacFarlane IA. Electrical spinal cord stimulation in the long-term treatment of chronic painful diabetic neuropathy. *Diabet Med.* 2005;22:393–398.
32. de Vos CC, Rajan V, Steenbergen W, et al. Effect and safety of spinal cord stimulation for treatment of chronic pain caused by diabetic neuropathy. *J Diabetes Complications.* 2009;23:40–45.
33. Kumar K, Taylor RS, Jacques L, et al. The effects of spinal cord stimulation in neuropathic pain are sustained: a 24-month follow-up of the prospective randomized controlled multicenter trial of the effectiveness of spinal cord stimulation. *Neurosurgery.* 2008;63:762–770, discussion 770.
34. van Eijs F, Stanton-Hicks M, Van Zundert J, et al. Evidence-based interventional pain medicine according to clinical diagnoses: 16. Complex regional pain syndrome. *Pain Pract.* 2010;10. [Epub ahead of print; 26 Aug 2010], DOI: 10.1111/j.1533-2500.2010.00388.x.

19 Carpal Tunnel Syndrome

Jacob Patijn, Ricardo Vallejo, Markus Janssen, Frank Huygen, Arno Lataster, Maarten van Kleef and Nagy Mekhail

Introduction

Carpal tunnel syndrome (CTS) is a neurological disorder characterized by paresthesias, pain and numbness in the hands due to lesions (compression) and/or dysfunction of the nervus medianus.

In the Netherlands, the prevalence of CTS is estimated to be 9% in females and 0.6% in male. Incidence figures elsewhere show an overall incidence of 276/100,000 man-years.[1] For females, the incidence amounts to 506/100,000 man-years, while for males, it is 139/100,000 man-years, with a male/female ratio of 1:3.6. Although uncommon in children or adolescents, the disorder could be caused by trauma or by an autosomal dominant hereditary factor and mucopolysaccharidoses in children. CTS is most prevalent between the ages of 40 to 60 years. Risk factors are obesity, diabetes, pregnancy, menopause, ovariectomy, and hysterectomy.[2] CTS is frequently accompanied by hypothyroidism and rheumatoid arthritis.[2]

The carpal tunnel is a passage at the palmar side of the wrist; its floor is defined by a row of carpal bones and its roof by the ligamentum carpi transversum. The nervus medianus travels between these structures. The nervus medianus may become trapped in the carpal tunnel as a result of edema, inflammation of synovial sheaths, tumors or the deposition of metabolic products. In addition, the nervus medianus may become compressed when the shape of the carpal tunnel changes.[3] This happens in conjunction with osteoarthritis, rheumatoid arthritis, acromegaly, or after trauma. CTS may also be related to repetitive strain injury (RSI), an injury caused by repeated movement of a particular body part often seen in workers whose physical routine is unvaried.

Treatment of RSI usually begins with attempts to change the conditions that caused the injury. Often, exercises and anti-inflammatory drugs are prescribed; in some cases surgery is necessary. Many workers' compensation cases and lawsuits relating to RSI have been brought against employers and product manufacturers. To avoid the high costs of RSI, some businesses have introduced ergonomic workstations and enforced rest periods.

In the majority of cases, the etiology of CTS is unknown; therefore, the pathophysiology of this disorder is also unclear. The same holds true for hormonal disorders related to CTS for example in patients with hypothyroidism and in postmenopausal patients. In pregnant women, fluid retention is thought to cause compression symptoms. Congenital and acquired structural changes of the carpal tunnel result in constriction and therefore in compression of the nervus medianus.

Diagnosis

History

In cases of CTS, the symptoms generally consist of unilateral nocturnal paresthesias in the dermatome of the nervus medianus (digits I to III including, and half of digit IV). In addition, there may be pain in the hand, wrist, and forearm. If a patient awakens because of CTS, waving the hand may bring some pain relief. Atypical localization of the tingling sensations (ulnar area) is also seen; in these cases, the diagnosis CTS may be supported by the intermittent nature of the symptoms and by factors that exacerbate or relieve it. CTS is mainly unilateral, but it may be bilateral as well. Later on, the symptoms may occur during the day and may be accompanied by a subjective loss of strength.

Physical examination

Generally, the diagnosis CTS can be based on the typical pattern of symptoms that emerges when the patient's history is taken.[4] With regard to physical examination, the neurological defects are often not definitive. The same applies to various provocation tests (Hoffmann–Tinel, Phalen's test, etc.).

Evidence-Based Interventional Pain Medicine: According to Clinical Diagnoses, First Edition. Edited by Jan Van Zundert, Jacob Patijn, Craig T. Hartrick, Arno Lataster, Frank J.P.M Huygen, Nagy Mekhail, Maarten van Kleef.

Additional tests

Nerve conduction examination of the nervus medianus at both hands of the patient can be considered[2] and is the best predictor of symptom severity and functional status in idiopathic CTS.[5] Presently, magnetic resonance imaging (MRI) of the wrist does not provide additional diagnostic information in cases of CTS,[2,6] but can predict surgical benefit independently of nerve conduction studies.[7] In patients with a clinical diagnosis of CTS, the accuracy of sonography is similar to that for EMG.[8] When structural defects in the wrist are suspected, a radiograph of the wrist, MRI scan, or ultrasound scan may be considered.[2]

Differential diagnosis

With respect to differential diagnosis in patients with CTS, the following disorders should be considered: compression of the nervi digitales of the nervus medianus, proximal trauma, neuropathy of the nervus ulnaris, defects of the plexus cervicalis, defects of cervical spinal roots, polyneuropathy, neurovascular compression syndromes in the shoulder, multiple sclerosis and processes in the spinal cord.

Treatment options

Conservative management

In the majority of CTS patients, the disorder has a benign course and/or causes little functional hindrance.[2] When CTS occurs during pregnancy the symptoms may resolve after birth.[9] The choice between conservative and surgical treatment is determined by the severity of the symptoms and physical limitations.[2] In pregnant women, conservative treatment by means of a splint is preferred.[2,10]

Recommended conservative treatments include behavior modification, medications including anti-inflammatory drugs and analgesics, immobilization via splinting or bracing, physical and occupational therapies, oral corticosteroids, and ultrasound.[11] There are indications that local injections with corticosteroids are less effective in the long-term than surgical interventions. The surgical option, open or endoscopic carpal tunnel surgery entails greater risks of complications.[2] However, if the symptoms are most severe and if daily activities have become limited, surgical intervention is indicated.[12]

Interventional management

Local injections of corticosteroids

The guidelines of the Dutch Institute for Health Care Improvement (CBO) recommend local injections with methylprednisolone 40 mg or a combination of 25 mg hydrocortisone and 10 mg lidocaine. The Cochrane review identified two good quality randomized controlled trials, which showed that local injections with corticosteroids were clinically more effective than placebo during study periods of 4 weeks or less. Local injections with corticosteroids also were more effective than oral corticosteroids.[13,14]

Table 19.1. Summary of the evidence for interventional management of carpal tunnel syndrome.

Technique	Evaluation
Local injections with corticosteroids	1B+
Pulsed radiofrequency treatment nervus medianus	0

Pulsed radiofrequency of the nervus medianus

A single case of pulsed radiofrequency (PRF) treatment of the nervus medianus has been described in a patient with recurring CTS due to scar formation after two previous operations for CTS symptoms. Symptoms decreased by 70%, and this effect lasted for 12 weeks.[15] PRF—possibly under ultrasound guidance—could be considered, preferably in a study context. Without further evidence regarding the efficacy PRF for CTS, no recommendation for PRF in the treatment of CTS can be advanced.

Complications of interventional management

One of the major complications of steroid injection in CTS is iatrogenic injury to the nervus medianus. The safest location for a CTS injection is unclear. Some authors recommend steroid injection to be performed through the retinaculum flexorum.[16]

Evidence for interventional management

The available evidence for interventional pain management techniques is summarized in Table 19.1.

Recommendations

In cases of CTS, the initial choice is conservative treatment, including behavior modification, medications including anti-inflammatory drugs and analgesics, immobilization via splinting or bracing, physical and occupational therapies, oral corticosteroids, and ultrasound. If the patient experiences hindrance of normal daily activity, interventional treatment with local injections with corticosteroids may be indicated. The longterm effect of this treatment has not been proven. PRF treatment of the nervus medianus should only be considered in a study context. In cases of severe physical limitations, surgical treatment of CTS is preferred.

Clinical practice algorithm

Figure 19.1 illustrates the clinical practice algorithm for the management of CTS.

Technique(s)

Injections with corticosteroids

The recommended techniques for corticosteroid injections have been described in the guidelines of the Dutch Institute for Health Care Improvement. The injections are administered in or just proximal of the carpal tunnel, 3 to 4 cm proximally of the distal wrist fold.[2]

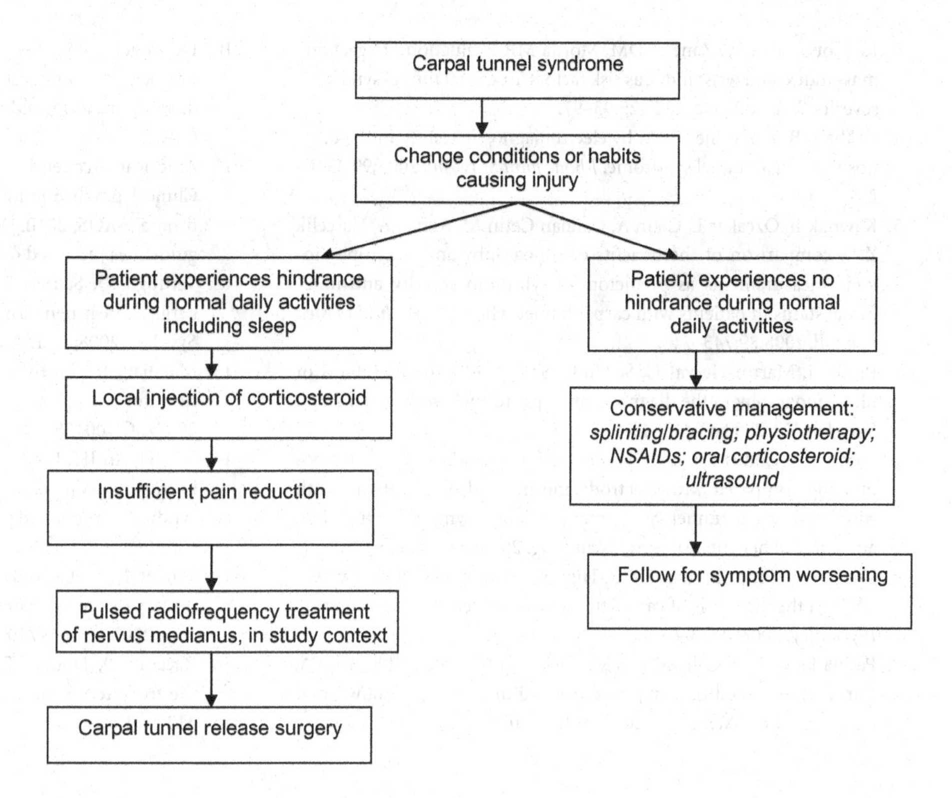

Figure 19.1. Clinical practice algorithm for the treatment of carpal tunnel syndrome.

Injection in the tunnel: in these cases, the needle is inserted near the distal wrist fold at the ulnar side of the tendon of the musculus palmaris longus. The wrist is kept in slight dorsiflexion. The needle is inserted in the direction of the base of the middle finger at an angle of approximately 45° so that it reaches the carpal tunnel through the ligamentum carpi transversum. The needle should be retracted and reinserted 1 cm more proximally if the patient's fingers start tingling.

Alternatively, the needle can be inserted initially either in a more ulnar position in the tendon of the musculus palmaris longus or between the tendons of the musculus palmaris longus and the musculus flexor carpi radialis. In the latter case, the needle should be inserted at an angle of 30°. When the needle tip is in the carpal tunnel, rather than in a tendon, the needle and injection will meet minimal resistance.[2]

During injection proximal of the carpal tunnel, the risk of damaging the nervus medianus is smaller if the needle is inserted 3 cm proximal of the distal wrist fold. This is because at that site the nerve is less fixated (more mobile) than it is inside the carpal tunnel. The 3-cm-long injection needle is inserted in a more ulnar position in relation to the tendon of the musculus palmaris longus or between the tendons of the musculus palmaris longus and the musculus flexor carpi radialis at an angle of 10° to 20°, toward the third interosseous space. The corticosteroid injected proximal to the tunnel reaches the tunnel through diffusion. Massaging the injection site is recommended as this facilitates spread.[2]

Pulsed radiofrequency treatment of the nervus medianus

In the only available case report, a patient received three ultrasound-guided PRF treatments, during the same session, at (1) the position of the anterior surface, (2) the medial aspect, and (3) the posterior surface of the nervus medianus. During each treatment, PRF current was applied for 90 seconds.

Summary

Carpal tunnel syndrome is a common disorder. In the majority of cases, patients with CTS can be diagnosed by means of appropriate history taking, and by physical / neurological examination. Nerve conduction tests of the nervus medianus are the most important additional examinations. Which treatment is preferred depends on the severity of the symptoms and the limitations they cause. If few limitations are present, treatment by means of a splint or through corticosteroid injections is preferred.

References

1. Becker J, Nora DB, Gomes I, et al. An evaluation of gender, obesity, age and diabetes mellitus as risk factors for carpal tunnel syndrome. *Clin Neurophysiol.* 2002;113:1429–1434.
2. Nederlandse Vereninging voor Neurologie. *Diagnostiek en behandeling van het carpale-tunnelsyndroom.* Alphen aan den Rijn: CBO; 2005.

3. Kouyoumdjian JA, Zanetta DM, Morita MP. Evaluation of age, body mass index, and wrist index as risk factors for carpal tunnel syndrome severity. *Muscle Nerve.* 2002;25:93–97.
4. Graham B. The value added by electrodiagnostic testing in the diagnosis of carpal tunnel syndrome. *J Bone Joint Surg Am.* 2008;90:2587–2593.
5. Kaymak B, Ozcakar L, Cetin A, Candan Cetin M, Akinci A, Hascelik Z. A comparison of the benefits of sonography and electrophysiologic measurements as predictors of symptom severity and functional status in patients with carpal tunnel syndrome. *Arch Phys Med Rehabil.* 2008;89:743–748.
6. Pinilla I, Martin-Hervas C, Sordo G, Santiago S. The usefulness of ultrasonography in the diagnosis of carpal tunnel syndrome. *J Hand Surg Eur Vol.* 2008;33:435–439.
7. Jarvik JG, Comstock BA, Heagerty PJ, et al. Magnetic resonance imaging compared with electrodiagnostic studies in patients with suspected carpal tunnel syndrome: predicting symptoms, function, and surgical benefit at 1 year. *J Neurosurg.* 2008;108:541–550.
8. Visser LH, Smidt MH, Lee ML. High-resolution sonography versus EMG in the diagnosis of carpal tunnel syndrome. *J Neurol Neurosurg Psychiatry.* 2008;79:63–67.
9. Padua L, Aprile I, Caliandro P, Mondelli M, Pasqualetti P, Tonali PA. Carpal tunnel syndrome in pregnancy: multiperspective follow-up of untreated cases. *Neurology.* 2002;59:1643–1646.
10. De Angelis MV, Pierfelice F, Di Giovanni P, Staniscia T, Uncini A. Efficacy of a soft hand brace and a wrist splint for carpal tunnel syndrome: a randomized controlled study. *Acta Neurol Scand.* 2009;119: 68–74.
11. American Academy of Orthopaedic Surgeon's Work Group Panel. Clinical practice guideline on the treatment of carpal tunnel syndrome. AAOS. 2010. [WWW document]. URL http://www.aaos.org/guidelines [accessed on October 23, 2010]
12. Verdugo RJ, Salinas RA, Castillo JL, Cea JG. Surgical versus nonsurgical treatment for carpal tunnel syndrome. *Cochrane Database Syst Rev.* 2008;4:CD001552.
13. Marshall S, Tardif G, Ashworth N. Local corticosteroid injection for carpal tunnel syndrome. *Cochrane Database Syst Rev.* 2007;2:CD001554.
14. Lee JH, An JH, Lee SH, Hwang EY. Effectiveness of steroid injection in treating patients with moderate and severe degree of carpal tunnel syndrome measured by clinical and electrodiagnostic assessment. *Clin J Pain.* 2009;25:111–115.
15. Haider N, Mekasha D, Chiravuri S, Wasserman R. Pulsed radiofrequency of the median nerve under ultrasound guidance. *Pain Physician.* 2007;10:765–770.
16. Racasan O, Dubert T. The safest location for steroid injection in the treatment of carpal tunnel syndrome. *J Hand Surg Br.* 2005;30: 412–414.

20 Meralgia Paresthetica

Jacob Patijn, Nagy Mekhail, Salim Hayek, Arno Lataster, Maarten van Kleef and Jan Van Zundert

Introduction

Meralgia paresthetica (MP) is a neurological disorder characterized by paresthesia and numbness in an anterolateral cutaneous area of the thigh due to a lesion (compression) and/or dysfunction of the nervus cutaneus femoris lateralis (lateral femoral cutaneous nerve, LFCN).

Even though MP can develop spontaneously at any age, the disease usually presents in the 30- to 40-year age group.[1] The incidence in children could be higher than originally assumed.[2] MP appears in one-third of children who have undergone surgery for an osteoid osteoma.[1] An incidence of 0.43 in 10,000 was found in a Dutch study of a population of first-line care of 173,375 patients.[3] There is a higher incidence of MP in males. In addition, there is a correlation with obesity, diabetes, and pregnancy related to increased intra-abdominal pressure.[4] However, MP is also seen in children of relatively slender build.[5]

Meralgia paresthetica can have many etiologies and can be subdivided into two main groups: spontaneous onset and iatrogenic.[6] Spontaneous MP occurs without previous surgical intervention and can be subdivided into an idiopathic, metabolic, and/or mechanical type.[6,7] In the case of the mechanical type, increased intra-abdominal pressure plays a role that appears with obesity and pregnancy.[4] External direct pressure on the LFCN from wearing belts, corsets, or tight pants can lead to MP. However, internal pressure, such as that caused by tumors of the uterus, can also present as MP.[8] Other causes for the spontaneous onset of MP are radiological degenerative defects of the symphysis pubica[9] and leg-length disparity.[10] L1 radiculopathy can also mimic MP.[11] Metabolic factors such as lead poisoning, alcoholism, hypothyroidism, and diabetes are considered in particular to correlate with MP.[7]

Surgery on the spinal column and the pelvis (osteotomy), in which a direct lesion to the LFCN occurs, is the most important iatrogenic cause for the onset of MP, and is seen in about 20% of cases.[12] Neurotmesis of the LFCN is frequently described in relation to autogenous bone graft harvesting from the crista iliaca in spondylodesis operations.[12] This is due to the fact that the LFCN has different anatomical variations, including the variant in which it runs across the crista iliaca.[13] Compression neuropraxia in patients who undergo spine surgery on a Hall–Relton frame and neuropraxia of the LFCN by traction on the musculus psoas major during retroperitoneal dissection are also described.[15] Many other operations are associated with the onset of an iatrogenic MP due to positioning, compression by restraining belts or devices, or direct surgical injury, such as total hip replacement surgery, laparoscopic cholecystectomy and myomectomy, transplantations for coronary bypass surgeries, stomach reductions, surgery for morbid obesity, and laparoscopic inguinal repair.[6] When surgery is performed in the area of the spina iliaca anterior superior (anterior superior iliac spine, ASIS), the patient has a 35% risk of sensory loss and a 5% risk of developing MP.[14]

The variable gross anatomical topography of the LFCN with regard to the surrounding bone structures and soft tissues is important, on the one hand, because it could possibly be a predictor of the onset of MP; and on the other, for the interpretation of the diagnostic blockade and for potential local treatment options. Anatomical variation of the LFCN appears in 25% of patients.[15]

Evidence-Based Interventional Pain Medicine: According to Clinical Diagnoses, First Edition. Edited by Jan Van Zundert, Jacob Patijn, Craig T. Hartrick, Arno Lataster, Frank J.P.M Huygen, Nagy Mekhail, Maarten van Kleef.

The progression of five different types of LFCN can be distinguished based on cadaver studies.[15]

Type A: LFCN runs posterior to the ASIS over the crista iliaca (4%).

Type B: LFCN runs anterior to the ASIS above the tendinous origin of the musculus sartorius, but is embedded in the tissue of the ligamentum inguinale (27%).

Type C: LFCN runs medial to the ASIS, embedded in the tendinous origin of the musculus sartorius (23%).

Type D: LFCN runs medial to the tendinous origin of the musculus sartorius, localized between the tendon of the musculus sartorius and a thick fascia of the musculus iliopsoas under the ligamentum inguinale (26%).

Type E: LFCN runs further medially and is embedded in the connective tissue under the ligamentum inguinale and lies on the thin fascia of the musculus iliopsoas where it branches off toward the ramus femoralis of the nervus genitofemoralis (20%).[9]

Types A, B, and C are the most sensitive to traumas.[16] Outside the above-mentioned anatomical variants, various branching pattern of the LFCN has been described with one or two vertebral origins of the nerve.[17,18] When the lesion is located around the ligamentum inguinale, the LFCN undergoes pathological changes, such as local demyelinization and Wallerian degeneration, mainly of the large fibres.

Diagnosis

History

Symptoms involving MP usually consist of unpleasant paresthesia on the exterior side of the thigh. This occurs unilaterally in most cases, but in 20% of cases it appears bilaterally.[14]

The patients complain of a typical burning, stabbing pain with a tingling sensation in the thigh. They usually localize the symptoms as occurring on the skin itself. Even though some MP patients report pain in the context of an allodynia in the area of the LFCN, most of them indicate that they have an unpleasant tingling sensation (dysesthesia) instead of pain. These MP symptoms can be provoked with postural change by extending the hip or by prolonged standing.[6] The symptoms sometimes disappear when the patient sits down.

Physical examination

During physical examination, palpation is usually painful on the lateral part of the ligamentum inguinale at the point where the nerve crosses the ligamentum inguinale. Some patients also present with hair loss in the areas of the LFCN because they constantly rub this area.[6]

Additional tests

Somatic: none.

Psychocognitive: none.

When indicated, pelvic radiography can be performed to rule out bone tumors. MRI or ultrasound examinations are indicated if pelvic tumor, including retroperitoneal tumor, is suspected. Blood tests and thyroid function tests are indicated if a metabolic cause is suspected.

When in doubt, neurophysiological evaluation using a somatosensory-evoked potential and a nerve conduction test of the LFCN can be carried out. As well as demonstrating MP, this test can simultaneously provide information and locate the lesion in the LFCN.[19]

A positive diagnostic blockade with 8 mL local anesthetic, performed by locating the LFCN using a nerve stimulator, can usually confirm the diagnosis. However, it should always be borne in mind that an abnormal course of the LFCN can also cause a negative diagnostic block.

Differential diagnosis

In general, diagnosis can be established from the typical medical history, physical examination, and general neurological examination. This is of great importance because other neurological, urogenital, and gastrointestinal symptoms are not usually part of the clinical diagnosis associated with MP.[6] It can provide the specialist with indications for the presence of other diseases that could account for the patient's symptom pattern. All patients with motor loss and/or reflex variations, or patients with loss of sensation in areas that are not supplied by the LFCN, require further testing. Differential diagnoses should rule out red flags such as metastases in the crista iliaca, lumbar disk herniation with radiculopathy, and avulsion fractures. Even chronic appendicitis can present as a syndrome similar to MP.[6]

Treatment options

Conservative management

The great majority of cases of MP have a favorable course and 85% will recover with conservative treatment.[20] The first choice of conservative treatment is always to tackle the underlying cause (when known), such as weight loss or the wearing of tight clothing and/or belts.[21] When pain predominates, tricyclic antidepressants, antiarrhythmics, and anticonvulsants can be administered to treat the neuropathic pain.[22] Capsaicin or lidocaine cream can be prescribed if there is dysesthesia of the epidermis.[23]

Interventional management

Local infiltration of the LFCN

Traditionally, local infiltration of the LFCN with an anesthetic, with or without corticosteroids, is administered in various dosages, but outcomes are rarely correctly reported in the literature.[6] Treatment success (>50% pain reduction and improvement in mobility) was reported after two injections under ultrasound guidance. Injections of bupivacaine 0.25%, 1:200 000 epinephrine and 40 mg methylprednisolone for the first injection and 20 mg methylprednisolone for the second injection were administered at a 3-week interval.[24]

Pulsed radiofrequency treatment of the LFCN

Pulsed radiofrequency (PRF) treatment of the LFCN was only reported in four case reports.[25–27] The first case, a 68-year-old patient diagnosed with MP of 4-month duration was treated with PRF in the area of the LFCN. The paresthesia disappeared 24 hours after treatment and the patient was still symptom-free after 6 months.[25] A positive effect was of PRF treatment of the LFCN in the other three case reports.[26,27]

Spinal cord stimulation

One case report mentions the use of spinal cord stimulation in a patient with 1-year history of MP confirmed by a positive diagnostic block of the LFCN. Conservative, pharmacological treatment yielded unsatisfactory pain relief and injection of local anesthetic with corticosteroid provided only 9-hour pain relief. A quadripolar lead was implanted at the mid-Th10 corpus vertebrae level. Eight months after implantation the patient was almost completely pain free, no longer used pain medication, and was working full time.[28]

Complications of interventional management

Local infiltration

The reports available do not mention complications or adverse effects; no conclusions can be drawn.

Pulsed radiofrequency treatment

No complications or adverse effects of PRF treatment were documented in the four case reports.[25–27]

In a review of the literature on PRF in more than 1,200 patients, no complications have been mentioned.[29]

Spinal cord stimulation

The patient discussed in the case report did not experience any side effect. The potential side effects and complications of spinal cord stimulation are described in the chapter on "Complex Regional Pain Syndrome".[30]

Surgical treatment options

Surgical intervention in painful MP should be reserved for very exceptionally serious cases that have been thoroughly examined and in which other psychocognitive factors have been ruled out.[4]

Evidence for interventional management

The summary of the evidence for the interventional management of MP is given in Table 20.1.

Recommendations

There is only limited documentation regarding the interventional treatment of MP. When conservative treatment provides inadequate results, local infiltration of the LFCN with anesthetics and corticosteroids can be considered. PRF treatment of the LFCN should only be performed in a study context. Spinal cord stimulation should be reserved for refractory cases, only in a study context.

Clinical practice algorithm

Figure 20.1 represents the treatment algorithm for the management of MP.

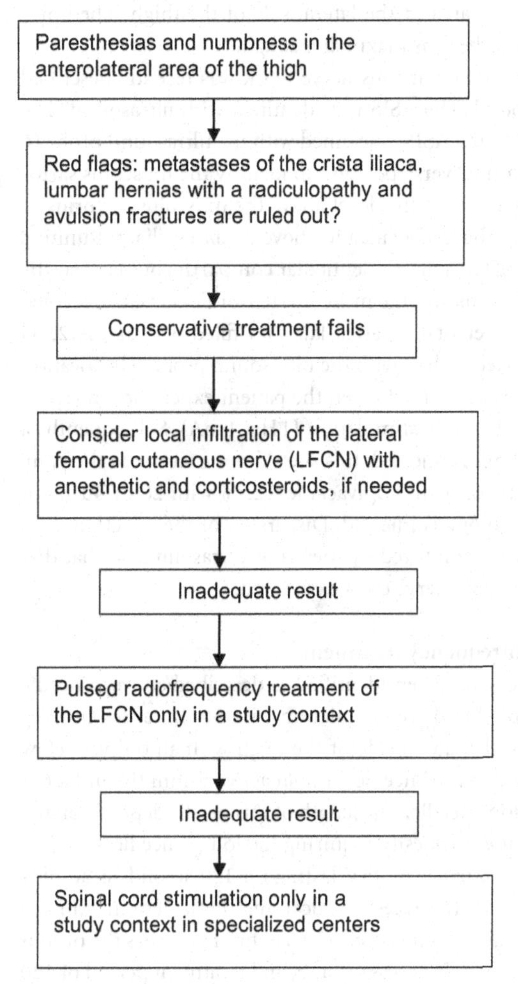

Figure 20.1. Clinical practice algorithm for the treatment of meralgia paresthetica.

Table 20.1. Summary of the evidence for interventional management of meralgia paresthetica.

Techniques	Evaluation
LFCN infiltration	2C+
Pulsed radiofrequency treatment of LFCN	0
Spinal cord stimulation	0

LFCN, lateral femoral cutaneous nerve.

Technique(s)

LFCN block

Lateral femoral cutaneous nerve block is carried out with the patient in the supine position. A pillow under the knees can increase the patient's comfort, especially if extension of the legs is painful. The LFCN can sometimes be identified by palpation. A point 2 cm medial and 2 cm caudal to the ASIS is selected as the injection site. The needle (22 to 25 G) is inserted past the deep fascia of the thigh (fascia lata) where a "pop" is noted when perforating the fascia. Thereafter, paresthesia can usually be quickly generated in the area of the lateral side of the thigh. The point where the paresthesia is maximal is sought.

Lateral femoral cutaneous nerve block was recently described using ultrasound. The ASIS was identified with ultrasound. The tissue caudal to the ASIS is scanned with the ultrasound probe (6 to 13 Hz) in a transverse position to identify the musculus sartorius. The LFCN lies at this level above the musculus sartorius in the area under the fascia lata and above the fascia iliaca. Running caudally the LFCN enters a lenticular compartment between the musculus sartorius and the musculus tensor fasciae latae, formed by a double layer of the fascia lata and filled with fat. A 22-G needle is inserted in-line with the ultrasound probe. The location of the LFCN is confirmed when the patient experiences a reproducible paresthesia by stimulation (1 Hz; 1 mA). Subsequently, a test dose of 1 mL is injected; this should not exacerbate the pain. A total volume of 9 mL bupivacaine 0.25% with 20 or 40 mg of methylprednisolone is injected. Dispersion of the injection fluid is continuously monitored by means of ultrasound, so that dispersion around the nerve can be observed.

Pulsed radiofrequency treatment

After the LFCN has been identified as described above, a needle location is sought where stimulation with 50 Hz causes tingling in the area of the lateral side of the thigh with an output below 0.6 V, using a 23-G RF needle with an active 5-mm tip and a 60- or 100-mm-long needle. The length of this needle depends on the size of the patient (obesity requiring the longer needles). Subsequently, a PRF current of 45 V lasting for 120 seconds is administered without any preceding local anesthetic. The maximum temperature should not exceed 42°C, but if this occurs the output should be reduced. If necessary, a second treatment period of 120 seconds can be administered if the impedance is above 500 Ω, prior to injection of 1 mL NaCl 0.9% solution.

Spinal cord stimulation

We refer to the chapter on "Complex Regional Pain Syndrome" for the technique.[30]

Summary

Meralgia paresthetica is a frequent complaint. An exact medical history and neurological examination are usually enough to establish its diagnosis. When using diagnostic blocks and local invasive treatment, it is important to realize that in 25% of patients anatomic variants of the nervus cutaneus femoris lateralis (lateral femoral cutaneous nerve, LFCN) may be present. Conservative treatment is always the first choice of therapy. Infiltration with corticosteroids and local anesthetics can be considered. PRF treatment and spinal cord stimulation are also an option, but should be performed only in the context of a study.

References

1. Goldberg VM, Jacobs B. Osteoid osteoma of the hip in children. *Clin Orthop Relat Res.* 1975;106:41–47.
2. Fernandez-Mayoralas DM, Fernandez-Jaen A, Jareno NM, Perez BC, Fernandez PM, Sola AG. Meralgia paresthetica in the pediatric population: a propos of 2 cases. *J Child Neurol.* 2010;25: 110–113.
3. van Slobbe AM, Bohnen AM, Bernsen RM, Koes BW, Bierma-Zeinstra SM. Incidence rates and determinants in meralgia paresthetica in general practice. *J Neurol.* 2004;251:294–297.
4. Williams PH, Trzil KP. Management of meralgia paresthetica. *J Neurosurg.* 1991;74:76–80.
5. Richer LP, Shevell MI, Stewart J, Poulin C. Pediatric meralgia paresthetica. *Pediatr Neurol.* 2002;26:321–323.
6. Harney D, Patijn J. Meralgia paresthetica: diagnosis and management strategies. *Pain Med.* 2007;8:669–677.
7. Grossman MG, Ducey SA, Nadler SS, Levy AS. Meralgia paresthetica: diagnosis and treatment. *J Am Acad Orthop Surg.* 2001;9:336–344.
8. Suber DA, Massey EW. Pelvic mass presenting as meralgia paresthetica. *Obstet Gynecol.* 1979;53:257–258.
9. Bierma-Zeinstra S, Ginai A, Prins A, et al. Meralgia paresthetica is related to degenerative pubic symphysis. *J Rheumatol.* 2000;27:2242–2245.
10. Goel A. Meralgia paresthetica secondary to limb length discrepancy: case report. *Arch Phys Med Rehabil.* 1999;80:348–349.
11. Yang SN, Kim DH. L1 radiculopathy mimicking meralgia paresthetica: a case report. *Muscle Nerve.* 2010;41:566–568.
12. Mirovsky Y, Neuwirth M. Injuries to the lateral femoral cutaneous nerve during spine surgery. *Spine.* 2000; 25:1266–1269.
13. van den Broecke DG, Schuurman AH, Borg ED, Kon M. Neurotmesis of the lateral femoral cutaneous nerve when coring for iliac crest bone grafts. *Plast Reconstr Surg.* 1998;102:1163–1166.
14. Ecker AD. Diagnosis of meralgia paresthetica. *JAMA.* 1985;253:976.
15. de Ridder VA, de Lange S, Popta JV. Anatomical variations of the lateral femoral cutaneous nerve and the consequences for surgery. *J Orthop Trauma.* 1999;13:207–211.
16. Aszmann OC, Dellon ES, Dellon AL. Anatomical course of the lateral femoral cutaneous nerve and its susceptibility to compression and injury. *Plast Reconstr Surg.* 1997;100:600–604.
17. Carai A, Fenu G, Sechi E, Crotti FM, Montella A. Anatomical variability of the lateral femoral cutaneous nerve: findings from a surgical series. *Clin Anat.* 2009;22:365–370.
18. Majkrzak A, Johnston J, Kacey D, Zeller J. Variability of the lateral femoral cutaneous nerve: an anatomic basis for planning safe surgical approaches. *Clin Anat.* 2010;23:304–311.
19. Seror P. Somatosensory evoked potentials for the electrodiagnosis of meralgia paresthetica. *Muscle Nerve.* 2004;29:309–312.

20. Dureja GP, Gulaya V, Jayalakshmi TS, Mandal P. Management of meralgia paresthetica: a multimodality regimen. *Anesth Analg.* 1995;80:1060–1061.
21. Craig E. Lateral femoral cutaneous neuropathy. In: Frontera W, Silver J, eds. *Essentials of Physical Medicine and Rehabilitation.* 1st ed. Philadelphia, PA: Hanley & Belfus, Inc.; 2002.
22. Massey EW. Sensory mononeuropathies. *Semin Neurol.* 1998;18: 177–183.
23. Devers A, Galer BS. Topical lidocaine patch relieves a variety of neuropathic pain conditions: an open-label study. *Clin J Pain.* 2000;16: 205–208.
24. Tumber PS, Bhatia A, Chan VW. Ultrasound-guided lateral femoral cutaneous nerve block for meralgia paresthetica. *Anesth Analg.* 2008;106:1021–1022.
25. Gofeld M. Pulsed radiofrequency treatment of intractable meralgia paresthetica: case study. In: INS, ed. *6th INS World Congress.* Madrid: International Neuromodulation Society; 25–28 Jun 2003, 58 abstr. 22.
26. Dalmau-Carola J. Treatment of meralgia paresthetica with pulsed radiofrequency of the lateral femoral cutaneous nerve. *Pain Physician.* 2009;12:1025–1026; author reply: 1026–1027.
27. Philip CN, Candido KD, Joseph NJ, Crystal GJ. Successful treatment of meralgia paresthetica with pulsed radiofrequency of the lateral femoral cutaneous nerve. *Pain Physician.* 2009;12:881–885.
28. Barna SA, Hu MM, Buxo C, Trella J, Cosgrove GR. Spinal cord stimulation for treatment of meralgia paresthetica. *Pain Physician.* 2005;8:315–318.
29. Cahana A, Van Zundert J, Macrea L, van Kleef M, Sluijter M. Pulsed radiofrequency: current clinical and biological literature available. *Pain Med.* 2006;7:411–423.
30. van Eijs F, Stanton-Hicks M, Van Zundert J, et al. 16. Complex regional pain syndrome. *Pain Pract.* 2011;11:70–87.

21 Phantom Pain

Andre Wolff, Eric Vanduynhoven, Maarten van Kleef, Frank Huygen, Jason E. Pope and Nagy Mekhail

Introduction

Complete or partial amputation of a limb does not always result in pain. It is termed phantom pain when the patient feels pain or dysesthesia in limbs that are no longer present (deafferentation). It is important to distinguish phantom pain from other amputation sequelae, including phantom sensation, telescoping, and stump pain. Phantom sensations are nonpainful and typically manifest as kinetic, kinesthetic, or exteroceptive perceptions. Telescoping is a progressive sensation resulting in the distal limb being perceived more proximally. Stump pain is residual limb pain, commonly localized to distal existing body part. If patients suffer from phantom pain, the onset is usually amputation secondary to trauma or surgical intervention. Ambrosius Paré described this type of pain in the sixteenth century.

It is estimated that over 1.5 million amputees live in the United States, where the majority have had amputations of the lower limbs below the knee.[1] The reported incidence of phantom limb pain varies widely from as low as 2% to 80%. More recent epidemiological studies report a much higher percentage of amputees having phantom limb pain. A retrospective study in patients with combat related traumatic amputations found that 78% of participants experienced phantom limb pain at some time since amputation, and 68% of them received treatment from their health care provider.[2] Patients prospectively followed after limb amputation due to peripheral vascular disease show a comparable incidence of phantom limb pain (78.8%), and stump pain (51.2%) 6 months after amputation.[3] In one study, probably the largest field survey performed in Europe, a questionnaire containing 62 questions was filled in by 537 out of 1,088 amputees. Of the amputees who responded, 14.8% were pain free, 74.5% had phantom limb pain, 45.2% had stump pain and 35.5% had a combination of both.[4]

Seventeen years after the war between Iraq and Iran, 64% of 200 soldiers who had lost limbs during this war suffered from phantom pain, 32% from phantom movement pain, while 24% suffered from stump pain.[5] Telephone interviews held between 1998 and 2000, in which 914 people participated, showed that the incidences during the past 4 weeks prior to the interview amounted to 79.9% for phantom pain and 67.7% for stump pain, respectively. A quarter of the people who were interviewed had a visual analogue scale (VAS) pain score ranging from 7 to 10.

Mechanism

It is assumed that every individual develops a proprioceptive, tactile and visual image of the body. For a long time, the cortical representation of these images was thought to remain unchanged after amputation. Although there are still many questions as to the underlying mechanisms, peripheral as well as central neuronal mechanisms seem to be involved.[6] There are also indications that neuroplastic changes take place including changes of the cortical representation.

Peripheral input can play a part in the perception of phantom pain. When peripheral nerves are cut or injured, regenerative sprouting of the injured axon occurs. The enlarged and disorganized endings of C fibers and demyelinated A-fibers show an increased rate of spontaneous activity. Spontaneous and abnormal activity has been perceived in neuromas at the nerve endings and in the spinal ganglia after peripheral mechanic or chemical stimulation as a consequence of up-regulation of the sodium channels. Ectopic discharge in the dorsal root ganglion has also been implicated as a potential mechanism. Ectopic discharge may be induced by emotional distress leading to increased circulating levels of epinephrine. Factors such as temperature, oxygenation,

Evidence-Based Interventional Pain Medicine: According to Clinical Diagnoses, First Edition. Edited by Jan Van Zundert, Jacob Patijn, Craig T. Hartrick, Arno Lataster, Frank J.P.M Huygen, Nagy Mekhail, Maarten van Kleef.

and local inflammation may play a role. Therefore, the sensitivity of these neuromas or ganglia may increase due to epinephrine or stress, in combination with increasing norepinephrine from sympathetic efferents, which are located in close proximity to afferent sensory nerve cells, for example in the case of sprouting. This results in exacerbation of phantom pain. Peripheral factors may be of varying importance in the origin and modulation of phantom limb pain, but also central factors play must play a role.[7]

The spinal cord may be involved as well. Changes in activity levels in neuromas and ganglia may result in long-term adaptations in the central projecting neurons in the posterior horn. This may lead to spontaneous neuronal activity, changes in RNA transcription, increased metabolic activity in the spinal cord and may cause the receptive fields to enlarge; all these factors result in central (spinal) sensitization.

Apart from functional changes, anatomical changes have been observed as well. Afferent C fibers of lamina II in the spinal cord may degenerate, so that the number of synapses with second-order neurons diminishes. Therefore, Aβ mechanosensitive afferents, normally present in deeper layers, may connect with the exposed nociceptive second-order neurons within lamina II which may induce sprouting of A-fiber terminals in these areas, where they are normally not represented. The incoming A-fiber input might then be interpreted as noxious and could be the anatomical substrate of allodynia. In this way, normal stimuli through Aβ neurons may lead to other sensations, such as pain. Eventually, neuroplastic changes will occur in the thalamus in subcortical and in cortical structures. It becomes clear that there is a relationship between the spinal cord and higher centres in cases where pain-free amputees had transient phantom pain after spinal anesthesia, while conversely patients with phantom pain became pain free after a focal cerebral infarction or a spinal cord lesion.

An especially relevant mechanism may be the invasion of regions of the spinal cord where the amputated limb was previously represented. Neuropeptides such as Substance P, normally expressed by nociceptor primary afferent Aδ- and C fibers may also become expressed by Aβ-fibers after peripheral nerve injury. Supraspinal changes related to phantom limb pain involve the brainstem, the thalamus and the cortex.[7]

Changes in the functional and structural architecture of primary somatosensory cortex after amputation and deafferentation in adult monkeys are demonstrated. Reorganizational changes in the sensory and motor maps were shown. Also in people with arm or hand amputations a shift of the mouth into the hand representation in primary somatosensory cortex was illustrated. The larger the shift of the mouth representation into the zone that formerly represented the amputated hand and arm, the greater the phantom limb pain.

Reorganization of the motor system was limited to the cortex; spinal changes were not observed. Thalamic stimulation and recordings in amputees have shown that reorganizational changes also occur at the thalamic level and are closely related to the perception of phantom limbs and phantom limb pain.[7] The loss of a limb may have a substantial psychological impact. Fear, depression and anger may follow sorrow and may affect the pain. Depression is a significant predicting factor for severe pain and distress.[8] Just as in other chronic pain syndromes, psychosocial factors play a potential part in prolonging the pain, but specific psychological factors related to amputation appear to have a minor role in this respect. However, studies have shown that patients with phantom pain are more likely to be rigid and show more controlling behavior.

Diagnosis

History

Most patients with phantom pain have intermittent pain, with intervals that range from 1 day to several weeks. Even intervals of over a year have been reported. Pain often presents itself in the form of attacks that vary in duration from a few seconds to minutes or hours. Patients usually describe the pain as shooting, stabbing, piercing, cramping, pinching, or burning. In most cases, the pain is experienced distally in the missing limb, in places with the most extensive innervation density and cortical representation. Examples are fingers or toes.[9]

Phantom pain often begins within 14 days after the amputation. Half of the patients, however, suffer from pain within the first 24 hours after amputation. Some patients will not have pain until several years after amputation; however, phantom pain only becomes manifest a year after the amputation in fewer than 10% of the cases. Two years after the onset of the phantom pain, the prevalence of phantom pain has hardly decreased.

Some studies suggest a relationship between phantom limb pain and the etiology of amputation, while other studies could not indicate a relationship between the patient's general health status and the incidence.[9] Two recently published studies tried to identify if gender has an influence on the occurrence of phantom pain.[10,11] The longitudinal study over 3½ years reveals that men are less prone to experience phantom pain than women. Phantom pain occurs more after arm amputation than after leg amputation.[10] Phantom pain occurs almost immediately after surgery.[12] A postal survey in persons with limb loss, on the contrary, showed that a greater proportion of males reported phantom limb pain. This difference disappeared when corrected for the cause of amputation. Several sex differences in the overall biopsychosocial experience of pain did emerge.[11] Phantom limb pain does not seem to depend on the nature of the cause: surgical or traumatic.[13] In children and in people who have been missing a limb from birth, the incidence of phantom pain is lower. Phantom pain is more common in cases of bilateral amputation, amputation of the legs and in cases where the limb was amputated in a more proximal site.[14]

There are indications that severe pre-amputation and postoperative pain are risk factors for chronic phantom pain.[15] However, the literature reports contradictory results in this respect. It is also unclear whether pre-amputation pain is experienced as the same pain that is felt after amputation as phantom pain: on the one hand retrospective results have been reported, where the number of cases in which pre-amputation pain is experienced as phantom pain, ranges from 12.5% to 80%, whereas a prospective study by Nikolajsen et al.[16] does not show a relationship.

Phantom pain has also been described in parts of the body other than the limbs. Phantom pain after mastectomy occurred in 9 of 39 patients with a bilateral mastectomy, phantom sensations in 20 of 39 patients.[17] Phantom pain has also been described in a quarter of patients who underwent enucleation of the eye after which orbital implants had been inserted. The risk in these patients may have been increased by perioperative headaches and pain in the eye.[18] Tinnitus is presumably related to phantom pain as well, due to changes in the afferent input in the auditory, central neural system caused by axonal sprouting and hyperexcitation.[19] Recent rat studies performed by Tritsch et al.[20] point to the role of supporting cells in the middle ear: when exposed to loud noises, adenosine tri phosphate may be released by supporting cells and thus stimulate hair cells, even though the sound stimulus has disappeared. Process changes in tonotopic receptive fields within auditory structures such as the dorsal cochlear nucleus, inferior colliculus nucleus, and auditory somatosensory areas may also be involved in central neuroplastic changes.

Phantom sensations are painless sensations such as sensations of heat, tingling, telescoping (notably in fingers or toes) and the sensation that the limb becomes shorter over time. Approximately 50% of the amputees have stump pain as well, while 50% to 88% of the patients with phantom pain also suffer from stump pain. In many cases myofascial trigger points are present in the stump that can evoke phantom sensations and phantom pain.[21]

Physical examination

As yet physical examination is not very useful in cases of phantom pain, because the pain is localized in the missing body part and the pain mechanisms predominantly involve the peripheral and the central nervous system.

In stump pain, however, there is clearly a local pain source. For example, in 20% of phantom pain patients skin pathology and circulatory disorders, infections and neuromas may prolong the disorder. Local trigger points may be localized in the stump, especially in patients who have a prosthesis. These trigger points may provoke phantom pain.

Differential diagnosis

Phantom pain is a painful sensation in a part of the body that is no longer present. Stump pain is pain in the remaining stump where the source of the pain is in the stump itself. Phantom sensations: any form of painless sensation that the patient experiences in the part of the body that is no longer present.

In over half of patients, the phantom pain decreases or disappears over time. In cases where the pain is exacerbated special causes should be sought. Apart from changes in autonomous regulation or sympathicotonia due to temperature or weather changes, radicular pain (because of a nucleus pulposus hernia or radiculitis), angina (in cases of pain in the upper phantom limb), and malignant growths (metastasis) may provoke symptoms that may be taken for phantom pain. Infections with herpes zoster (shingles) should also be considered, especially in patients with reduced immunity.

Treatment options

Phantom pain is generally quite therapy resistant. Treatments of phantom pain are rarely successful. In their review article Nikolajsen and Jensen point out that a literature search performed in 1980 identified 68 different treatment methods of which 50 are still in use.[9] Although many caregivers present more favorable reports of their results, fewer than 10% of patients indicate permanent pain relief. The various systematic reviews that have been published indicate that most treatments have no or only limited succes.[22–24] In addition, there are only a few sound studies that deal with phantom pain specifically. Since the systematic review of Sherman[24] was published in 1980, no groundbreaking therapeutic developments have been reported, and the systematic review by Halbert et al.[23] shows that epidural analgesia, regional nerve blocks, treatment with calcitonin, or ketamine do not provide any consistent results. There are, however, three positive studies that show that nerve blocks could have some effect. The analgesic effectiveness of transcutaneous electrical nerve stimulation for the treatment of phantom and/or stump pain was assessed in a Cochrane review. No randomized controlled studies (RCTs) were found thus preventing any conclusions.[25]

However, even if there are still many questions that remain open, there is greater insight into the underlying mechanism of phantom pain. It has been suggested that the focus of treatment should be specifically aimed at preventing chronicity by intervening sooner with respect to the structural and functional changes in the central and peripheral nervous system; these changes are a consequence of the deficient or detrimental somatosensory input and deafferentation after amputation. Unfortunately, in this respect the results of pre- and postoperative epidural blocks are ambiguous. There is much to be learnt about effective interventions with respect to neuroplasticity. It seems that a multimodal approach is essential, in which nociception, inflammation, hormonal, physiological, and mental changes all play an important part. Adequate information, proper surgical indications and techniques for amputation, if possible effective mental preparation and aftercare, long-term rehabilitation and optimum pain treatment are integral elements.

Another problem is that not all phantom pain patients receive treatment. A study by Hanley et al.[26] shows that 53% of patients with phantom pain ($n = 183$), 38% of whom with a severe form of phantom pain, never received treatment for the disorder. Those who did receive treatment suffered from severe pain and experienced considerable distress from the disorder. These patients were mostly treated with analgesics: paracetamol, morphine-like substances and non-steroidal anti-inflammatory drugs. In the perception of the patients, only opioids and chiropractic therapy were effective to some extent.

Conservative management

Drug therapy

Because phantom limb pain is classified as neuropathic pain, an approach to the pharmacological treatment according to published guidelines could be envisioned. Little is known, however, about the specific effectiveness of these medications in phantom pain. In a study by Wilder-Smith et al.,[27] tramadol as well as amitriptyline appear to be more effective than placebo treatment in phantom pain patients. Although the benefit of amitriptyline was not supported in a recent randomized placebo controlled trial of 39 patients,[28] carbamazepine, one of the older drugs used to treat neuropathic pain, proved to have favorable effects.[29,30] Studies that compared gabapentin with placebo did not show a difference for amputation patients with respect to the incidence and intensity of the phantom pain.[31] Another study, however, did demonstrate diminished pain intensity with gabapentin in comparison to placebo patients.[32]

A prospective study in 42 cancer patients assessed the value of treatment according to the World Health Organization analgesic ladder and found that the addition of opioids to antidepressants and anticonvulsants reduces the incidence of phantom pain from 60% 1 month post surgery to 32% 2 years after amputation.[33]

Oral morphine was compared to placebo in a double-blind crossover study in 12 patients with unilateral arm or leg amputation with phantom pain. The results suggested that pain was improved with oral morphine, with a concurrent potential reduction in cortical reorganization as determined by magnetoencephalographic recordings.[34]

A comparison between intravenous lidocaine and morphine in 31 patients with postamputation pain (either phantom pain combined with stump pain or phantom pain or stump pain exclusively) showed that stump pain responds well to both treatments, whereas phantom pain could only be relieved by morphine.[35] A recent randomized controlled crossover trial in patients with postamputation pain of 6 months or longer, having a pain intensity of at least 3 on a 10 point numeric rating scale, compared the efficacy of morphine, mexiletine and placebo. Therapy with morphine but not mexiletine resulted in a decrease in intensity of post-amputation pain but was associated with higher rates of side effects and no improvement in self-reported levels of overall functional activity and pain-related interference in daily activity.[36]

In one RCT where intravenously administered ketamine was compared with placebo, pain and hyperalgesia decreased in patients with stump pain and phantom pain with ketamine in comparison with the control patients.[37] Conversely, in a placebo controlled RCT memantine, another *N*-methyl-D-aspartate receptor antagonist, proved not to be effective,[38–40] while more recent case reports continue to anecdotally support its use.[41] Benzodiazepines do not seem to be effective in cases of phantom pain. The effects of other drugs such as beta-blockers, calcitonin and capsaicin and mexiletine are anecdotal as yet.

Calcitonin, ketamine and their combination were tested in a randomized, double-blind crossover study for the management of chronic phantom limb pain. Ketamine, but not calcitonin, reduced phantom limb pain. The combination was not superior to ketamine alone.[42] Perioperatively ketamine maintained for 72 hours compared to placebo administration did not result in significant differences in subsequent post-amputation pain severity over a 6-month period.[43]

The inflammatory cytokine tumor necrosis factor alpha (TNF-α) plays an important role in neuropathic pain conditions; systemic drugs that block TNF-α alleviate pain and pain-related behavior. A report of six patients with phantom limb pain who were treated with a series of perineural injections of etanercept, a TNF-α antagonist, describes a significant improvement in 5 of 6 patients' residual limb pain at rest and with activity, phantom limb pain, functional capacity, and psychological well-being 3 months after injections.[44]

Interventional management

Epidural anesthesia, applied before, during or after amputation, seems to decrease the severity of phantom pain while the actual incidence does not decrease at all.[45] Various studies have examined the effectiveness of epidural anesthesia. Unfortunately, these studies have different designs and the results are variable and inconsistent.

Many studies have been performed examining pre- and post-operative nerve blocks, with and without catheter techniques. Lambert performed a randomized prospective study comparing preoperative epidural and intraoperative perineural analgesia for the prevention of postoperative stump pain and phantom limb pain and found preoperative epidural block 24 hours before amputation was not superior to intraoperative perineural infusion of local anesthetic in reducing phantom limb pain up to 1 year later, but was more effective in reducing immediate postoperative stump pain.[46] In spite of early pain reduction, the results for patients treated were no better than control patients and the same applied to the patients treated with epidural anesthesia. Favorable results that have been reported are mainly based on case reports.

The use of echographic controlled phenol instillation into neuroma was prospectively assessed in 82 patients. All patients had marked improvement and 12% were pain free after 1 to 3 instillations. The low complication rate (5% minor and 1.3% major complications) is attributed to the use of high resolution sonography.[47] Pre- peri- and postoperative continuous nervus ischiadicus (sciatic) block was assessed in 18 patients who were prospectively followed for 24 months. In this population, an incidence of phantom pain of 25% to 30% was observed.[48]

A case report on a patient with phantom pain treated with pulsed radiofrequency (PRF) of the nervus ischiadicus showed pain relief and reduction of the need of analgesic medication for 4 months.[49] Another patient underwent pulsed radiofrequency of the proximal and distal ends of a sciatic neuroma with treatment at 42°C for 120 seconds under ultrasound guidance with VAS reduction of 90%, 90%, and 70% at 1, 3, and 6 months, respectively.[50] Two patients with primarily stump pain after lower limb amputation and difficulty tolerating the limb prosthesis were treated with PRF adjacent to the L4–L5 ganglion spinale (dorsal root ganglion, DRG). Both patients experienced at least 50% pain reduction for 6 months and tolerated better the prosthesis.[51]

The long-term effect of spinal cord stimulation in a patient with complex regional pain syndrome (CRPS) after two amputations of the right leg has been reported.[52] Katayama et al. investigated spinal cord stimulation, deep brain stimulation of the nucleus thalamicus ventralis caudalis, and the motor cortex for treatment of phantom limb pain. Of the 19 patients, six had long-term pain control with spinal cord stimulation, defined as at least 80% pain reduction for at least 2 years.[53] More recently, a case series of four patients with postcancer resection lower extremity phantom limb pain experienced >80% pain reduction immediately postoperatively, while only 75% had statistically significant reduction in VAS and total symptom score at a minimum of 8 months follow-up.[54]

Other invasive treatments have often been applied as well, including stump injections, trigger point injections, blocks of the sympathetic nervous system and intrathecal injections. In the case of myofascial trigger points, injections with botulinum A have been described. In several of these case studies, a reduction of the pain by 60% to 80% was claimed. In the 1980s, lesions in the dorsal root entry zone were applied. However, no long-term favorable results based on good quality studies have been mentioned in the literature since.

Other forms of therapy

Neuroimaging studies could indicate a cortical reorganization that may influence phantom limb pain. Animal work on stimulation-induced plasticity suggests that extensive behaviorally relevant stimulation of a body part leads to an expansion of its representation zone.[55] These observations have led to the development of treatment strategies based on active stimulation of the phantom limb. The use of myoelectric prosthetics was positively associated with both less phantom limb pain and less cortical reorganization.[56] A recent sham controlled crossover trial showed that mirror therapy is better than mental visualization or covered mirror therapy.[57]

Cases have been described in which mirror therapy was applied with success. The principle of this treatment is based on the idea that the central representation of the missing hand of the phantom could be recovered. This could relieve or eliminate the phantom pain.[58] The added value of the "virtual limb" was studied in a randomized controlled trial where patients who had undergone lower limb amputation were studied before, during and after repeated attempts to simultaneously move both intact and phantom legs. Subjects were randomly assigned to a condition in which they only viewed the movements of their intact limb (control) or a mirror condition in which they additionally viewed the movements of a "virtual limb". The mirror condition elicited a significantly greater number of phantom limb movements than the control condition. Both conditions resulted in a significant attenuation of phantom sensations and pain. Both, the control and the mirror condition reduced phantom limb pain. The use of mirror condition as a prolonged treatment of phantom limb pain may be favorable because a significantly greater number of phantom limb movements may reverse the chronic cortical reorganization.[59]

Some case reports with favorable results from the application of deep brain stimulation have been described. Patients with phantom pain appear to respond favorably. Here, the periventricular gray matter is treated by electrostimulation, in some cases in combination with the somatosensory thalamus. This technique is reported to have been especially effective in reducing the burning pain, the use of opioids, and improving the quality of life.[60] In another study 38 of 47 patients responded favorably to the experimental stimulation. Fifty-three percent of them had a lasting favorable effect from stimulation of the gray matter around the aqueduct, 13% from stimulation of the thalamus and 34% from stimulation of both these structures.

Some studies examining the application of transcranial magnetic stimulation show that this treatment has an inadequate effect on phantom pain.

Preventive strategies

Theoretically the preventive strategy should be built upon two main pillars: surgical technique and pre-emptive analgesia. Despite the obligatory transection of major nerves in leg amputation, no attention has been paid in phantom limb studies to intra-operative handling of the nerves. This lack of attention is particularly surprising given that various nerve ligature models have been used to study chronic neuropathic pain in experimental studies. A survey among Danish orthopedic surgeons showed a surprisingly high use (about 30%) of ligation of the large diameter nerves during leg amputation[61] which, according to experimental preclinical data, may precipitate the development of chronic neuropathic pain.[62] Major orthopedic textbooks recommend ligation of the nerves during amputation. Since a clean nerve cut may lead to less persistent pain compared to a ligature or crush nerve injury, there is an urgent need for clinical studies investigating the role of nerve handling as a risk factor for phantom limb pain after limb amputation.[62]

Several pre-emptive analgesic strategies have been tested with variable results. Detailed discussion of these findings is beyond the scope of this review. It must, however, be stressed that a multimodal approach seems to generate better outcome. Such a multimodal approach can consist of: psychological counseling and treatment; cognitive behavioral therapy and pharmacological treatment using molecules with different mode of action in order to target the different mechanisms of phantom pain.[1,63]

A recently published series of case reports suggests that preventive mirror therapy reduces phantom limb pain.[64]

Complications of interventional management

In a review on the available literature regarding PRF over more than 1,200 patients no side effects have been reported.[65]

The potential complications of spinal cord are described in the chapter on CRPS.[66]

Evidence for interventional management

The summary of the evidence for interventional management of phantom pain is given in Table 21.1.

Recommendations

Based on the available evidence with respect to phantom pain the following recommendations can be made:

Initially phantom pain should be treated with drugs. PRF treatment and spinal cord stimulation can be considered, but should only take place within an experimental framework.

Clinical practice algorithm

Figure 21.1 represents the treatment algorithm for phantom pain.

Techniques

For PRF treatment the neuroma can be identified by means of ultrasound, thus allowing precise needle placement.

The technique of spinal cord stimulation is described in the chapter on CRPS.[66]

Table 21.1. Summary of evidence for interventional management of phantom pain.

Technique	Evaluation
Pulsed radiofrequency treatment of the stump neuroma	0
Pulsed radiofrequency treatment adjacent to the ganglion spinale (DRG)	0
Spinal cord stimulation	0

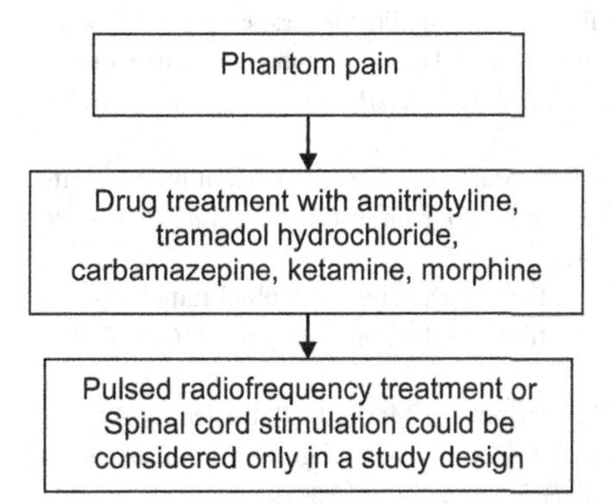

Figure 21.1. Clinical practice algorithm for the treatment of phantom pain.

Summary

The number of cases of phantom pain after amputation ranges from 60% to 80%. Over half the patients with phantom pain have stump pain as well. Myofascial trigger points often occur in stump pain. There are indications that neuroplastic changes also occur, including changes in cortical representation. Generally, phantom pain is fairly therapy resistant. Results reported in literature relating to the effectiveness of the interventional treatment are inconsistent. In the long term, these treatments are not very effective. Based on the available evidence some effect may be expected from drug treatment. PRF and spinal cord stimulation can only be considered in a study design.

References

1. Cohen SP, Christo PJ, Moroz L. Pain management in trauma patients. *Am J Phys Med Rehabil.* 2004;83:142–161.
2. Ketz AK. The experience of phantom limb pain in patients with combat-related traumatic amputations. *Arch Phys Med Rehabil.* 2008;89:1127–1132.
3. Richardson C, Glenn S, Nurmikko T, Horgan M. Incidence of phantom phenomena including phantom limb pain 6 months after major lower limb amputation in patients with peripheral vascular disease. *Clin J Pain.* 2006;22:353–358.
4. Kern U, Busch V, Rockland M, Kohl M, Birklein F. [Prevalence and risk factors of phantom limb pain and phantom limb sensations in Germany. A nationwide field survey]. *Schmerz.* 2009;23: 479–488.
5. Ebrahimzadeh MH, Fattahi AS, Nejad AB. Long-term follow-up of Iranian veteran upper extremity amputees from the Iran-Iraq war (1980–1988). *J Trauma.* 2006;61:886–888.
6. Nikolasjen L, Jensen TS. Postamputation pain. In: Melzack R, Wall P, eds. *Handbook of Pain Management.* 4th ed. Edinburgh: Churchill Livingstone; 2003:247–257.
7. Flor H. Phantom-limb pain: characteristics, causes, and treatment. *Lancet Neurol.* 2002;1:182–189.
8. Ephraim PL, Wegener ST, MacKenzie EJ, Dillingham TR, Pezzin LE. Phantom pain, residual limb pain, and back pain in amputees: results of a national survey. *Arch Phys Med Rehabil.* 2005;86: 1910–1919.
9. Nikolajsen L, Jensen TS. Phantom limb pain. *Br J Anaesth.* 2001;87:107–116.
10. Bosmans JC, Geertzen JH, Post WJ, van der Schans CP, Dijkstra PU. Factors associated with phantom limb pain: a 31/ 2-year prospective study. *Clin Rehabil.* 2010;24:444–453.
11. Hirsh AT, Dillworth TM, Ehde DM, Jensen MP. Sex differences in pain and psychological functioning in persons with limb loss. *J Pain.* 2010;11:79–86.
12. Weeks SR, Anderson-Barnes VC, Tsao JW. Phantom limb pain: theories and therapies. *Neurologist.* 2010;16:277–286.
13. Jensen TS, Krebs B, Nielsen J, Rasmussen P. Phantom limb, phantom pain and stump pain in amputees during the first 6 months following limb amputation. *Pain.* 1983;17:243–256.

14. Dijkstra PU, Geertzen JH, Stewart R, van der Schans CP. Phantom pain and risk factors: a multivariate analysis. *J Pain Symptom Manage.* 2002;24:578–585.
15. Hanley MA, Jensen MP, Smith DG, Ehde DM, Edwards WT, Robinson LR. Preamputation pain and acute pain predict chronic pain after lower extremity amputation. *J Pain.* 2007;8:102–109.
16. Nikolajsen L, Ilkjaer S, Kroner K, Christensen JH, Jensen TS. The influence of preamputation pain on postamputation stump and phantom pain. *Pain.* 1997;72:393–405.
17. Rothemund Y, Grusser SM, Liebeskind U, Schlag PM, Flor H. Phantom phenomena in mastectomized patients and their relation to chronic and acute pre-mastectomy pain. *Pain.* 2004;107: 140–146.
18. Gerding H, Vo O, Husstedt IW, Evers S, Soros P. [Phantom pain after eye enucleation]. *Ophthalmologe.* 2003;100:943–949.
19. Bartels H, Staal MJ, Albers FW. Tinnitus and neural plasticity of the brain. *Otol Neurotol.* 2007;28:178–184.
20. Tritsch NX, Yi E, Gale JE, Glowatzki E, Bergles DE. The origin of spontaneous activity in the developing auditory system. *Nature.* 2007;450:50–55.
21. Kern KU, Martin C, Scheicher S, Muller H. [Referred pain from amputation stump trigger points into the phantom limb]. *Schmerz.* 2006;20:300, 302–306.
22. Manchikanti L, Singh V. Managing phantom pain. *Pain Physician.* 2004;7:365–375.
23. Halbert J, Crotty M, Cameron ID. Evidence for the optimal management of acute and chronic phantom pain: a systematic review. *Clin J Pain.* 2002;18:84–92.
24. Sherman RA. Published treatments of phantom limb pain. *Am J Phys Med.* 1980;59:232–244.
25. Mulvey MR, Bagnall AM, Johnson MI, Marchant PR. Transcutaneous electrical nerve stimulation (TENS) for phantom pain and stump pain following amputation in adults. *Cochrane Database Syst Rev.* 2010;5:CD007264.
26. Hanley MA, Ehde DM, Campbell KM, Osborn B, Smith DG. Self-reported treatments used for lower-limb phantom pain: descriptive findings. *Arch Phys Med Rehabil.* 2006;87:270–277.
27. Wilder-Smith CH, Hill LT, Laurent S. Postamputation pain and sensory changes in treatment-naive patients: characteristics and responses to treatment with tramadol, amitriptyline, and placebo. *Anesthesiology.* 2005;103:619–628.
28. Robinson LR, Czerniecki JM, Ehde DM, et al. Trial of amitriptyline for relief of pain in amputees: results of a randomized controlled study. *Arch Phys Med Rehabil.* 2004;85:1–6.
29. Patterson JF. Carbamazepine in the treatment of phantom limb pain. *South Med J.* 1988;81:1100–1102.
30. Elliott F, Little A, Milbrandt W. Carbamazepine for phantom-limb phenomena. *N Engl J Med.* 1976;295:678.
31. Nikolajsen L, Finnerup NB, Kramp S, Vimtrup AS, Keller J, Jensen TS. A randomized study of the effects of gabapentin on postamputation pain. *Anesthesiology.* 2006;105:1008–1015.
32. Bone M, Critchley P, Buggy DJ. Gabapentin in postamputation phantom limb pain: a randomized, double-blind, placebo-controlled, cross-over study. *Reg Anesth Pain Med.* 2002;27:481–486.
33. Mishra S, Bhatnagar S, Gupta D, Diwedi A. Incidence and management of phantom limb pain according to World Health Organization analgesic ladder in amputees of malignant origin. *Am J Hosp Palliat Care.* 2007;24:455–462.
34. Huse E, Larbig W, Flor H, Birbaumer N. The effect of opioids on phantom limb pain and cortical reorganization. *Pain.* 2001;90: 47–55.
35. Wu CL, Tella P, Staats PS, et al. Analgesic effects of intravenous lidocaine and morphine on postamputation pain: a randomized double-blind, active placebo-controlled, crossover trial. *Anesthesiology.* 2002;96:841–848.
36. Wu CL, Agarwal S, Tella PK, et al. Morphine versus mexiletine for treatment of postamputation pain: a randomized, placebo-controlled, crossover trial. *Anesthesiology.* 2008;109:289–296.
37. Willoch F, Rosen G, Tolle TR, et al. Phantom limb pain in the human brain: unraveling neural circuitries of phantom limb sensations using positron emission tomography. *Ann Neurol.* 2000;48:842–849.
38. Wiech K, Kiefer RT, Topfner S, et al. A placebo-controlled randomized crossover trial of the N-methyl-D-aspartic acid receptor antagonist, memantine, in patients with chronic phantom limb pain. *Anesth Analg.* 2004;98:408–413.
39. Nikolajsen L, Gottrup H, Kristensen AG, Jensen TS. Memantine (a N-methyl-D-aspartate receptor antagonist) in the treatment of neuropathic pain after amputation or surgery: a randomized, double-blinded, cross-over study. *Anesth Analg.* 2000;91:960–966.
40. Maier C, Dertwinkel R, Mansourian N, et al. Efficacy of the NMDA-receptor antagonist memantine in patients with chronic phantom limb pain–results of a randomized double-blinded, placebo-controlled trial. *Pain.* 2003;103:277–283.
41. Hackworth RJ, Tokarz KA, Fowler IM, Wallace SC, Stedje-Larsen ET. Profound pain reduction after induction of memantine treatment in two patients with severe phantom limb pain. *Anesth Analg.* 2008;107:1377–1379.
42. Eichenberger U, Neff F, Sveticic G, et al. Chronic phantom limb pain: the effects of calcitonin, ketamine, and their combination on pain and sensory thresholds. *Anesth Analg.* 2008;106:1265–1273.
43. Hayes C, Armstrong-Brown A, Burstal R. Perioperative intravenous ketamine infusion for the prevention of persistent post-amputation pain: a randomized, controlled trial. *Anaesth Intensive Care.* 2004;32:330–338.
44. Dahl E, Cohen SP. Perineural injection of etanercept as a treatment for postamputation pain. *Clin J Pain.* 2008;24:172–175.
45. Gehling M, Tryba M. [Prophylaxis of phantom pain: is regional analgesia ineffective?] *Schmerz.* 2003;17:11–19.
46. Lambert A, Dashfield A, Cosgrove C, et al. Randomized prospective study comparing preoperative epidural and intraoperative perineural analgesia for the prevention of postoperative stump and phantom limb pain following major amputation. *Reg Anesth Pain Manag.* 2001;26:316–321.
47. Gruber H, Glodny B, Kopf H, et al. Practical experience with sonographically guided phenol instillation of stump neuroma: predictors of effects, success, and outcome. *AJR Am J Roentgenol.* 2008;190: 1263–1269.
48. Becotte A, de Medicis E, Martin R, Gagnon V. Continuous sciatic nerve block in phantom limb pain prevention. *Can J Anaesth.* 2008;55(Suppl 1):464294.
49. Wilkes D, Ganceres N, Solanki D, Hayes M. Pulsed radiofrequency treatment of lower extremity phantom limb pain. *Clin J Pain.* 2008;24:736–739.
50. Restrepo-Garces CE, Marinov A, McHardy P, Faclier G, Avila A. Pulsed radiofrequency under ultrasound guidance for persistent stump-neuroma pain. *Pain Pract.* 2011;11:98–102.

51. Ramanavarapu V, Simopoulos TT. Pulsed radiofrequency of lumbar dorsal root Ganglia for chronic postamputation stump pain. *Pain Physician.* 2008;11:561–566.
52. Enggaard TP, Scherer C, Nikolajsen L, Andersen C. [Long term effect of spinal cord stimulation in a patient with complex regional pain syndrome and phantom pain syndrome type 1 after amputation]. *Ugeskr Laeger.* 2008;170:460.
53. Katayama Y, Yamamoto T, Kobayashi K, Kasai M, Oshima H, Fukaya C. Motor cortex stimulation for phantom limb pain: comprehensive therapy with spinal cord and thalamic stimulation. *Stereotact Funct Neurosurg.* 2001;77:159–162.
54. Viswanathan A, Phan PC, Burton AW. Use of spinal cord stimulation in the treatment of phantom limb pain: case series and review of the literature. *Pain Pract.* 2010;10:479–484.
55. Jenkins WM, Merzenich MM, Ochs MT, Allard T, Guic-Robles E. Functional reorganization of primary somatosensory cortex in adult owl monkeys after behaviorally controlled tactile stimulation. *J Neurophysiol.* 1990;63:82–104.
56. Lotze M, Flor H, Grodd W, Larbig W, Birbaumer N. Phantom movements and pain. An fMRI study in upper limb amputees. *Brain.* 2001;11:2268–2277.
57. Chan BL, Witt R, Charrow AP, et al. Mirror therapy for phantom limb pain. *N Engl J Med.* 2007;357:2206–2207.
58. Rosen B, Lundborg G. Training with a mirror in rehabilitation of the hand. *Scand J Plast Reconstr Surg Hand Surg.* 2005;39:104–108.
59. Brodie EE, Whyte A, Niven CA. Analgesia through the looking-glass? A randomized controlled trial investigating the effect of viewing a 'virtual' limb upon phantom limb pain, sensation and movement. *Eur J Pain.* 2007;11:428–436.
60. Bittar RG, Otero S, Carter H, Aziz TZ. Deep brain stimulation for phantom limb pain. *J Clin Neurosci.* 2005;12:399–404.
61. Rasmussen S, Kehlet H. Management of nerves during leg amputation–a neglected area in our understanding of the pathogenesis of phantom limb pain. *Acta Anaesthesiol Scand.* 2007;51:1115–1116.
62. Kehlet H. Persistent postsurgical pain: surgical risk factors and strategies for prevention. In: Castro-Lopes J, Raja SN, Schmetz M, eds. *IASP Refresher Course on Pain Management held in Conjunction with the 12th World Congress on Pain.* Vol. Glasgow: IASP Press; 2008: 153–158.
63. Hartrick CT. Multimodal postoperative pain management. *Am J Health Syst Pharm.* 2004;61(Suppl 1):S4–S10.
64. Hanling SR, Wallace SC, Hollenbeck KJ, Belnap BD, Tulis MR. Preamputation mirror therapy may prevent development of phantom limb pain: a case series. *Anesth Analg.* 2010;110:611–614.
65. Cahana A, Van Zundert J, Macrea L, van Kleef M, Sluijter M. Pulsed radiofrequency: current clinical and biological literature available. *Pain Medicine.* 2006;7:411–423.
66. van Eijs F, Stanton-Hicks M, Van Zundert J, et al. 16. Complex regional pain syndrome. *Pain Pract.* 2011;11:70–87.

22 Traumatic Plexus Lesion

Robert van Dongen, Steven P. Cohen, Maarten van Kleef, Nagy Mekhail and Frank Huygen

Introduction

Traumatic plexus brachialis lesions are the most common form of plexus injuries. This syndrome is frequently the result of high-impact trauma in young male adults, as is often observed following a motorcycle accident or industrial injury. It can be caused by damage of the cervical vertebrae, the clavicula, and the humerus.

An injury due to trauma of the plexus lumbosacralis may also result from a serious accident, but this occurs less frequently. The plexus lumbosacralis can also be involved after a hemorrhage in the pelvic retroperitoneum, or as a result of tumor spread. The symptoms mainly occur in the thigh and around the knee region. Due to the low incidence of the latter, only plexus brachialis lesions will be addressed here.

Anatomically, the plexus brachialis consists of the five roots (radices) stemming from the (C5 to T1 dermatomes, which ultimately form the five major peripheral nerves of the arm (nervus muscolocutaneus, nervus axillaris, nervus radialis, nervus medianus, and nervus ulnaris). Therefore, clinical and anatomical distinctions exist between superior (C5 to C7) and inferior (C8 to Th1) plexus brachialis lesions. Majority of brachial plexus injuries result from a combination of traction and avulsion caused by the trauma itself. Penetrating trauma and surgical interventions can also lead to a disruption of the nerves. Anatomically, plexus brachialis injuries can be stratified according to location: preganglionic (ie, nerve root avulsion from the spinal cord), postganglionic, or combination lesions. Postganglionic lesions can be further classified into nerve disruption and lesions in continuity. Lesions located between the spinal cord and (proximal) ganglion can result in particularly debilitating pain complaints.[1,2]

Diagnosis

History

In addition to the (often severe) neurologic impairment, neuropathic pain in the arm/hand area is the main complaint in 30% to 90% of people with a traumatic plexus brachialis lesion (de-afferentation pain) (Figure 22.1). In the presence of a "preganglionic lesion," the incidence of serious pain increases to approximately 90%.[1] In one observational study involving 22 patients with signs of postconcussion syndrome, in the absence of severe brain damage secondary to whiplash injury, half had neurologic evidence of plexus brachialis injury.[3]

In those patients where the radices of the nerves are disconnected from the spinal cord (root avulsion), severe pain usually occurs immediately following the injury, although in some cases it can arise after a painfree interval.[4,5] The initial continuous "background pain" is often described as "burning," "shooting," or "stabbing" in quality, but may later be exacerbated by superimposed paroxysms. The pain is usually worst in the distal parts of the arm and hand, typically in a nondermatomal distribution. The use of validated questionnaires designed to distinguish between neuropathic and nociceptive pain may be useful for diagnostic, prognostic, and therapeutic purposes.[6] Serious sensory and/or motor loss confirms the diagnosis (MRC scale) (Medical Research Council; see Table 22.1). Psychosocial problems in the context of chronic pain and disability can also be influenced by cognitive disorders secondary to head trauma.

Physical examination

The results of neurologic examination depend on the location of the lesion (Table 22.2).[2,7] Injury to the upper region of the plexus brachialis generally results in extensive loss of function in the

Evidence-Based Interventional Pain Medicine: According to Clinical Diagnoses, First Edition. Edited by Jan Van Zundert, Jacob Patijn, Craig T. Hartrick, Arno Lataster, Frank J.P.M Huygen, Nagy Mekhail, Maarten van Kleef.

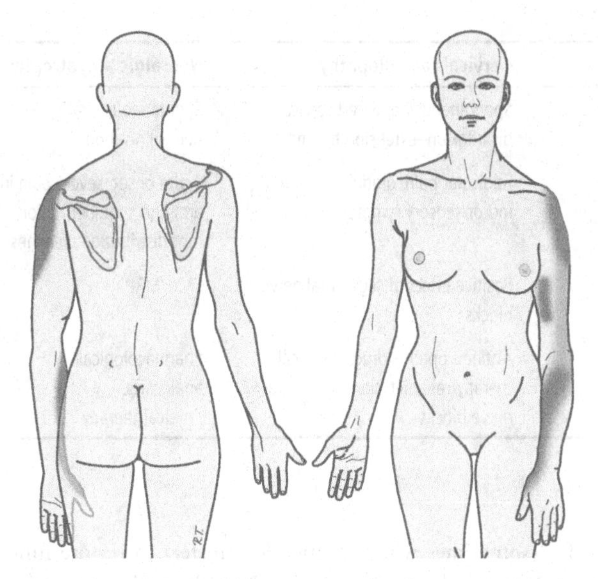

Figure 22.1. Clinical examination after a traumatic lesion of the plexus brachialis; changed muscle contour and changes in sensitivity. Illustration: Rogier Trompert, Medical Art, www.medical-art.nl.

Table 22.1. MRC grading for muscle strength.

0	Total paralysis, no contraction
1	Flicker contraction, no movement in joint
2	Muscle contraction with active motion with gravity eliminated
3	Full range of motion against gravity
4	Full range of motion against gravity with some resistance
5	Full range of motion against gravity with maximum resistance for that muscle

Table 22.2. Neurologic symptoms which may occur with a brachial plexus lesion (Adapted from Kuks et al.[2]).

Brachial plexus lesion	Dermatome	Motor	Sensory
Impairment in the upper part	C5–C6–C7	Reduced abduction of the upper arm, endorotation of the elbow and pronation of the hand (policeman's tip position)	±Extensor side of the forearm
Impairment in the lower part	C8–Th1	Paralysis of the small intrinsic hand muscles, flexors of the hand and fingers	Reduced sensation in the ulnar part of the forearm

proximal part of the arm and shoulder girdle, with motor function in the hand remaining unaltered or partially intact. By contrast, damage to the lower part of the plexus brachialis typically leads to serious loss of hand function, while the sensory losses are less extensive. Muscle strength can be determined by the MRC grading scale, with a correlation existing between the degree of motor dysfunction and the severity of injury (Table 22.1). Vegetative changes in the arm and hand often arise because of the trauma. A Horner's symptom on the affected side is indicative of a plexus brachialis lesion in the proximal region of roots C8 to T1. Combined damage to the plexus brachialis and spinal cord may lead to a difficult and time-consuming diagnostic process.[8,9]

Additional tests

In cases of major trauma, imaging can differentiate preganglionic from postganglion lesions, a distinction that serves a vital role in guiding treatment. Conventional magnetic resonance imaging (MRI) can detect signal changes in the spinal cord (present in approximately 20% of preganglionic injuries), which may indicate edema or hemorrhage in the acute phase and myelomalacia in the chronic phase. Contrast enhancement of intradural nerve roots may signify functional impairment despite morphological continuity. Abnormal enhancement of paraspinal muscles on MRI can also serve as a sensitive indicator of root avulsion.

Computed tomographic (CT)-myelography facilitates visual separation of ventral and dorsal nerve roots, and identification of intradural neuropathology. At upper levels (eg, C5 to C6), CT-myelography may be a more sensitive diagnostic tool than MRI for preganglionic lesions. Diffusion-weighted neurography may be a valuable tool for evaluating postganglionic plexus lesions, where neural structures can be difficult to distinguish from adjacent tissues using conventional MRI.[10]

Neurophysiological testing like EMG (electromyogram)/Nerve Conducting Studies (NCS) and somatosensory evoked potential can lead to better identification of the site of the lesion. This is especially important if surgical reconstruction is being considered.[7] Traditionally, EMG has been performed 3 to 4 weeks after injury, although some experts advocate earlier (1 to 2 weeks) testing, arguing that a normal sensory evoked potential from an anesthetic finger suggests preganglionic pathology. One of the drawbacks in performing EMG too early is that it cannot reliably distinguish between axonotmesis (nerve lesion within an intact perineurium) and neurotmesis (complete cutting of the nerve and perineurium). A neuropsychological examination should be considered if there is concomitant brain damage caused by the accident.

Differential diagnosis

The medical history in trauma patients is often conclusive. If pain and weakness develop suddenly without any inciting traumatic event, one should consider neuralgic amyotrophy of the plexus brachialis.

Table 22.3. Differential diagnosis, clinical signs, and general treatment of brachial plexopathy.

Syndrome	Brachial plexus lesion	Thoracic outlet syndrome	Cervical radiculopathy	Neuralgic amyotrophy
Cause	Traumatic/surgical stretch/sharp	Spontaneous, repetitive movements	Spontaneous/herniated cervical disk/flexion–extension trauma	Spontaneous/viral?; demyelinisation
Symptoms	Functional loss, paresthesias, pain	Pain, paresthesias, weakness in hand, cold intolerance; vascular signs	Radicular pain, gradual onset and motor/sensory symptoms	Acute onset, severe pain in arm and shoulder region, root distribution weakness
Diagnosis	MRI/CT-myelography/EMG	Clinical neurophysiologic testing	Positive effect of segmental nerve blocks	EMG/MRI
Treatment	Physical therapy/operative-reconstructive	Physical therapy, local infiltration	Antineuropathic drugs. Physical therapy/rehabilitation. Segmental nerve blocks	Pharmacological/ analgesics. Physical therapy

MRI, magnetic resonance imaging; EMG, electromyogram.

Table 22.3 gives an overview of potential differential diagnoses, clinical signs, and general treatment of brachial plexopathy.

Treatment options

Conservative, surgical, and interventional management

Extensive physical therapy is a first-line treatment strategy for a traumatic strain or avulsion injury. This is necessary to prevent the development of contractures and secondary pain.

Due to the complexity of problems and the disability that frequently ensues, an individually tailored rehabilitation program is indicated in most patients. Besides physical support and the use of orthoses, psychosocial interventions also play an important role. Drug therapy depends primarily on the type and quality of pain (eg, nociceptive vs. neuropathic, spontaneous vs. evoked). Recent clinical trials have demonstrated synergistic effects when two different adjuvants (eg, nortriptyline and gabapentin), or an adjuvant and opioid (gabapentin and morphine) are used to treat neuropathic pain.[11,12] Some experts advocate a mechanistic-based treatment approach based on response to a series of prognostic infusion tests.[13]

Most surgical therapies are initiated 3 to 6 months after injury, although some literature suggests that early intervention may improve outcomes.[14] Especially in cases of sharp, lacerating injuries, urgent exploration within the first 72 hours and repair by-end-to-end anastomoses appear to be necessary.[7] Surgical intervention is also usually considered if there has been no improvement (signs of re-innervation) in 3 to 6 months. A prolonged follow-up with delayed intervention carries the risk of severe muscular atrophy. These surgical interventions ostensibly reduce the risk of persistent serious pain, and may be particularly compelling if there is a chance to restore motor function.[1] The technique employed depends on the type and extent of injury. Preganglionic injuries are generally not amenable to repair, and may be treated with nerve (eg, intercostal nerves) transfer (sometimes with free muscle transfer) to restore function in denervated muscle(s). For postganglionic injuries, nerve grafting and nerve repair can improve function in 40% to 75% of patients.[15]

Our knowledge of the mechanisms responsible for pain in these patients is still very limited. Not surprisingly then, neurostimulation techniques have been reported to have wide-ranging and unpredictable effects.[16,17] Injuries characterized by complete de-afferentation are unlikely to respond positively to spinal cord stimulation (SCS). Although there is a zone of spinal hyperactivity in the dorsal part of the spinal cord, which could theoretically be amenable to SCS, disinhibition in the tractus spinothalamicus with changes in the spinoreticular fibers can lead to a more centralized disinhibition. In theory, motor cortex stimulation (MCS) should have a positive effect on de-afferentation pain, which has been borne out in clinical practice.[17–19]

Sometimes, there are other anatomical defects that can account for pain. The co-prevalence rate of pseudomeningocele has been estimated to range between 21% and 57% in patients with nerve avulsion,[20] and may be treated conservatively or surgically. A traumatic lesion due to traction can cause intramedullary bleeding with focal gliosis and the formation of microscopic cystic changes. Spinal cord herniation has also been reported following plexus brachialis avulsion injury,[20,21] and typically manifests as Brown-Séquard syndrome.

The literature does not provide sufficient data regarding the effects of various pain treatments in patients with a brachial plexus lesion. However, it is well-documented that a large percentage of patients will have persistent symptoms refractory to conventional therapy. In these individuals, surgical interruption of the afferent sensory input into the spinal cord can be considered in patients. In the DREZ (dorsal root entry zone) procedure,[1] also known as MDT (microsurgical DREZotomy), a 2 mm deep, 35° incision is made ventromedially in the sulcus dorsolateralis of the cornu posterior. The level(s) at which this intervention takes place depend(s) on the location of the radicular avulsion.

Table 22.4. Summary of the evidence for interventional management of traumatic plexus lesion.

Technique	Evaluation
Spinal cord stimulation	0

Results following DREZ have been mostly positive. Thomas and Kitchen[22] reported that 79% of 44 patients with brachial plexus avulsion achieved good or fair results at the mean 63-month follow-up. Sindou et al.[1] found that 66% of 55 patients with preganglionic plexus brachialis injuries experienced excellent or good pain relief lasting more than a year (mean follow-up: 6 years), with 71% obtaining significant functional improvement. Chen and Tu[23] reported more modest results. Although 80% of 40 patients with plexus brachialis avulsion reported good pain relief postoperatively after thermocoagulation DREZ lesions, success rates declined to 60% at 5-year follow-up, and 50% at 10-year follow-up. Potential complications of surgical treatment include motor weakness and ataxia. Theoretically, so-called MCS could have a positive effect on this pain.

Complications of interventional management

The complications of SCS have been described in the chapter on complex regional pain syndrome.[24]

Evidence for interventional management

The summary of the evidence for interventional pain management is given in Table 22.4.

Recommendations

In patients with pain resulting from a traumatic brachial plexus lesion who respond inadequately to drug treatment and physical therapy, SCS should only be considered in a study context after a positive trial period and in specialized centers.

Clinical practice algorithm

Figure 22.2 represents the treatment algorithm for traumatic plexus brachialis lesion.

Techniques

The techniques for neurostimulation were described in the chapter on complex regional pain syndrome.[24]

Summary

After high-impact trauma, damage to the plexus brachialis can lead to neurologic impairment a neuropathic pain. Extensive physical therapy and rehabilitation treatment are initiated first, particularly to prevent contractures, secondary pain, and atrophy. The cornerstone of treatment is pharmacotherapy, although the

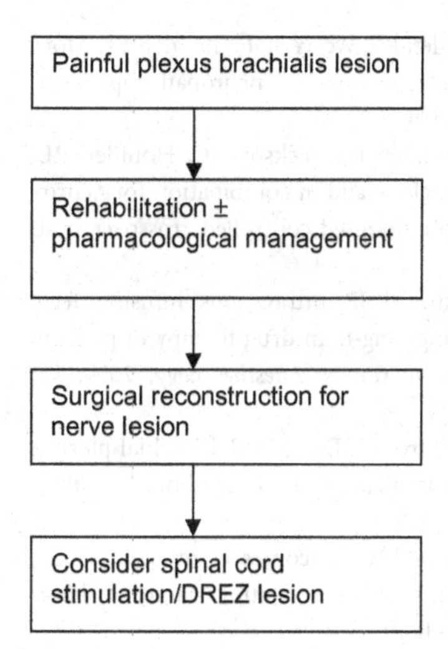

Figure 22.2. Clinical practice algorithm for the treatment of painful plexus brachialis lesion.

evidence supporting different drug regimens is typically extrapolated from clinical trials conducted for other neuropathic pain disorders. Surgical correction of brachial plexus injuries is generally attempted before SCS is used. SCS should only be considered as part of a multimodal regimen when more conventional treatment strategies have failed.

References

1. Sindou MP, Blondet E, Emery E, Mertens P. Microsurgical lesioning in the dorsal root entry zone for pain due to brachial plexus avulsion: a prospective series of 55 patients. *J. Neurosurg.* 2005;102:1018–1028.
2. Kuks J, Snoek J, Oosterhuis H. *Klinische Neurologie.* Houten: Bohn Stafleu en van Loghum; 2004.
3. Bring G, Westman G. Chronic posttraumatic syndrome after whiplash injury. A pilot study of 22 patients. *Scand. J. Prim. Health Care.* 1991;9:135–141.
4. Kim KK. Acute brachial neuropathy—electrophysiological study and clinical profile. *J. Korean Med. Sci.* 1996;11:158–164.
5. Guenot M, Bullier J, Sindou M. Clinical and electrophysiological expression of deafferentation pain alleviated by dorsal root entry zone lesions in rats. *J. Neurosurg.* 2002;97:1402–1409.
6. Bennett MI, Smith BH, Torrance N, Lee AJ. Can pain can be more or less neuropathic? Comparison of symptom assessment tools with ratings of certainty by clinicians. *Pain.* 2006;122:289–294.
7. Kandenwein JA, Kretschmer T, Engelhardt M, Richter HP, Antoniadis G. Surgical interventions for traumatic lesions of the brachial plexus: a retrospective study of 134 cases. *J. Neurosurg.* 2005;103:614–621.
8. Akita S, Wada E, Kawai H. Combined injuries of the brachial plexus and spinal cord. *J. Bone Joint Surg. Br.* 2006;88:637–641.
9. Chillemi C, Marinelli M, Galizia P. Fracture-dislocation of the shoulder and brachial plexus palsy: a terrible association. *J. Orthop. Traumatol.* 2008;9:217–220.
10. Yoshikawa T, Hayashi N, Yamamoto S, et al. Brachial plexus injury: clinical manifestations, conventional imaging findings, and the latest imaging techniques. *Radiographics.* 2006;26(suppl 1):S133–S143.

11. Gilron I, Bailey JM, Tu D, Holden RR, Weaver DF, Houlden RL. Morphine, gabapentin, or their combination for neuropathic pain. *N. Engl. J. Med.* 2005;352:1324–1334.
12. Gilron I, Bailey JM, Tu D, Holden RR, Jackson AC, Houlden RL. Nortriptyline and gabapentin, alone and in combination for neuropathic pain: a double-blind, randomised controlled crossover trial. *Lancet.* 2009;374:1252–1261.
13. Cohen SP, Kapoor SG, Rathmell JP. Intravenous infusion tests have limited utility for selecting long-term drug therapy in patients with chronic pain: a systematic review. *Anesthesiology.* 2009;111: 416–431.
14. Wilberg M, Backman C, Wahlstrom P, Dahlin LB. [Brachial plexusz injuries in adults. Early reconstruction for better clinical results]. *Lakartidningen.* 2009;106:586–590.
15. Terzis JK, Vekris MD, Soucacos PN. Outcomes of brachial plexus reconstruction in 204 patients with devastating paralysis. *Plast. Reconstr. Surg.* 1999;104:1221–1240.
16. Cruccu G, Aziz TZ, Garcia-Larrea L, et al. EFNS guidelines on neurostimulation therapy for neuropathic pain. *Eur. J. Neurol.* 2007;14: 952–970.
17. Brill S, Aryeh IG. Neuromodulation in the management of pain from brachial plexus injury. *Pain Physician.* 2008;11:81–85.
18. Lefaucheur JP, Drouot X, Cunin P, et al. Motor cortex stimulation for the treatment of refractory peripheral neuropathic pain. *Brain.* 2009;132:1463–1471.
19. Saitoh Y, Yoshimine T. Stimulation of primary motor cortex for intractable deafferentation pain. *Acta Neurochir. Suppl.* 2007;97: 51–56.
20. Tanaka M, Ikuma H, Nakanishi K, et al. Spinal cord herniation into pseudomeningocele after traumatic nerve root avulsion: case report and review of the literature. *Eur. Spine J.* 2008;17(suppl 2): S263–S266.
21. Yokota H, Yokoyama K, Noguchi H, Uchiyama Y. Spinal cord herniation into associated pseudomeningocele after brachial plexus avulsion injury: case report. *Neurosurgery.* 2007;60:E205; discussion: E205.
22. Thomas DG, Kitchen ND. Long-term follow up of dorsal root entry zone lesions in brachial plexus avulsion. *J. Neurol. Neurosurg. Psychiatr.* 1994;57:737–738.
23. Chen HJ, Tu YK. Long term follow-up results of dorsal root entry zone lesions for intractable pain after brachial plexus avulsion injuries. *Acta Neurochir. Suppl.* 2006;99:73–75.
24. van Eijs F, Stanton-Hicks M, Van Zundert J, et al. 16. Complex Regional Pain Syndrome. *Pain Pract.* 2011;11:70–87.

23 Pain in Patients with Cancer

Kris C. P. Vissers, Kees Besse, Michel Wagemans, Wouter Zuurmond, Maurice J.M.M. Giezeman, Arno Lataster, Nagy Mekhail, Allen W. Burton, Maarten van Kleef and Frank Huygen

Introduction

The treatment of pain in patients with cancer is a delicate balance, affected by a range of interfering factors, such as the patient's general condition, the co-medication, and the nature of the pain, which is usually a mixture of nociceptive and neuropathic pain. Interventional pain management techniques have a specific role in the treatment of pain in patients with cancer.[1] Until recently, mainly because of potential complications and special requirements of aftercare and the need for specific devices, these techniques have been mostly used as a last resort among the arsenal of pain treatment options in patients with cancer. Several recent publications, however, as well as the new guidelines on the management of pain in patients with cancer of the Dutch association of anesthesiologists (NVA), the society of Dutch comprehensive cancer centers VIKC and the Dutch Institute for Health Care Improvement (CBO), have recommended the use of certain interventional techniques at earlier stages, possibly even at the stage, where opioid treatment is first being considered.[2] Reserving the use of these techniques until the last few days of life is certainly not a good idea. All interventional pain management techniques impose a certain burden on the patient, which must be taken into account when considering these treatment options. In addition, correct performance of these techniques requires one or more days of hospitalization. This information must be communicated to the patient to allow for an informed decision-making process.

The interventional pain management techniques can be classified into two main categories:

1 Intrathecal/epidural administration of medication, used to treat pain refractory to oral and transdermal pharmacologic therapy.

2 Specific targeted nerve blocks; in this article the following techniques will be discussed: cervical cordotomy, plexus coeliacus block, nervus splanchnicus block, plexus hypogastricus block, and lower end (saddle) block.

Another treatment modality that is becoming more popular is spinal cord and peripheral nerve stimulation, which, however, has not (or at least not yet) played an important role in oncologic pain management.

Epidural and intrathecal administration of analgesics

Epidural and intrathecal administration of analgesics directly targets the receptors or pain transmission pathways in the spinal cord. The use of these techniques is mainly proposed in situations, where oral or transdermal analgesics have insufficient effect or produce unacceptable side effects. Central administration of the analgesics is then expected to increase the analgesic effect and reduce the risk of side effects. In addition, this administration route allows simultaneous administration of other analgesics, such as bupivacaine and clonidine. The analgesic is administered via a catheter into the cerebrospinal fluid (intrathecal or spinal) or outside the dura mater (epidural).

The use of epidural and intrathecal drug administration has not increased, despite considerable progress in our understanding of the safety, effectiveness, and side effects of epidural and intrathecal opioid administration techniques, and further optimization of the logistics that allow its use in the home situation. This may be attributed to the fact that various new opioids have become available, and average individual dosages have increased, allowing the switch to epidural and intrathecal opioids to be postponed.

Evidence-Based Interventional Pain Medicine: According to Clinical Diagnoses, First Edition. Edited by Jan Van Zundert, Jacob Patijn, Craig T. Hartrick, Arno Lataster, Frank J.P.M Huygen, Nagy Mekhail, Maarten van Kleef.

The increasing use of subcutaneous opioids at patients' homes has also reduced the use of intrathecal and epidural administration. There is still an indication for intrathecal and epidural analgesics, however, provided that optimal use has been made of all options for oral and transdermal opioids.[2]

Diagnosis

History

There are two major reasons to switch to epidural or intrathecal analgesia, when the pain cannot be sufficiently relieved despite suitable dosages of opioids, where indicated co-analgesics, and when side effects prove intolerable despite aggressive treatment.

Physical examination

Physical examination of patients who are suffering pain that is refractory to oral or transdermal analgesics and for whom intrathecal or epidural analgesia is being considered should focus on:

1 Inspecting the painful area, concentrating on local problems of infection, skin abnormalities or open wounds, as well as on possible causes of the pain, such as a tumor compressing a nerve tract. It is important to estimate the consequences of the presence of such a tumor.

2 Detailed neurologic examination and tests of skin sensitivity by means of pinprick, ice cube or cold roller and ether test, to allow the difference in response to be evaluated after the catheter has been placed and local analgesics and opioids have been delivered.

3 Inspection of the entire spinal column, focusing on the sites, where the catheter is to be inserted and tunneled.

4 Clinical examination of mobility and motor function of the patient's lower limbs, which might be affected by the use of the spinal or epidural catheter.

5 Consulting with patient and nurse to decide on the best exit site for the catheter in terms of nursing convenience, and the advantages and disadvantages of the treatment.

Indications for the use of an epidural or intrathecal catheter

1 Pain resistant to very high dosages of oral, transdermal, or systemic opioids.

2 Pain that is responsive to systemic opioids but accompanied by intolerable side effects like nausea, vomiting, constipation, or allergic reactions.

3 Pain that cannot be treated with other modalities such as neurolytic blocks, cordotomy, or other neuroablative of neuromodulatory techniques.

4 Refractory pain of oncologic origin occurring in a localized and well-defined area.

Contraindications for the use of an epidural or intrathecal catheter

1 Elevated intracranial pressure.

2 Generalized or localized infections at the spinal level corresponding to the painful area.

3 Suspected tumor mass at the level of the insertion site.

4 Hemorrhagic diatheses.

5 Allergic reaction to the epidural or intrathecal agents to be used.

6 Agitation or cognitive disorders that may induce the patient to unexpectedly pull out the catheter, which are not expected to subside after the administration of locoregional analgesics.

7 Expected problems in nursing the exit or insertion site of the catheter or exchanging the medication supply.

Epidural and spinal drug delivery

In a 2005 Cochrane review, Ballantyne was only able to include 1 RCT comparing intrathecal morphine delivery and conventional (oral and transdermal) administration of opioids in patients with pain due to cancer.[3] The clinical success rates were 85% and 71%, respectively. The group receiving intrathecal morphine reported less pain and fewer side effects, and survived longer. The other studies included in the review were cohort studies of patients exclusively treated with epidural or intrathecal opioids. The effectiveness of epidural opioids has been reported on in 31 uncontrolled studies involving a total of 1,343 patients. Intrathecal opioid delivery was studied in 28 cohort studies involving a total of 722 patients, the most frequently used opioid being morphine. Good to excellent analgesic effect was achieved in 87% and 89% of the intrathecal and epidural groups, respectively.

Addition of a local anesthetic has been most extensively studied using bupivacaine. One RCT and several cohort studies found that the addition of bupivacaine is effective for those patients who fail to achieve sufficient pain relief with intrathecal and epidural morphine.

A prospective observational study on the effect of intrathecal morphine and levobupivacaine, included 55 cancer patients who were highly opioid tolerant. Complete data with adequate follow-up until death were available for 45 patients. The initial morphine dose was calculated from the previous opioid consumption. During treatment the doses of morphine and levobupivacaine were adjusted according to the clinical needs and balanced with adverse effects. Statistical significant differences in pain intensity were noted at all time intervals until death. Significant improvement in drowsiness and confusion was found until 1 month after starting intrathecal therapy. The daily morphine dose was threefold increased at the time of hospital discharge. Subsequent dose increases were not significant. The use of systemic opioids decreased significantly until death.[4]

Administration of clonidine has been investigated in one RCT and several cohort studies. Clonidine proved more effective than placebo (56% and 5%, respectively) especially for patients with neuropathic pain.[2]

For an audit in a tertiary centre medical records of 29 patients who received intrathecal drug administration were reviewed. Eighty-six percent of those patients had metastatic cancer. The main reason for intrathecal drug administration was poor pain control. The pain intensity decreased significantly at the time of hospital discharge. The number of opioid side effects decreased.[5]

Epidural and intrathecal medication

The most frequently used types of medication for epidural or intrathecal delivery are morphine, hydromorphone, fentanyl, bupivacaine, ropivacaine, and clonidine. These drugs are often combined; a commonly used mixture consists of morphine 1 mg/mL and bupivacaine 2 to 3 mg/mL. Intrathecal delivery starts at a continuous rate of 0.5 to 2 mL/hour, with a bolus option of 0.1 to 0.3 mL per 20 minutes. If the infusion rate is below 0.5 mL/hour, the concentration of the morphine and bupivacaine solution must be adjusted. When using morphine, it is important to remember that this compound is metabolized to morphine-6 glucuronide, and morphine-3 glucuronide. There is a limit to the amount of latter that can be processed in a long-term spinal administration (maximum 16 mg intrathecal morphine per day), and excess administration may cause opioid-induced hyperalgesia.

Higher doses of local anesthetics may induce motor weakness and sensory deficiencies. In addition, urinary retention may occur, as well as transient arterial hypotension. There are no literature reports on toxic effects on the nervous system in case of long-term administration of local anesthetics on nerve tracts. Intrathecal clonidine can be added to the opioids and/or local anesthetics if required, at doses of 150 to 600 μg/day.

Ziconotide, the synthetic analog of the omega-conotoxin, has been used in both chronic nonmalignant pain and pain due to cancer. A randomized controlled trial found intrathecal ziconotide to be effective in relieving pain in patients with cancer or AIDS over a short follow-up period.[6] In the recently published Italian registry, ziconotide was used for the management of chronic pain, in general. In those patients with cancer, a significant improvement in pain intensity was achieved faster than in noncancer patients.[7]

In U.S., in refractory cases the use of intrathecal ziconotide starting at low dose 1 to 2 μg/day with a slow titration up to 8 to 10 μg/daily or higher seemed successful in several cases. However, the side effects are the major limitation of this drug.

Additional considerations

The choice between implantable drug delivery systems and external pumps depends mainly on the patient's life expectancy. When the patient's condition and life expectancy justifies the use of an implantable pump, because of the complexity and dynamic state of cancer pain preference should be given to a programmable pump that allows patient controlled bolus administration.[8] A cost-effectiveness analysis has shown that implantable systems are to be preferred over external pumps if the patient has a life expectancy of at least 3 months.[9]

Epidural delivery will be preferred if the treatment goal is focal analgesia and a short treatment period is expected. The catheter tip is then inserted at the level of vertebra corresponding to the dermatome, where analgesia is required. Intrathecal delivery will be preferred if the painful area to be treated is large, if a disorder of the epidural space precludes the insertion of a catheter, or if the patient has a life expectancy of more than a few weeks.[10]

Side effects and complications

Side effects like nausea, urinary retention, pruritus, and headaches are common in the start-up phase of intrathecal treatment. A study found that infections occurred in 1% (epidural), or 2% (intrathecal) of cases. In the epidural group, 16% of the patients had to have their catheter exchanged or removed because of catheter-related complications (such as fibrosis). The corresponding figure in the intrathecal group was 5%. Other catheter-related complications, like infections and mechanical obstruction, have been reported with varying incidence rates (1% to 44%).[11]

A recent study into safety and complications found a relation between the occurrence of an inflammatory mass around an intrathecal catheter and the concentrations and dosages of morphine used.[12] Previously, a relation had been found between high dosages of intrathecal morphine and the occurrence of myoclonias and hyperpathia. Long-term intrathecal morphine administration also results in hormonal changes: hypogonadotropic hypogonadism, and hypocorticism.[13]

A systematic review and meta-analysis investigated the infection rates associated with epidural catheters in place for at least 7 days. Of the 12 studies, 9 were published after 1990. Eight were retrospective (3,893 patients) and 4 studies were prospective (735 patients). There were 6.1% catheter-related infections, 4.6% superficial and 1.2% deep infections. The incidence of catheter-related infections was calculated to be 0.4/1,000 catheter days.[14]

Another systematic review and meta-analysis on the serious complications with external intrathecal catheters identified 10 articles, including a total of 821 patients. Twenty catheter-related infections; 10 superficial and 10 deep infections were noted. The risk for bleeding was calculated to be 0.9% and for neurologic injury 0.4%. The authors concluded that the risks for serious complications are low in both hospitalized and homebound patients with intrathecal catheters.[14] Aprili, et al. in their meta-analysis on the related topic specifically looking at tunnelled intrathecal catheters, found a rate of superficial infection of 2.3%, with deep infection rate of 1.4%, bleeding at 0.9%, and neurologic injury 0.4%. They further calculated that every 71st patient would get an infection after 54 days of therapy through statistical means.[15]

Other therapeutic options

Spinal drug delivery is usually considered as a final option when all other treatment modalities produce insufficient results. If spinal drug delivery is contraindicated or impossible for a particular patient, treatment may include of a combination of therapeutic modalities involving subcutaneous or intravenous administration of analgesics. If a patient in the terminal stages is suffering from a refractory pain syndrome, palliative sedation can be considered, in consultation with the patient and their caregivers.

Evidence for epidural and intrathecal medication delivery for cancer pain relief

The evidence for epidural and intrathecal medication delivery for cancer pain is listed in Table 23.1.

Table 23.1. Summary of the evidence for epidural and intrathecal medication delivery.

Technique	Evaluation
Intrathecal medication delivery	2B+
Epidural medication delivery	2C+

Recommendations

Use of intrathecal medication delivery is recommended for patients with refractory pain due to cancer especially when they have a significant neuropathic pain component. To this end, morphine should preferably be combined with a local anesthetic. Epidural delivery may be considered for short treatments or for a quick assessment of the required dosage; in all other circumstances, intrathecal delivery is to he preferred.

In some locations of the U.S., home catheter care is virtually unavailable, and an implanted pump can be used with a 40 mL reservoir, and maximal medication concentration fill prior to sending a patient to a home hospice situation with a remote geographical location. Often, this reservoir will outlast the patient's life expectancy with fair certainty. Also, in many practices, the patient therapy manager device (PTM) with the Medtronic brand implanted pump will allow the patient to deliver "as needed" boluses, simplifying the home care programming needs significantly.

Technique

Preparing the patient

1 Discuss the method and the consequences of placing an epidural or intrathecal catheter with the patient and their family or caregivers.

2 Ensure that a suitable treatment facility is available, equipped with all the materials required for normal anesthesia, resuscitation, and sterile procedures. If the patient is to be given anesthesia, he will need to be fasted. Note that with some tumors of the gastrointestinal tract, the patient can never be regarded as fasted.

3 Ensure the availability of a radiographic image intensifier to check the specific position of the catheter or to inspect the cause of unexpectedly difficult insertion, especially when inserting an epidural or intrathecal catheter near the tumor or extensive metastases.

4 Evaluate the patient's physical condition to determine the most suitable position for the treatment: cervical and thoracic catheters are best inserted with the patient sitting upright, unless the physical condition does not allow this or extensive sedation or anesthesia is required. Lumbar catheters are preferably inserted with the patient in lateral recumbent position, unless the patient is unable to lie down due to, eg, extreme dyspnea.

Preparation for the intervention

The insertion site for the needle should be 10 to 15 cm from the intended catheter tip position. In the case of *epidural* analgesia, the following levels should be chosen for the following types of pain:

1 Lumbar insertion (Th12 to L5) for sub-diaphragmatic pains and pains in the pelvis and lower limbs.

2 Low thoracic approach (Th8 to Th12) for patients with lymphedema of the lower half of the body, previous lower back surgery, a tumor in the lumbar spine, presence of pyelostomy catheters or high upper abdominal tumors.

3 Mid-thoracic approach (Th4 to Th8) for patients with thoracic pain due to tumors of the thorax (rib metastases, oncologic rib fractures, mesotheliomas, or pulmonary tumors).

4 High thoracic approach (Th1 to Th4) for patients with a Pancoast tumor, severe neuropathic pain from mammary tumors or brachial plexopathy (due to tumor infiltration or radiotherapy) and refractory angina pectoris.

5 A spinal (*intrathecal*) catheter should always be inserted at the lumbar level, below the level of the presumed lower end of the conus medullaris (L1 to L2).

Inserting the needle and introducing the catheter

1 Apply local anesthesia to the skin and underlying subcutaneous tissues at the insertion site of the epidural or spinal needle and along the tunneling pathway. If required, the patient may also be sedated using propofol, ketamine, or other agents.

2 Place a 17G Tuohy needle preferably on the midline, as a paramedian approach is associated with a greater risk of accidental puncture of epidural blood vessels, paresthesias or radicular pain. Use the "loss of resistance" technique with a specially adapted syringe to detect the epidural space.

3 For epidural pain control, the epidural catheter can now be introduced, ensuring that the catheter tip ends up at the intended level for effective pain relief.

4 For spinal (intrathecal) pain control, the Tuohy needle is placed transversely and inserted until CSF reflex is obtained. Although the "dural click" can be felt in some cases, this is frequently not the case, and the surgeon should check regularly whether CSF is flowing from the needle. As patients who have only been given local anesthesia are usually able to well indicate when the spinal space has been accessed, their reactions should be observed. When CSF flows from the needle (positive glucose test can confirm if necessary) the catheter is advanced through the spinal space to the required level, guided by the patient's reactions. Avoid excessive CSF leakage. Initial insertion of the catheter through the spinal space may be somewhat difficult. If necessary, check the position of the spinal catheter radiographically with a contrast medium.

5 Check whether CSF is flowing from the catheter, preferably by allowing the catheter to hang downward and letting any fluid drain out by gravity.

6 Withdraw the Tuohy needle by 1 to 2 cm, but do not remove it until an incision has been made and the first tunneling device has been introduced (see below).

7 Delivering a bolus of morphine and/or a local anesthetic after the catheter has been inserted may result in rapid pain relief.

8 Tunnel the epidural/intrathecal catheter.
9 Make a 4 to 6 mm incision down to the fascia around the Tuohy needle, to free the needle from the surrounding skin.
10 If tunneling cannot be completed in one movement, make incisions along the intended course of the tunneled catheter, except at the exit site (to prevent any CSF leakage along the catheter).
11 If patients prefer to have a full immersion bath, apply paravertebral tunneling across the shoulder to the ipsilateral parasternal area.
12 If the paravertebral route is contraindicated, for instance due to paravertebral metastases, extensive tumor growth or skin damage due to radiotherapy along the intended course of the catheter, abdominal tunneling in a ventral direction may be used.
13 Ensure that the catheter is not accidentally retracted during the tunneling procedure; if in doubt, check by means of radiography.
14 Use a second Tuohy needle or a special tunneling needle to guide the catheter subcutaneously. The tunneling device should always be inserted from peripheral to central.
15 With each manipulation of the catheter, check whether CSF is still spontaneously flowing by gravity from the end of the catheter when held below the level of insertion.
16 Finally, connect the catheter to the special connector and fasten the connector onto the skin to prevent the catheter being dislocated and accidentally withdrawn from the spinal space.
17 The catheter may also be connected to a permanent access port system, which is fastened subcutaneously over a hard substrate. This requires a pocket to be made on the fascia of the thoracic wall.
18 Check whether the catheter is sufficiently embedded in the subcutaneous adipose tissue at all incision sites, to avoid fistula formation.
19 Cover all incision sites with aseptic bandaging;, while covering the catheter exit site with separate bandaging for easy nursing access. Connect a micropore bacterial filter and connect this to a medication pump from which all air has been removed. Ensure that the catheter is free of air from the point, where it leaves the pump to the micropore filter.
20 Try to avoid traction on the catheter by providing extra loops on the skin or in the tunneling channel, as this reduces the risk of dislocation.
21 After the incisions have healed and a semipermeable bandage has been applied to the catheter exit site, the patient will be able to take a shower or use a hip bath.
22 If a subcutaneous central venous access device is used, the needle insertion should always be checked.

Instructions

Instructions must be provided:
1 To the patient about the correct way to use the pump (possible bolus option).
2 To the patient's family about the care required by the patient and any special concerns.
3 To the nursing staff about programming, exchanging batteries and medication cassettes, pain assessment, and advice for correct usage (Instructions should preferably be given in writing or by referring to printed guidelines for this treatment available at the clinic).
4 To the patient's family doctor and other medical staff involved, about preferred dosage, possible side effects, aspects to be observed and possible adjustments.

Observation

After an epidural or spinal catheter has been installed, the patient should be observed at the postoperative care department for a few hours, after which they should stay on a hospital ward for further observation for at least two to three days, which time can be used:
1 To teach the patient how to use the pump correctly.
2 To find the correct dosage for optimum pain relief.
3 To identify and treat possible side effects.
4 To dress the wounds correctly.

For permanent implantable pumps specific surgical techniques are used.

Unilateral pain with limited life expectancy

Introduction

Unilateral oncologic pains situated below the shoulder or dermatome C5, such as may occur with Pancoast, pleural mesothelioma or invasion of the plexus brachialis, or plexus lumbalis, may be eligible for treatment with cordotomy, if they prove refractory to other techniques.

Cordotomy involves creating a lesion of the tractus spinothalamicus lateralis at the C1 to C2 level of the spinal cord with the aim of relieving unilaterally localized pain below the level of dermatome C5. The technique was first described by Mullan in 1963.[16] Although the treatment was originally applied for nononcologic pain, because of the potential side effects, it is now mainly reserved for the management of patients with refractory pain due to cancer whose maximum life expectancy is 1 year.[17,18]

Diagnosis

History

Unilateral refractory pains due to cancer located under the dermatome C5 are eligible for treatment with cordotomy. Best results are obtained for the treatment of neuropathic pain and incident pain, occurring by some form of strain. Visceral pain, especially abdominal pain, is not an indication for cordotomy. It is also important to assess whether pain elsewhere in the body is well-controlled. The patient must be informed that successful cordotomy may unmask other pain.

Physical examination

Clinical neurologic examination results obtained before and after treatment should be compared to identify any neurologic deficits.

This includes pain perception and/or temperature perception on both sides, as well as motor function.

Additional tests

The referring doctor must have completed the technical examination that is required to accurately identify the causes of the pain, to provide a detailed picture of the situation before any interventional pain management techniques are applied.

Differential diagnosis

All causes of unilateral pain of nononcologic, neurologic, osteogenic, or myofascial origin must be excluded.

Treatment options

Cordotomy

The effects of cordotomy on patients have been described in one nonrandomized study and a number of observational studies. A study comparing cordotomy with subarachnoid phenol found that both techniques yielded similar pain control at lower opioid dosages.[19] Seven of the 10 cordotomy patients developed pain on the contralateral side of the body, whereas 4 of the 10 patients developed complications, which resulted in functional deterioration. Since 1990, 6 case series have been described in which a total of 677 patients with cancer were treated with unilateral cordotomy.[20–25] The authors reported considerable or even complete pain reduction in 82% to 98% of the patients, whereas opioid consumption was reduced by 50%. The best results were obtained in the treatment of unilateral pain.

A number of patients (31% to 88%) experienced recurrence of the pain, which can usually be effectively treated with opioids. Two studies described 3 patients who survived for considerably longer than 2 years.[21,25] These patients did not develop neuropathic pain as a result of the procedure. However, this number is too small to allow conclusions about the long-term safety of cordotomy. A recent report describes a patient who survived 5 years after right-sided cervical cordotomy. Sensory dysfunction was observed in the left side of the body, but no motor neuron or autonomic dysfunction was observed. There was limited influence on the patient's daily activities.[26]

Cordotomy is only used for cancer patients suffering severe pain, which is refractory to pharmacologic treatment. The Dutch CBO guidelines for the treatment of pain from cancer recommend that these therapeutic options should only be considered for patients with a limited life expectancy (1 year).[2]

The immediate results of the treatment are evaluated by applying the pinprick test to the patient's thorax. We recommend regular evaluation of the pain (at least weekly). In view of the complexity of the pain syndrome and the risk of other (masked) pains becoming manifest, we recommend that the pharmacologic treatment be adjusted on the basis of the patient's complaints.

There have been contradictory reports about the value of bilateral cordotomy to relieve pain due to cancer. Amano et al.[20] found that 95% of the 60 patients who had a bilateral cordotomy reported (virtually) complete pain reduction, vs. 82% of the patients who had a unilateral cordotomy. In this study, however, both groups were suffering from bilateral pain. In contrast, Sanders et al.[23] found no advantage of bilateral cordotomy, whereas the risk of complications appeared greater.

Computer tomography-guided radiofrequency (RF) treatment was also described for ablation of the upper spinal cord pain pathways. Of a series of 55 patients, 42 underwent a unilateral cervical cordotomy. Patients reported initial and 6 months pain relief of 98% and 80%, respectively.[27]

Another series of 207 patients treated with CT-guided cordotomy over 20 years reports an initial success rate of 92.5%. The success rate was higher in patients suffering with pain due to malignancies. In this group, selective cordotomy (pain sensation denervated only in the painful region of the body) was achieved in 83%. Bilateral cordotomy was successfully applied in 12 cases.[28]

Side effects and complications

The localization of the tractus spinothalamicus lateralis and the size of the thermolesion relative to the spinal cord, explains the risk of damage to adjoining nerve tracts. Reported complications include pareses (up to 10%), bladder dysfunction (up to 15%), and respiratory depression (up to 10%),[29] as well as head and neck pain and dysesthesias. These side effects proved to be permanent in a number of cases.[23] In addition, there is a risk of other, previously masked pains becoming manifest, or of developing "mirror pain," that is, pain on the contralateral side. The incidence of such pain syndromes is between 9% and 63%.[29] Interestingly, none of the studies reported neuropathic pain due to the treatment. The risk of major complications is larger with bilateral cordotomy.[23]

Other treatment options

If patients are not eligible for cordotomy, epidural or intrathecal analgesics may be considered. Surgical neuroablation techniques have been abandoned because they were insufficiently selective.

Evidence for cordotomy

The evidence for cervical cordotomy is given in Table 23.2.

Recommendations for cordotomy

Cordotomy may be considered for patients with unilaterally localized refractory oncologic pain below the level of dermatome C5, with a maximum life expectancy of 1 year, who obtain insufficient relief from conventional treatment. Cordotomy should only be carried out at centers, where staffs have extensive experience with this treatment.

Table 23.2. Summary of the evidence for interventional management of unilateral pain with limited life expectancy.

Technique	Evaluation
Cervical cordotomy	2C+

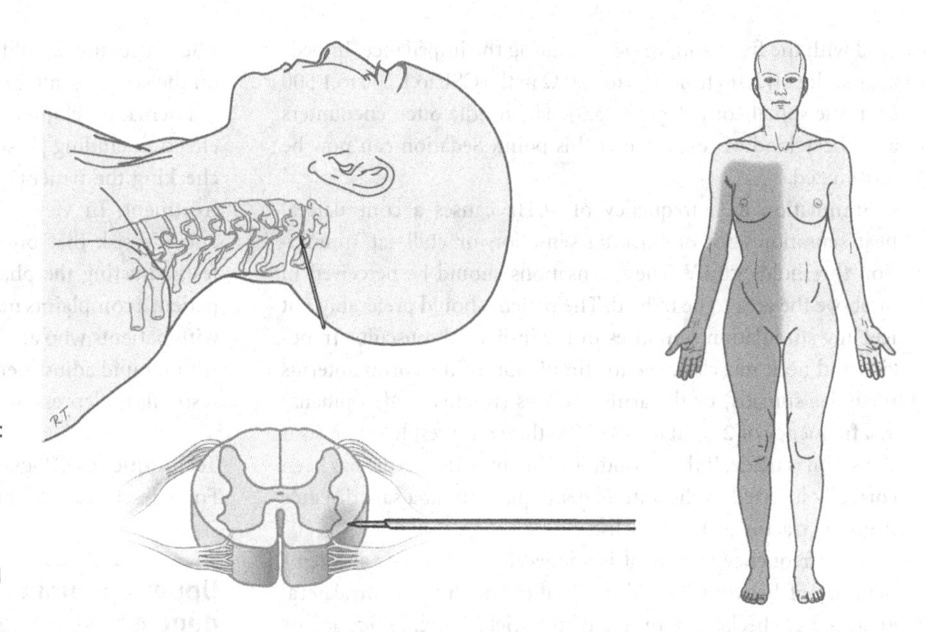

Figure 23.1. Anatomic representation of cordotomy: (a) needle placement between C1 and C2, (b) location of the tractus spinothalamicus lateralis in the anterolateral part of the spinal cord, (c) maximum extent of the area, where pain can be treated by left-sided cordotomy. Illustration: Rogier Trompert, Medical Art, www.medical-art.nl.

Technique for fluoroscopy guided cordotomy

Cordotomy is applied at cervical level, between C1 and C2, where the fibers of the tractus spinothalamicus lateralis run close together in the anterolateral quadrant. The fibers are somatotopic, with the most cervical fibers in the most anterior position and the most sacral fibers in most posterior position. The treatment is applied on the contralateral side of the pain (Figure 23.1).

All aspects of the procedure should be thoroughly discussed with the patient beforehand, including the fixation of the head, the unpleasant effects that may be caused by stimulating the spinal cord and the potentially lengthy duration of the procedure. During the intervention, a nurse should always be at hand to reassure the patient if necessary. The patient will need to cooperate to check the correct placement of the electrode in the spinal cord.

The radiofrequency treatment is performed using a thermocouple cordotomy electrode (eg, Levin) with a 2 mm noninsulated tip. The patient is placed in supine position and the head firmly fixed.

The arcus posterior atlantis (posterior arch of C1) is projected as a line in lateral fluoroscopy. The angles of the jaw and the meatus acusticus externus must also be projected over it as a reference. This ensures the best visibility of the space between C1 and C2, which is projected as an arrow shape with its tip pointing ventrally.

Treatment is carried out under sedation, while monitoring ECG and blood pressure. It starts with a 20G spinal needle being inserted into the subarachnoid space between the first and second cervical vertebrae. The direction should be as ventral as possible. Its position should be checked by means of lateral fluoroscopy. As soon as the CSF is reached, a mini-myelogram is made, using emulsified contrast medium (lipiodol with NaCl 0.9% 2:6, or with CSF 1:1 after very thorough shaking) to visualize "3 lines": the ventral side of the spinal cord, the ligamentum denticulatum and the posterior surface of the dural sac (Figure 23.2).

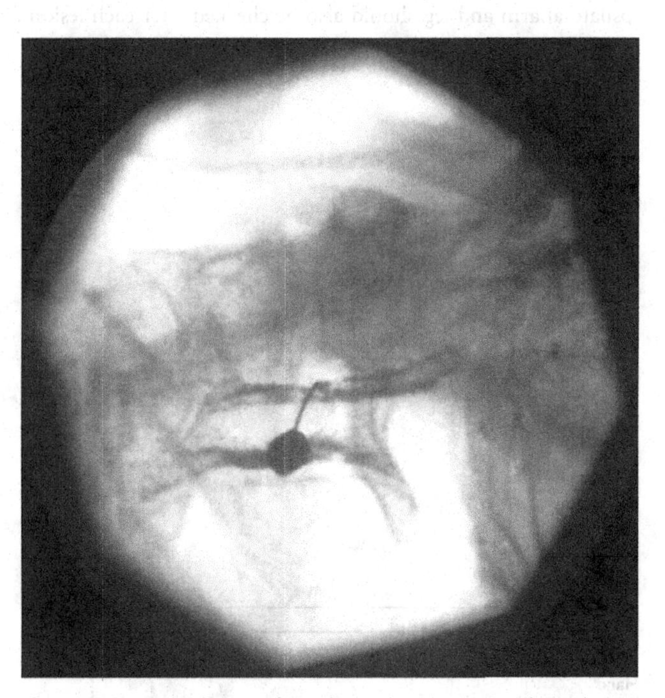

Figure 23.2. Needle placement for cordotomy: lateral view. Note the myelogram at the level of the ligamentum denticulatum.

Depending on the position of the needle, a second spinal needle may be introduced. This should be inserted, using a stylet, 1 to 2 mm ventral to the ligamentum denticulatum, at a right angle to the spinal cord, where the tractus spinothalamicus lateralis is situated.

The (Levin) thermocouple electrode is inserted after the stylet has been removed. It is connected to the radiofrequency generator, after which the tip of the electrode is inserted into the spinal cord with the free hand, while measuring the impedance. Impedance suddenly rises from 150 to 300 Ω in the CSF to 1,200 to 1,500 Ω in the spinal cord (Figure 23.3). The needle often encounters a rubbery kind of resistance at this point. Sedation can now be terminated.

Stimulation at a frequency of 50 Hz causes a contralateral heat sensation (hot or burning sensation or chill) at stimulation thresholds <0.1 V. These sensations should be perceived in or above the area to be treated. The patient should preferably not feel any stimulation responses in the ipsilateral musculus trapezius and neck muscles (due to stimulation of the cornu anterius medullae spinalis) or the arms and legs (tractus corticospinalis) at a frequency of 2 Hz at 0.5 to 2 V, as this could result in paresis if the lesion is made. If these conditions are met, the needle has been correctly inserted in the anterolateral quadrant at a safe distance from the tractus corticospinalis.

Radiofrequency treatment is applied for 10 seconds at a temperature of between 80 and 90°C, after which the contralateral analgesia is checked by means of pinprick. Muscle force in the ipsilateral arm and leg should also be checked after each lesion.

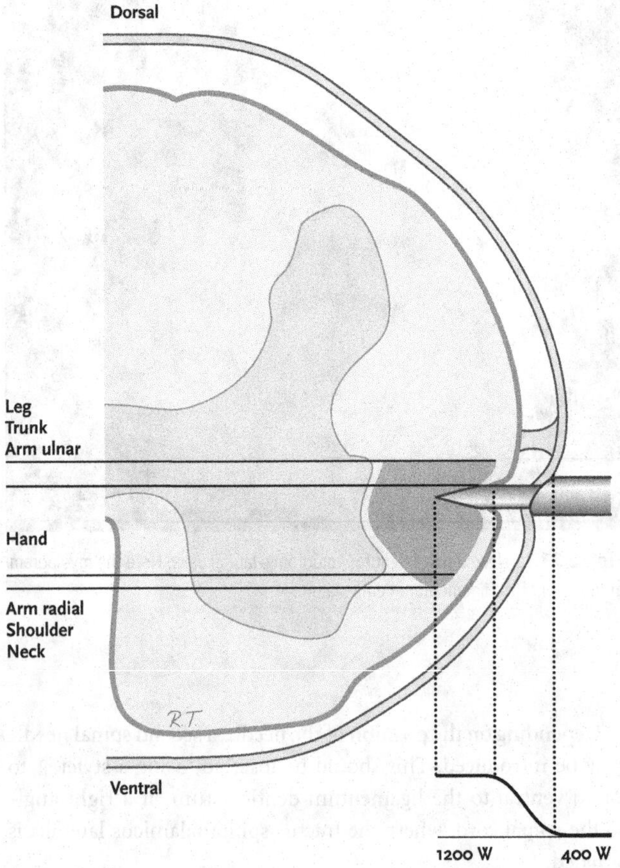

Figure 23.3. Definitive needle position for percutaneous cordotomy: note the increase in impedance as the needle is advanced into the spinal cord. Illustration: Rogier Trompert, Medical Art, www.medical-art.nl.

The procedure should be repeated one or two times, depending on the size and intensity of the analgesic area.

Edema development in the spinal cord may result in side effects, including persistence or increase of the pain, so regularly checking the patient's pain level is a precondition for optimum treatment. In view of the complexity of the pain syndrome, and the risk that previously masked pains may become manifest, adjusting the pharmacologic treatment on the basis of the patient's complaints may be required. Special care should be taken with patients who are being treated with high opioid dosages, for whom rapid adjustment of the dosage is often required to prevent respiratory depression.

Technique for CT-guided cordotomy

For a description of this technique we refer to Kanpolat et al.[28]

Upper abdominal pain due to cancer of the pancreas/stomach

Introduction

Pancreatic carcinoma usually leads to death within a relatively short time, as the diagnosis is often established at a time when cancer is already in an advanced stage, where tumor resection is no longer an option. Patients often first present with upper abdominal pain, although in the advanced stages they also frequently complain of back pain. Cancer of the pancreas is also associated with anorexia, loss of appetite, sleeping problems and weight loss.

Upper abdominal pain may also be caused by metastases of stomach cancer.

The plexus coeliacus is the network of orthosympathetic (sympathetic) nerve fibers located in front of the aorta at the level of truncus coeliacus. The plexus is formed from the nervi splanchnici, which arise from the thoracic truncus sympathicus. Plexus coeliacus block was first described by Cappis in 1914 for the treatment of upper abdominal pain after abdominal surgery. It is most currently applied in patients with cancer, usually due to pancreatic carcinoma.

Diagnosis

History taking and clinical symptoms

If a patient presents with severe upper abdominal pain and also complains of loss of appetite, sleeping problems and unexplained weight loss, the doctor should first seek to confirm the cause of the pain.

The pain is worse when the patient lies down and subsides as he or she sits up or bends forward.

Patients will report indistinctly localized, deep-seated pain, which resembles pinching, cramps or colic. Other symptoms include referred pain, such as shoulder pain, which occurs as the tumor invades the diaphragm, and is caused by stretching, compression or invasion of visceral structures.

Physical examination

Although physical examination is irrelevant to the pain syndrome, it is important to ascertain whether the pain is indeed situated in the upper abdomen. Additional radiation of the pain to the lower abdomen or back due to a primary upper abdominal process is not a contraindication for nerve blocks/neurolysis. Patients should also be checked for local anatomic abnormalities (severe scoliosis) and infections at the level of the intended puncture site. In addition, the patient must be able to lie in prone position for the duration of the procedure.

Additional testing (multidimensional)

Basic additional examination includes medical imaging, whether or not followed by laparoscopic examination, during which any obstructive symptoms can be treated. The technical examination required for accurate assessment of the cause of the pain should have been completed by the referring doctor. The examination should yield an accurate understanding of the situation before interventional pain control techniques are applied.

Differential diagnosis

Pain related to nononcologic problems are not eligible for neurolytic plexus coeliacus block.

Treatment options

Interventional management

A meta-analysis of 24 studies assessing the effectiveness of plexus coeliacus block among a total of 1,145 patients with various types of cancer was published in 1995.[30] This analysis showed that 89% of the patients report reduced pain after 2 weeks, with complete relief reported by 58% of the patients. The corresponding figures after 3 months were 90% and 56%, respectively. Later publications based on double-blind RCTs have confirmed the conclusions of the meta-analysis that plexus coeliacus block leads to reduced pain scores and/or reduced opioid consumption. Reported effects on quality of life have been variable. A meta-analysis evaluating the effect size of the treatment showed that plexus coeliacus block reduces the pain, but does not remove the need for opioids.[31] It concluded that plexus coeliacus block is not a substitute for pharmacologic treatment.

A double-blind randomized controlled trial compared the efficacy of conventional analgesic treatment and sham intervention with plexus coeliacus block and analgesic treatment. Pain reduction was greater in the group receiving active plexus coeliacus block at 1 week and over time. Opioid consumption and quality of life were not significantly different between groups. One year after randomization 16% of patients in the plexus coeliacus block group were still alive compared with 6% in the conventional treatment group, this difference was, however, not significant.[32]

The efficacy of CT-guided neurolytic plexus coeliacus block was compared with pharmacological treatment of pain due to pancreatic cancer. In the short term (1 to 14 days after the intervention) the VAS score of patients in the group having received a neurolytic block were significantly lower than in the group receiving pharmacological treatment. In the longer term up to 90 days after randomization, the difference in VAS pain score disappeared. The opioid consumption, however, remained significantly lower in the neurolytic block group over the complete follow-up period. There were no differences in quality of life between the two groups.[33]

An open randomized comparison of clinical effectiveness of protocol-driven opioid analgesia, plexus coeliacus block, or thoracoscopic splanchnicectomy in patients with pancreatic and other abdominal malignancies showed no differences in outcome between the 3 groups at 2 months follow-up.[34] The results of this latter study differ from previous findings. The reported mortality rate within the 2 months follow-up suggests that the population studied consists of patients whose cancer is in a far advanced stage.

A comparative study found that ethanolization of the nervus splanchnicus was superior to plexus coeliacus block in terms of pain relief and quality of life in patients with a pancreatic tumor.[35] Therefore, this technique may be recommended, although further research is required to confirm the results.

Complications

Although there have been reports of transient hypotension or diarrhea, as well as local pain, percutaneous plexus coeliacus block appears to be a relatively safe technique. There have been only a few reports of serious complications like pareses, paresthesias (1%), hematuria, pneumothorax, and shoulder pain (1%).[30] There are case reports of paraplegia due to plexus coeliacus block.[36–38]

A recently published case report described hemorrhagic gastritis and duodenitis following plexus coeliacus neurolysis. The patient had a known history of gastritis and duodenitis and developed severe upper GI bleeding immediately following the plexus coeliacus neurolysis. It was speculated that inhibition of the sympathetic tone caused increased blood flow to the GI system, which resulted in active bleeding from previously indolent hemorrhagic gastritis and duodenitis.[39]

Relieving abdominal pain may cause other pains to become manifest. Although this means that it is often not possible to completely terminate analgesic treatment, considerable dosage reductions may be achieved.

Contraindications for plexus coeliacus or nervus splanchnicus block

1 hemorrhagic diatheses.
2 local infections.
3 patient's inability to lie in prone position.
4 tumor invasion into the insertion site.

Other treatment options

Initial treatment of upper abdominal pain due to pancreatic carcinoma consists of analgesics like nonsteroidal anti-inflammatory drugs and opioids, which may be administered in various forms.

Table 23.3. Summary of evidence for interventional treatment of upper abdominal pain due to cancer.

Technique	Evaluation
Neurolytic plexus coeliacus block	2A+
Neurolytic nervus splanchnicus block	2B+

Evidence for interventional management

The evidence for interventional management of upper abdominal pain due to cancer is summarized in Table 23.3.

Recommendations

We recommend the use of plexus coeliacus block or nervus splanchnicus block to reduce pain or opioid use in patients with upper abdominal pain due to malignancy. This treatment may be considered as soon as opioid treatment is started. Plexus coeliacus or nervus splanchnicus block may be repeated if necessary. The choice between these two techniques depends on the preferences and experience of the attending physician.

Technique

Plexus coeliacus block

Various techniques to approach the plexus coeliacus have been described. Literature reports do not indicate one to be superior to the others, although the results of nervus splanchnicus block at the Th11 level appear to be better than those of the transaortal approach.[35] The sections below discuss the posterior transaortal, paravertebral (retrocrural), and transdiscal techniques for plexus coeliacus block and nervus splanchnicus block.

Plexus coeliacus plexus block can also be implemented surgically and endoscopically (by a gastroenterologist), but these techniques are beyond the scope of this article. Also, there is a growing experience with anterior, ultrasound-guided techniques.

Posterior transaortal technique

The patient is lying in prone position, with support under the abdomen to achieve thoracolumbar kyphotic position. This increases the distance between the ribs and crista iliaca and between the processus transversus of the adjoining vertebral bodies. For the sake of comfort, the patient's head is turned sideways with the arms hanging down along the body or placed above the head.

It may be useful to mark the following reference points on the skin with a marking pen: the crista iliaca, the 12th rib, the dorsal midline, the corpora vertebrae, and the lateral limit of the paraspinal muscles. It is also useful to mark the intersection of the 12th rib and the lateral border of the paraspinal muscles on the left side (which usually corresponds to the L2 level). A steel ruler can then be used to draw bilateral lines parallel to the lower edge of the 12th rib. These lines, which cross the L1 corpus vertebrae, serve to indicate the direction of the needle. The surgery site is prepared and covered with sterile drapes.

The skin, subcutaneous tissues and muscles are anesthetized with a local anesthetic at the site, where the needles will be inserted. For the sake of patient comfort, spinal anesthesia with a short-acting local anesthetic may be considered.

A 20 or 22G, 15 cm stylet needle is inserted from the left. The needle is initially oriented at an angle of 45° to the midline and about 15° cranially to make contact with the L1 corpus vertebrae. As soon as the needle touches the bone, its depth of insertion is noted, after which the needle is retracted to the subcutaneous tissue. It is then repositioned slightly laterally (at about 60° to the midline) to pass along the lateral surface of the L1 corpus vertebrae. All this is carried out under fluoroscopic guidance. The needle is now cautiously advanced until aortic pulsations are felt in the needle. The stylet is then removed from the needle, and the needle is advanced so as to perforate the aortic wall. Blood emerging from the needle indicates it is in intraaortic position. The needle is advanced until no more blood emerges, indicating that the needle tip is in preaortic position. A "click" may be felt as the needle perforates the aortic wall. It is important to use anteroposterior as well as lateral views to ensure correct needle placement.

After the needle has reached its correct position, the stylet is removed and the hub is checked for blood and CSF, lymph fluid and urine. A small amount of contrast medium is then injected and its distribution pattern is checked with the help of the C-arm. If the contrast medium shows insufficient dispersion bilaterally, it may be necessary to introduce another needle from right side for the instillation of the neurolytic agent.

In the anteroposterior view, the contrast medium should show up in the midline, concentrated around the Th12 to L1 corpora vertebrae. The contrast medium should not spread beyond the contours of the corpora vertebrae on the fluoroscopic image. The lateral view of the corpus vertebrae should show a smooth posterior outline. The contrast medium should not spread dorsally toward the nerve roots.

Alternatively, if the procedure is carried out under CT-guidance, the contrast medium should appear laterally and behind the aorta. If the contrast medium is present only in the retrocrural space, the needles should be advanced deeper, to reduce the risk of local anesthetic or the neurolytic agent spreading to the somatic nerves.

Paravertebral (retrocrural) approach

The Th12 corpus vertebrae is identified in a posteroanterior view and marked. The C-arm is then rotated to an oblique position (about 45°) on the side, where the needle is to be inserted. The image should show the side of the diaphragm lateral to the corpus vertebrae. Observe the diaphragm movements as the patient breathes in and out. If the diaphragm obscures the Th12 vertebra and rib, identify the Th11 rib. For both levels, the needle insertion site on the skin is located at the point, where the connection between rib and vertebral body cross each other.

After the skin at this site has been anesthetized, a 14G, 5 cm extracath (as an introducer) is inserted under fluoroscopic guidance, in such a way that the catheter moves toward the target

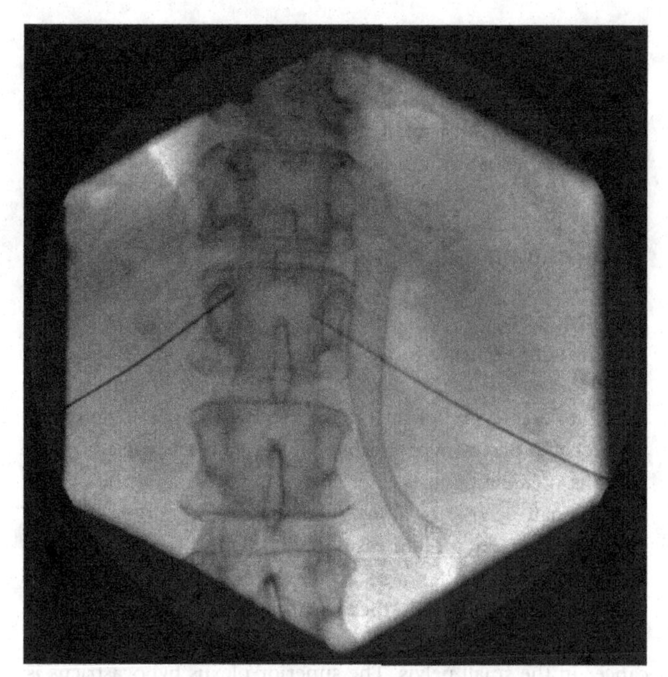

Figure 23.4. Neurolytic plexus coeliacus block: needle position in anteroposterior view. The needles enter at the L2 level and point obliquely upward toward L1 (a stent is present in the ductus choledochus).

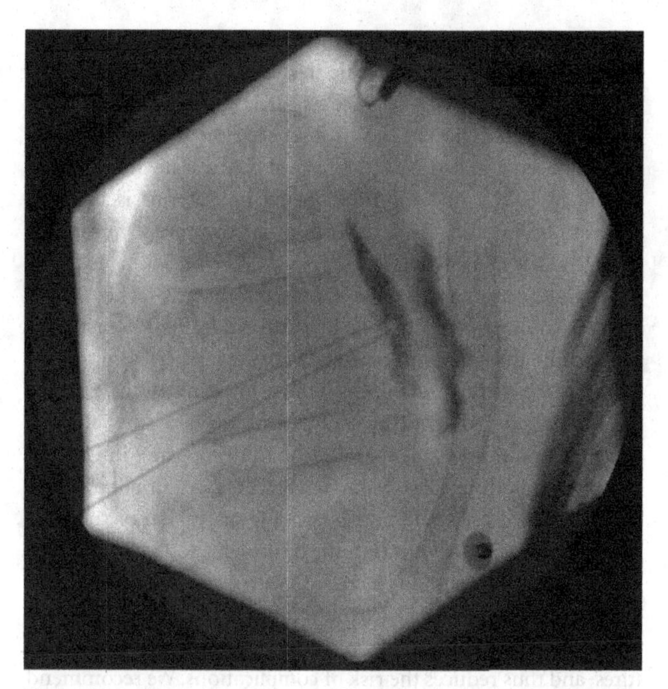

Figure 23.5. Neurolytic coeliacus plexus block: lateral view showing dispersion of contrast medium around Th12 to L1, both pre- and retro-aortic.

like the head of a needle. After the extracath has been inserted to two-third of its length, the stylet is removed and replaced by a 20 or 22G, 15 cm stylet needle. The C-arm is kept in oblique position. An extension tube is connected to the needle. The needle tip is advanced anteriorly in short (0.5 cm) increments, with the needle tip continuing to slide along the corpus vertebrae. Both needles are advanced further, under fluoroscopic guidance, past the Th12 to L1 corpus vertebrae. Check for blood or CSF by means of aspiration. The final needle location is checked on lateral views. After the contrast medium has been injected, the lateral view should show it in prevertebral position, whereas the anteroposterior view should show it within the contours of the spine (Figures 23.4–23.6). A neurolytic agent can now be gradually injected (see below).

Transdiscal technique

This approach was first described by R. Plancarte,[40] but needs to be further assessed for efficacy and safety.

The transdiscal procedure is also carried out under fluoroscopic or CT-guidance. The patient lies in prone position with a support underneath the crista iliaca to widen the access to the intradiscal space. Fluoroscopy is used to identify the Th12 to L1 level. The C-arm is then rotated obliquely to the left at an angle of 15 to 20°. It is important to align the inferior endplates using a cranio-caudal projection. The needle insertion site is 5 to 7 cm from the midline. After the skin and subcutaneous tissues have been locally anesthetized, the needle is advanced under tunnel view to the inferior aspect of the facet joint. After the disk has

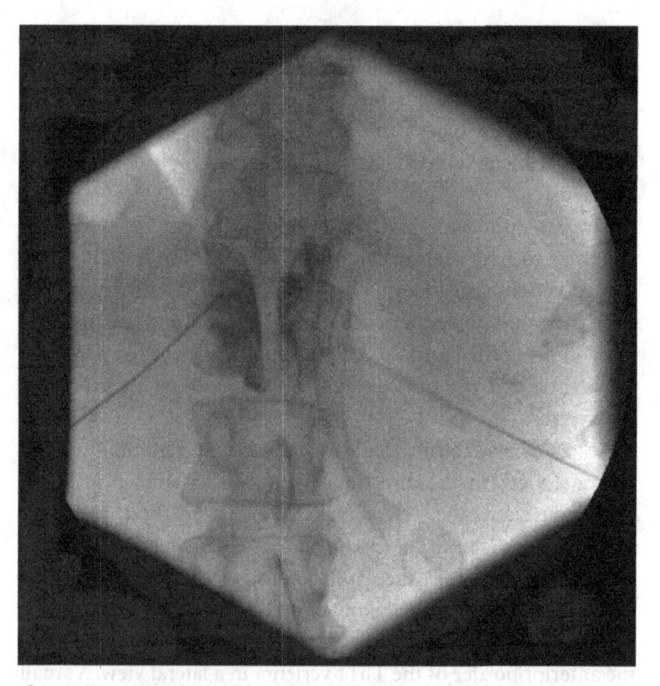

Figure 23.6. Neurolytic plexus coeliacus block: anteroposterior view showing dispersion of contrast medium within the spinal contours. Note the characteristic vacuole-like bright areas indicating correct placement.

been penetrated, 0.5 mL contrast medium (iohexol) is injected to check the position of the needle in the disk. The needle is then advanced until "loss of resistance" is perceived, indicating that the needle has exited the Th12 to L1 disc. After the final needle position has been checked with the help of contrast medium, 10 mL phenol in 10% saline (or 10% phenol in glycerin) is injected, followed by injection of 2 to 3 mL of air to prevent intradiscal leakage of the neurolytic agent.

Diagnostic prognostic blocks with the retrocrural technique are carried out by injecting 12 to 15 mL lidocaine 1% or 0.25% ropivacaine through both needles. Most researchers recommend carrying out therapeutic blocks by first injecting 10 to 16 mL of local anesthetic, followed by 10 to 16 mL of 96% ethyl alcohol, or a 10% solution of phenol in telebrix (10% phenol in glycerin in U.S.) via both needles. Many researchers have simultaneously injected a contrast medium to check the dispersion of the neurolytic agent. Before injecting the neurolytic solution, the area around the needle should be covered with wet gauze, followed by fractionated injection of the solution in 1 mL aliquots. This prevents the neurolytic agent from spreading to surrounding structures, and thus reduces the risk of complications. We recommend the use of 10% phenol in telebrix or in glycerin as a reference. After the neurolytic agent has been injected, each needle should be flushed with physiologic serum, or a local anesthetic to prevent fistula formation.

Nervus splanchnicus block

An alternative to the paravertebral (retrocrural) approach is the nervus splanchnicus block technique proposed by Abram and Boas.[41] This blocks the nervi splanchnici, branches of the thoracic truncus sympathicus and the nerve supply to the plexus coeliacus.

The patient is lying in prone position with support under the abdomen to achieve thoracolumbar kyphotic position. The Th11 corpus vertebrae is identified, after which the C-arm is rotated from the anteroposterior orientation in a caudal and lateral direction, allowing the concave mice-portion of the corpus vertebrae to be visualized without being obscured by ribs or the processus transversus.

A 20 or 22G, 15 cm needle is inserted paravertebrally, using a tunnel view, in the direction of the concave mid-portion of the corpus vertebrae. Try to make contact with the corpus vertebrae. Under lateral fluoroscopy, the needle is advanced to the anterolateral aspect of the Th11 corpus vertebrae. Radiographic imaging should show the tip of the needle just within the contour of the Th11 corpus vertebrae in an anteroposterior view, just at the anterior border of the Th11 vertebra in a lateral view. A small volume of contrast medium is injected to check dispersion along the anterolateral aspect of the corpus vertebrae. Before the neurolytic agent is injected (as described above), the area around the needle is covered with wet gauze, after which the neurolytic solution can be injected in fractions, preferably together with contrast medium. The same procedure is repeated on the other side. The needles then have to be flushed with saline, or a local anesthetic.

Aftercare

After the procedure, patients may experience pain at the insertion site, (orthostatic) hypotension or diarrhea. Patients should therefore be sufficiently hydrated and hospitalized for a night to check for signs of hypotension.

Visceral pain due to pelvic tumors

Introduction

Patients with extensive tumors in the small pelvis often perceive little benefit from oral or parenteral analgesics, or may experience intolerable side effects at the required dosages. This may necessitate a plexus hypogastricus block. Pain relief in the small pelvis is possible because afferent tracts innervating the organs in the small pelvis run along the sympathetic nerves, bundles and ganglia, making them easily accessible to neurolytic blocks. As visceral pain is often a major component of the pain due to tumors in the small pelvis, these neurolytic techniques deserve to be more commonly used for patients in the advanced stages of cancer in the small pelvis. The superior plexus hypogastricus is located bilaterally in the retroperitoneum, along the 3rd to 5th lumbar vertebrae, often extending to the upper third part of the first sacral vertebra.

Diagnosis

History taking and clinical symptoms

Plexus hypogastricus block may be considered for patients with a tumor in the small pelvis and pain in the lower abdomen. Patients with mostly visceral pain report ill-defined, dull, indistinctly localized pain.

Physical examination

Examination should concentrate on the anatomy of the lower back and os sacrum, and try to detect signs of infection and superficial tumor growth. Areas to which the pain radiates should be assessed to identify secondary and primary pains. The examiner should also assess whether the patient is able to lie in prone position for the duration of the treatment without the risk of collapse.

Additional testing

The location of the pain must be very carefully identified. If the patient suffers from radicular pain or very extensive painful zones in the lower abdomen or lower body, the preferred treatment option is epidural or intrathecal pain control. Pain in the higher parts of the upper abdomen should preferably be treated with plexus coeliacus block.

The technical examination requires accurate assessment of the cause of the pain and should have been completed by the referring doctor. This examination should yield an accurate understanding of the situation before interventional pain control techniques are applied.

Before deciding to carry out a neurolytic block, the physician should apply a diagnostic block with a local anesthetic, which should produce a 50% reduction of the pain for the normal duration of action of the anesthetic.

Contraindications

1 Hemorrhagic diatheses.
2 Serious infections in the area, where the needle is to be inserted.
3 Extensive tumor invasion in the area, where the needle is to be inserted.

Diff\erential diagnosis

Pain complaints related to nononcologic problems are not eligible for treatment with plexus hypogastricus block.

Treatment options

Interventional management

Plexus hypogastricus block

Plexus hypogastricus block has only been evaluated in observational studies. The study with the largest number of patients was that by Plancarte et al.[42] Of the 277 patients included in their study, 51% reported satisfactory pain relief. One study compared the effects of plexus hypogastricus block with those of pharmacologic treatment,[43] and found a favorable effect of plexus hypogastricus block on both pain and opioid consumption. The data provided, however, do not allow the specific effectiveness of plexus hypogastricus block to be evaluated. All studies involving more than 10 patients reported at least 60% of patients showing considerable pain reduction.[2]

Complications

Plexus hypogastricus block is a relatively safe technique provided it is carried out under X-ray or CT-guidance. Neurolysis of somatic nerves or intravascular injection of neurolytic agent is possible.

Bilateral superior plexus hypogastricus block can cause sexual dysfunction in men.[44] There are several cases of lumbar plexopathy with hip flexor weakness (AW Burton and B Hamid, unpublished data) due to injection into the musculus psoas major laterally, and the operator must be careful to inject the neurolytic solution medially enough to avoid the psoas compartment.

Evidence for interventional management

The evidence for interventional management of visceral pain due to cancer is summarized in Table 23.4.

Table 23.4. Summary of the evidence for interventional management of visceral pain due to pelvic tumors.

Technique	Evaluation
Neurolytic plexus hypogastricus block	2C+

Recommendations

We recommend the use of plexus hypogastricus block for patients with visceral pain due to pelvic tumors.

Technique

The patient is lying in prone position on a radio transparent table, with a support underneath the pelvis to reduce lumbar lordosis. It might be useful to apply lumbar spinal or epidural anesthesia before starting the plexus hypogastricus block procedure, to reduce the discomfort caused by the puncture. Alternatively, the deep paravertebral muscles may be infiltrated with local anesthetics.

The fluoroscopy tube is positioned in such a way as to allow the promontory or the concave mid-portion of the L5 corpus vertebrae to be seen in tunnel view from the needle insertion point 5 to 7 cm lateral of the midline, at the L4 level. This means that the tube has to be angulated by about 45°, both in anteroposterior and cranial view.

A 20 or 22G, 15 cm needle is positioned at the front of the L5 to S1 intervertebral space, under radiographic guidance (tunnel view). Use aspiration to check its position, to avoid injecting into the iliac blood vessels. The radiographic images should show the tip of the needle paravertebrally at the level of the L5 to S1 intervertebral space in anteroposterior view, whereas a lateral view should show the tip just touching the anterior border of the L5 to S1 vertebra (Figures 23.7–23.9). At this point, it is useful to inject a water-soluble contrast agent to confirm the correct position of the needle and avoid intravascular injection. The contrast medium should not disperse beyond the lateral confines of the L5 corpus vertebrae, or in a dorsal direction toward the nerve roots. A diagnostic plexus hypogastricus block can be carried out using 6 to 8 mL bupivacaine 0.25% to 0.5%. A therapeutic block is carried out using 6 to 8 mL 10% phenol solution in telebrix (in glycerin in U.S.) on each side of the vertebra. The safety of the

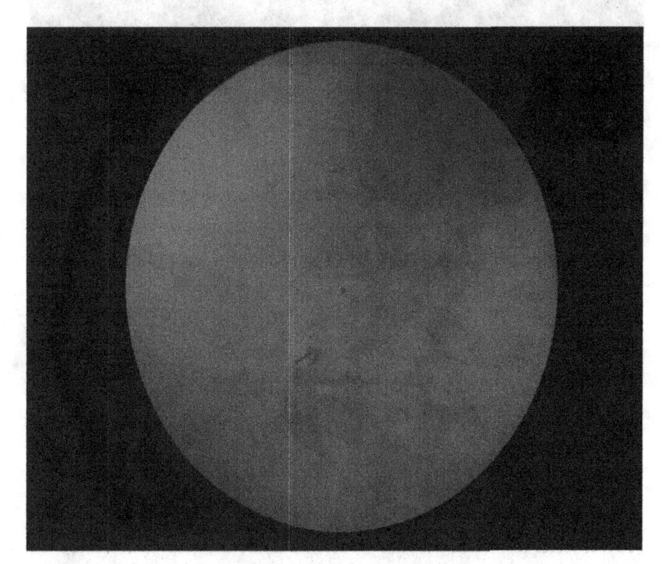

Figure 23.7. Needle position for plexus hypogastricus block: oblique view.

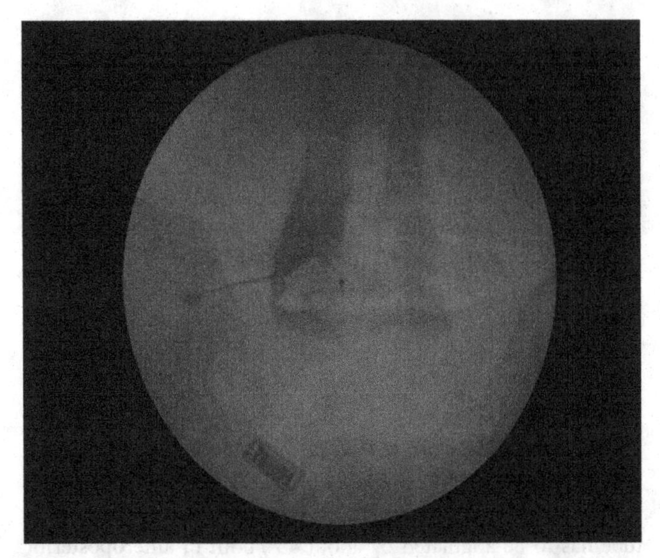

Figure 23.8. Needle position for plexus hypogastricus block: anteroposterior view.

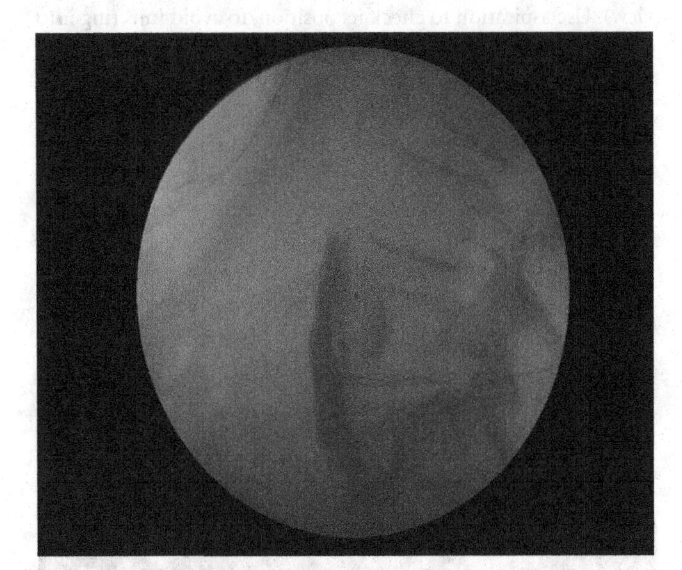

Figure 23.9. Plexus hypogastricus block: lateral view.

procedure can be improved by fractionated injection, with continuous monitoring of the dispersion of the phenol by means of contrast medium. Care must be taken to avoid the psoas compartment laterally at L5 to S1 level.

Perineal pain due to pelvic tumors

Introduction

Perineal pain caused by tumors may be treated with intrathecal phenolization of the lower sacral roots of the cauda equina (lower end block or saddle block). Physicians have hesitated to use this technique, however, because of the risk of permanent damage to the nerves controlling bladder and rectum function, with potentially serious consequences. That is why the technique is usually considered only as a last resort, after all other forms of oral or parenteral pain control have been tried and either proved ineffective or have caused intolerable side effects.

Diagnosis

History taking and clinical symptoms

Lower end block may be considered for patients with perineal pain due to tumors of the small pelvis. The technique is often considered only after the anus has already been surgically removed and the patient has been fitted with a stoma and a permanent bladder catheter.

Physical examination

The lower back and sacral zone must he carefully inspected to check for any infections or tumor invasion. Check whether the patient is able to sit up during the procedure and is cooperative. The patients must be able to accurately report sensory perceptions in the lower limbs.

Additional testing

Perineal pain should be of mainly somatic origin, and no other suitable therapy should be available. A precondition for the use of this technique is pre-existing urinary and fecal incontinence or the presence of a bladder catheter and an artificial anus.

Treatment options

Interventional management

Although lower end block is described in textbooks,[45,46] no high-quality studies on the subject have been published in the past 20 years. Three recent case reports included a limited number of patients. The results in these reports were variable: the median duration of the effect was 3 months, but opioid dosages could be reduced to 60%.[47–49]

Complications

1 Loss of sensory function, sometimes with dysesthesias of the lower limbs and/or the buttocks.
2 Loss of urinary or anal sphincter function.
3 Muscle weakness.

Contraindications

1 Life expectancy >6 months.
2 Blood coagulation deficiencies.
3 Extensive tumor invasion.
4 Extensive infection in the needle insertion area.

Evidence for interventional management

The evidence for interventional management of perineal pain due to pelvic tumors is summarized in Table 23.5.

Table 23.5. Summary of the evidence for interventional management of perineal pain due to pelvic tumors.

Technique	Evaluation
Intrathecal phenolization of lower sacral roots of cauda equina	0

Recommendations

A lower end block should only be considered for the treatment of cancer patients who experience pain in the small pelvis and have lost normal bladder or rectal function. As there have been no formal studies of the effectiveness of the treatment and the duration of the effect, we recommend using this technique only in the context of an experimental study or in cases of compassionate use with no other available forms of effective pain relief available with good informed consent.

Technique

The patient should be able to respond normally when being spoken to or asked questions during the procedure. There should be enough nursing staff present to place and hold the patient in the correct position and to change the patient's position during the procedure. All regulations for implementing aseptic procedures must be strictly observed. An intravenous line must be inserted to allow medication to be administered, and precautions for resuscitation must be in place.

The lower lumbar spinal segments must be in kyphotic position, so as to achieve maximum curvature. A large area should be disinfected and covered with a sterile surgical drape with an opening. The skin is anesthetized. A 22G spinal needle is inserted in the L5 to S1 intervertebral space at median level (midline approach), and carefully advanced until CSF flows from the needle. The phenol solution (6% in glycerin) is then freshly drawn into a 2 mL syringe with accurate volume graduation lines. The phenol syringe is connected to the spinal needle. The patient's position must now be adjusted. The patient is asked (assisted by the nursing staff) to lean backward at an angle of 45°, so that the back is at a 45° angle to horizontal. This requires considerable effort on the part of nursing staff. Phenol is now injected in 0.2 mL aliquots into the intrathecal space, to a total volume of 1 mL over a period of 5 minutes. Infiltration should be immediately stopped if the patient indicates sensory changes in the lower limbs, or the buttocks. In some cases, injection must be continued to a maximum total volume of 1.5 mL. The spinal needle is then removed and the patient should remain seated at a backward angle of 45° for the next 6 hours. Their blood pressure must be regularly checked, and some fluid replacement may be required.

Changes in pain perception should be checked by monitoring the VAS score for pain. Oral or parenteral analgesics should only be gradually reduced in the course of the following days, if the treatment has an analgesic effect. It is rarely possible to end analgesic use completely, as successful treatment often causes other pains to become manifest.

Spinal pain related to vertebral compression fracture (with or without pathologic tumor invasion)

Introduction

Many cancer patients suffer morbidity due to skeletal metastasis, pain, and vertebral compression fractures. Skeletal complications are very common in multiple myeloma regardless of stage, and in metastatic breast, prostate, and other solid tumors.

Extradural metastases account for some 95% of secondary spinal tumors. The primary sources of metastatic neoplasms to the spinal axis vary among the published series with 65% coming from carcinoma of the breast, lung, and prostate. Renal cell carcinoma and myeloma also occur and together account for 10% of spinal metastases.[50]

Diagnosis

History taking and clinical symptoms

Patients with cancer who develop significant axial spinal pain merit imaging studies via their oncologist to rule out metastatic disease or pathological fracture. Focal spinal pain in a cancer patient nearly always mandates some sort of radiological workup. Vertebral compression fracture pain is typically incidental, and nonradiating. Patients with neurologic deficit, band-like pain, or any loss of bowel and bladder control may have spinal cord compression and merit an immediate neurosurgical evaluation to include imaging studies.

Physical examination

Patients with cancer-related vertebral fracture should have a complete neurologic exam to ensure that the spinal cord is not compromised prior to consideration of these techniques. Furthermore, the pain should be concordant with the level of pathology.

Treatment options

Interventional management

Pathologic spinal involvement without fracture is usually treated with conventional radiotherapy. A spinal vertebral compression fracture with tumor is often treated with the same way, but the mechanical pain can be refractory to the radiation therapy. In these cases, percutaneous vertebroplasty (PV) or kyphoplasty can be helpful. In cases involving neurologic compromise or significant epidural disease, open surgical treatment may be indicated.

Percutaneous vertebroplasty and kyphoplasty

Indications for PV have expanded to include osteoporotic compression fractures and painful vertebral metastasis. Kyphoplasty is a modification of PV; it involves the percutaneous placement of balloons (called "tamps") into the corpus vertebrae with an inflation/deflation sequence to create a cavity prior to the cement injection. Percutaneous kyphoplasty (PK) may restore

Table 23.6. Indications and contraindications for percutaneous vertebroplasty.

Indications
Painful osteoporotic vertebral compression fracture refractory to 3 weeks of analgesic therapy
Painful vertebrae due to benign or malignant primary or secondary bone tumors
Painful vertebral compression fracture with osteonecrosis (Kummel's disease)
Reinforcement of vertebral body prior to surgical procedure*
Chronic traumatic vertebral compression fracture with nonunion*
Absolute contraindications
Asymptomatic vertebral compression fracture
Patient improving on medical therapy
Ongoing Infection
Prophylaxis in osteoporotic patient
Uncorrectable coagulopathy
Myelopathy due to retropulsion of bone/canal compromise
Allergy to PMMA or opacification agent
Relative contraindications
Radicular pain
VCF > 70% height loss*
Severe spinal stenosis, asymptomatic retropulsion of bony fragment
Tumor extension into canal/epidural space
Lack of surgical backup*

Modified from McGraw et al.[54] and updated by Gangi et al.[53]. Recommendations from the more recent update (Gangi 2006 are marked with *).

corpus vertebrae height and reduce the kyphotic angulation of the compression fracture prior to bone cement injection. [51,52] A recent prospective trial in noncancer VCF's shows good efficacy, with significant reduction in pain and improved function.[53] Several smaller case series show good pain improvement with these procedures.[54]

Complications

Complications are rare, but can be serious and the exact incidence is unknown. Most case series report *asymptomatic* polymethyl methacrylate (PMMA) extravasation rates of around 10% to 15%.[52,55] The Society for Interventional Radiology (SIR) divides complications for these techniques into minor and major. Minor complications are those considered to require no therapy and having no consequence, such as PMMA extravasation into the disk. Major complications are those requiring therapy, including an unplanned increase in the level of care needed, or having ongoing permanent sequelae (eg, PMMA into the spinal canal with neurologic deficit). SIR noted published complication rates for *major* complications to be less than 1%, except in those with neoplastic involvement of the vertebrae, where the reported level of major complications is less than 5%.[56,57]

Indications/relative and absolute contraindications

The indications and contraindications are summarized in Table 23.6. This table is based on the different guidelines from the SIR and Cardiovascular and Interventional Radiological Society of Europe. First published by McGraw et al.[56] and updated by Gangi et al.[57]

Table 23.7. Summary of the evidence for interventional management of vertebral compression fractures with or without pathologic tumor invasion.

Technique	Evaluation
Vertebroplasty	2B+
Kyphoplasty	2B+

Evidence for vertebroplasty or kyphoplasty

Recent reviews and editorials have called for a more critical evaluation of these procedures in view of some recent studies questioning the efficacy of these procedures in noncancer situations.

Table 23.7 summarizes the level of evidence.

Recommendations for vertebroplasty or kyphoplasty

In summary, we view PV/PK as valuable adjunctive therapies for cancer patients with painful vertebral compression fractures from all etiologies. The overall complication rate is low and efficacy acceptable.

Technique

The technique of both vertebroplasty and balloon kyphoplasty has been described in Peh et al.[51]

Summary

Interventional pain management techniques in the treatment of refractory oncologic pain syndromes are indicated if oral or parenteral analgesics cause such severe side effects that a satisfactory quality of life and satisfactory pain relief cannot he reached.

All of the techniques described in this article should only be considered in a specific multidisciplinary pain centre, with all capacities of a thorough clinical follow-up.

These Interventional techniques require high attention, great care and thorough specialist knowledge as well as extensive expertise. The clinical center needs to meet all requirements for the safe implementation of interventional techniques.

Effective nursing assistance, a specially equipped operating area and effective aftercare are required to satisfy all safety regulations.

References

1. Christo PJ, Mazloomdoost D. Interventional pain treatments for cancer pain. *Ann N Y Acad Sci.* 2008;1138:299–328.
2. Landelijke richtlijnwerkgroep Pijn bij kanker. Pijn bij kanker. Landelijke richtlijn. In: Landelijke richtlijnwerkgroep Pijn bij kanker. 2008:1–168. ISBN: 978-90-8523-168-4.

3. Ballantyne JC, Carwood CM. Comparative efficacy of epidural, subarachnoid, and intracerebroventricular opioids in patients with pain due to cancer. *Cochrane Database Syst Rev.* 2005;1: CD005178.
4. Mercadante S, Intravaia G, Villari P, Ferrera P, Riina S, David F, et al. Intrathecal treatment in cancer patients unresponsive to in mutiple trials of systemic opioids. *Clin J Pain.* 2007;23: 793–798.
5. Pasutharnchat K, Tan KH, Abdul Hadi M, Ho KY. Intrathecal analgesia in patients with cancer pain—an audit in a tertiary institution. *Ann Acad Med Singapore.* 2009;38:943–946.
6. Staats PS, Yearwood T, Charapata SG, et al. Intrathecal ziconotide in the treatment of refractory pain in patients with cancer or AIDS: a randomized controlled trial. *JAMA.* 2004;291:63–70.
7. Raffaeli W, Sarti D, Demartini L, Sotgiu A, Bonezzi C. Italian registry on long-term intrathecal ziconotide treatment. *Pain Physician.* 2011;14:15–24.
8. Stearns L, Boortz-Marx R, Du Pen S, et al. Intrathecal drug delivery for the management of cancer pain: a multidisciplinary consensus of best clinical practices. *J Support Oncol.* 2005;3:399–408.
9. Krames ES. Practical issues when using neuraxial infusion. *Oncology (Williston Park).* 1999;13:37–44.
10. De Pinto M, Dunbar PJ, Edwards WT. Pain management. *Anesthesiol Clin.* 2006;24:19–37 vii.
11. Mercadante S. Problems of long-term spinal opioid treatment in advanced cancer patients. *Pain.* 1999;79:1–13.
12. Yaksh TL, Horais KA, Tozier NA, et al. Chronically infused intrathecal morphine in dogs. *Anesthesiology.* 2003;99:174–187.
13. Abs R, Verhelst J, Maeyaert J, et al. Endocrine consequences of long-term intrathecal administration of opioids. *J Clin Endocrinol Metab.* 2000;85:2215–2222.
14. Ruppen W, Derry S, McQuay HJ, Moore RA. Infection rates associated with epidural indwelling catheters for seven days or longer: systematic review and meta-analysis. *BMC Palliat Care.* 2007;6:3.
15. Aprili D, Bandschapp O, Rochlitz C, Urwyler A, Ruppen W. Serious complications associated with external intrathecal catheters used in cancer pain patients: a systematic review and meta-analysis. *Anesthesiology.* 2009;111:1346–1355.
16. Mullan S, Lichtor T. Percutaneous microcompression of the trigeminal ganglion for trigeminal neuralgia. *J Neurosurg.* 1983;59:1007–1012.
17. Boersma F, Van Kleef M, Rohof O, Stolker R, Touw P, Zuurmond W. *Richtlijnen anesthesiologische pijnbestrijding. Groningen*, The Netherlands: Drukkerij van Denderen BV; 1996. ISBN: 90-71353-06-0.
18. Zuurmond WW, Perez RS, Loer SA. Role of cervical cordotomy and other neurolytic procedures in thoracic cancer pain. *Curr Opin Support Palliat Care.* 2010;4:6–10.
19. Nagaro T, Amakawa K, Yamauchi Y, Tabo E, Kimura S, Arai T. Percutaneous cervical cordotomy and subarachnoid phenol block using fluoroscopy in pain control of costopleural syndrome. *Pain.* 1994;58:325–330.
20. Amano K, Kawamura H, Tanikawa T, et al. Bilateral vs. unilateral percutaneous high cervical cordotomy as a surgical method of pain relief. *Acta Neurochir Suppl (Wien).* 1991;52:143–145.
21. Crul BJ, Blok LM, van Egmond J, van Dongen RT. The present role of percutaneous cervical cordotomy for the treatment of cancer pain. *J Headache Pain.* 2005;6:24–29.
22. Jackson MB, Pounder D, Price C, Matthews AW, Neville E. Percutaneous cervical cordotomy for the control of pain in patients with pleural mesothelioma. *Thorax.* 1999;54:238–241.
23. Sanders M, Zuurmond W. Safety of unilateral and bilateral percutaneous cervical cordotomy in 80 terminally ill cancer patients. *J Clin Oncol.* 1995;13:1509–1512.
24. Slavik E, Ivanovic S, Grujisic D, Djurovic B, Nikolic I. Microsurgical spinothalamic chordotomy in the treatment of cancer pain. *J Buon.* 2005;10:223–226.
25. Stuart G, Cramond T. Role of percutaneous cervical cordotomy for pain of malignant origin. *Med J Aust.* 1993;158:667–670.
26. Meeuse JJ, Vervest AC, van der Hoeven JH, Reyners AK. Five-year follow-up of a cordotomy. *Pain Res Manag.* 2008;13:506–510.
27. Raslan AM. Percutaneous computed tomography-guided radiofrequency ablation of upper spinal cord pain pathways for cancer-related pain. *Neurosurgery.* 2008;62:226–233 discussion 233–224.
28. Kanpolat Y, Ugur HC, Ayten M, Elhan AH. Computed tomography-guided percutaneous cordotomy for intractable pain in malignancy. *Neurosurgery.* 2009;64:187–193 discussion 193–184.
29. Jones B, Finlay I, Ray A, Simpson B. Is there still a role for open cordotomy in cancer pain management? *J Pain Symptom Manage.* 2003;25:179–184.
30. Eisenberg E, Carr DB, Chalmers TC. Neurolytic celiac plexus block for treatment of cancer pain: a meta-analysis. *Anesth Analg.* 1995;80:290–295.
31. Yan BM, Myers RP. Neurolytic celiac plexus block for pain control in unresectable pancreatic cancer. *Am J Gastroenterol.* 2007;102:430–438.
32. Wong GY, Schroeder DR, Carns PE, et al. Effect of neurolytic celiac plexus block on pain relief, quality of life, and survival in patients with unresectable pancreatic cancer: a randomized controlled trial. *JAMA.* 2004;291:1092–1099.
33. Zhang CL, Zhang TJ, Guo YN, et al. Effect of neurolytic celiac plexus block guided by computerized tomography on pancreatic cancer pain. *Dig Dis Sci.* 2008;53:856–860.
34. Johnson CD, Berry DP, Harris S, et al. An open randomized comparison of clinical effectiveness of protocol-driven opioid analgesia, celiac plexus block or thoracoscopic splanchnicectomy for pain management in patients with pancreatic and other abdominal malignancies. *Pancreatology.* 2009;9:755–763.
35. Suleyman Ozyalcin N, Talu GK, Camlica H, Erdine S. Efficacy of coeliac plexus and splanchnic nerve blockades in body and tail located pancreatic cancer pain. *Eur J Pain.* 2004;8:539–545.
36. Abdalla EK, Schell SR. Paraplegia following intraoperative celiac plexus injection. *J Gastrointest Surg.* 1999;3:668–671.
37. Kumar A, Tripathi SS, Dhar D, Bhattacharya A. A case of reversible paraparesis following celiac plexus block. *Reg Anesth Pain Med.* 2001;26:75–78.
38. van Dongen RT, Crul BJ. Paraplegia following coeliac plexus block. *Anaesthesia.* 1991;46:862–863.
39. Pello S, Miller A, Ku T, Wang D. Hemorrhagic gastritis and duodenitis following celiac plexus neurolysis. *Pain Physician.* 2009;12: 1001–1003.
40. Plancarte-Sanchez R, Mayer-Rivera F, del Rocio Guillen Nunez M, Guajardo-Rosas J, Acosta-Quiroz CO. Transdiscal percutaneous approach of splanchnic nerves. *Cir Cir.* 2003;71:192–203.
41. Abram SE, Boas R. Sympathetic and visceral nerve blocks. In: Benumof J, ed. *Clinical Procedures in Anesthesia and Intensive Care.* Philadelphia: Lippincott; 1992:787.

42. Plancarte R, de Leon-Casasola OA, El-Helaly M, Allende S, Lema MJ. Neurolytic superior hypogastric plexus block for chronic pelvic pain associated with cancer. *Reg Anesth.* 1997;22:562–568.
43. de Oliveira R, dos Reis MP, Prado WA. The effects of early or late neurolytic sympathetic plexus block on the management of abdominal or pelvic cancer pain. *Pain.* 2004;110:400–408.
44. Plancarte RS, Mayer-Rivera FJ. Radiofrequency procedures for sacral and pelvic region pain. *Pain Practice.* 2002;2:248–249.
45. Cousins M, Bridenbaugh P. *Neural Blockade in Clinical Anesthesia and Management of Pain.* 3rd ed. Philadelphia: Lippincott Williams & Wilkins; 1998.
46. deLeon Casasola O. *Cancer Pain: Pharmacological, Interventional, and Palliative Approaches.* 1st ed. Philadelphia: Saunders Elsevier; 2006.
47. Candido K, Stevens RA. Intrathecal neurolytic blocks for the relief of cancer pain. *Best Pract Res Clin Anaesthesiol.* 2003;17: 407–428.
48. Rodriguez-Bigas M, Petrelli NJ, Herrera L, West C. Intrathecal phenol rhizotomy for management of pain in recurrent unresectable carcinoma of the rectum. *Surg Gynecol Obstet.* 1991;173: 41–44.
49. Slatkin NE, Rhiner M. Phenol saddle blocks for intractable pain at end of life: report of four cases and literature review. *Am J Hosp Palliat Care.* 2003;20:62–66.
50. Dahan A, Yassen A, Bijl H, et al. Comparison of the respiratory effects of intravenous buprenorphine and fentanyl in humans and rats. *Br J Anaesth.* 2005;94:825–834.
51. Peh WC, Munk PL, Rashid F, Gilula LA. Percutaneous vertebral augmentation: vertebroplasty, kyphoplasty and skyphoplasty. *Radiol Clin North Am.* 2008;46:611–635 vii.
52. Kvarstein G, Mawe L, Indahl A, et al. A randomized double-blind controlled trial of intra-annular radiofrequency thermal disc therapy—a 12-month follow-up. *Pain.* 2009;145:279–286.
53. Bae H, Shen M, Maurer P, et al. Clinical experience using Cortoss for treating vertebral compression fractures with vertebroplasty and kyphoplasty: twenty-four-month follow-up. *Spine (Phila Pa 1976).* 2010;35:E1030–E1036.
54. Lim BS, Chang UK, Youn SM. Clinical outcomes after percutaneous vertebroplasty for pathologic compression fractures in osteolytic metastatic spinal disease. *J Korean Neurosurg Soc.* 2009;45:369–374.
55. McKiernan F, Faciszewski T, Jensen R. Quality of life following vertebroplasty. *J Bone Joint Surg Am.* 2004;86A:2600–2606.
56. McGraw JK, Cardella J, Barr JD, et al. Society of Interventional Radiology quality improvement guidelines for percutaneous vertebroplasty. *J Vasc Interv Radiol.* 2003;14:S311–S315.
57. Gangi A, Sabharwal T, Irani FG, Buy X, Morales JP, Adam A. Quality assurance guidelines for percutaneous vertebroplasty. *Cardiovasc Intervent Radiol.* 2006;29:173–178.

24 Chronic Refractory Angina Pectoris

Maarten van Kleef, Peter Staats, Nagy Mekhail and Frank Huygen

Introduction

Angina pectoris is severe chest pain that is often accompanied by a heavy oppressive feeling. Angina pectoris occurs because of insufficient blood supply to the heart muscle. In most cases, this is caused by a constriction of the coronary arteries. It often coincides with physical exertion or emotional strain, which causes the heart to beat more rapidly and is associated with higher oxygen consumption. The pain occurring in case of a sudden occlusion of a coronary artery because of a thrombus or embolus is usually more severe. A complete occlusion eventually leads to a myocardial infarction. Risk factors of angina pectoris include smoking, obesity, hypertension, diabetes mellitus, and hypercholesterolemia. Besides coronary obstruction, coronary spasms may also cause symptoms of angina pectoris.

Angina pectoris can be treated with vasodilating drugs or by the reduction of exertion. A reduction of the blood pressure also leads to a lower cardiac workload and to decreased angina symptoms. Presently, a large number of pharmacological therapies are available. In addition, revascularization procedures, such as percutaneous coronary angioplasty and coronary artery bypass grafting (CABG), can help with angina attacks if a single or several discrete areas of obstruction can be identified.

Angina pectoris is termed refractory if the conventional therapies mentioned above have insufficient or no effect. Patients with refractory angina pectoris generally have a long history of coronary disease and are usually clearly limited in their physical activities. In addition to extensive anti-anginal pharmacological treatment, these patients have often undergone one or more percutaneous coronary angioplasties or even CABG. Strikingly, most patients with refractory angina pectoris are relatively young, predominantly male, and sometimes have a limited ejection fraction.[1,2]

In Europe, the annual prevalence of class III and class IV Canadian Cardiovascular Society (CCS; angina pectoris upon mild exertion and at rest,) symptoms are estimated to be approximately 100,000.[3]

Spinal cord stimulation (SCS) is considered a reasonable treatment option for patients with chronic angina not responsive to more conservative strategies who are not candidates for coronary revascularization surgery. Since its first publication in 1987, several publications have demonstrated the safety and efficacy in patients with severe coronary artery disease.[4]

Diagnosis

History

The clinical signs of angina pectoris are typical. They are provoked by exertion and disappear at rest. Patients with severe coronary disease may experience various symptoms during exertion, usually located substernally and sometimes radiating to adjacent areas, especially on the left side, such as the arms, neck, throat, jaw, or even the teeth. The pain sensation is often accompanied by other symptoms such as perspiration, nausea, and, sometimes, vomiting. Some patients suffering from angina pectoris are able to estimate the amount of exertion that will cause an attack of angina pectoris. The maximum exercise tolerance is closely related to the degree of coronary constriction in the main vessels. At rest, the angina pectoris threshold is clearly influenced by emotional stress, exposure to cold, meals, and smoking. These aspects of pain sensation suggest a dynamic stenosis of the coronary artery. The variability of the angina pectoris threshold suggests that a combination of fixed and variable obstructions of the coronary vessels plays a role. Therefore, it can generally be stated that angina pectoris is not a specific indicator of the degree of coronary constriction but that angina pectoris can be an

Evidence-Based Interventional Pain Medicine: According to Clinical Diagnoses, First Edition. Edited by Jan Van Zundert, Jacob Patijn, Craig T. Hartrick, Arno Lataster, Frank J.P.M Huygen, Nagy Mekhail, Maarten van Kleef.

inconsistent, nonspecific phenomenon, determined by a variety of causes.

Angina pectoris is considered refractory if constant reversible myocardial ischemia and pain occur despite optimal anti-anginal therapy in cases with substantial stenosis of a significant coronary artery (more than 75% stenosis in one or more of the main coronary arteries).

Physical examination

Physical examination is mainly directed at excluding other disorders in the differential diagnosis. By the time the pain physician is involved, the patient will have had an extensive workup by a cardiologist.

Additional tests

Angina pectoris can be diagnosed when ischemia is identified on an electrocardiogram when the patient is experiencing symptoms. Exercise stress tests, such as a bicycle ergometer test or a stress echo test and angiography, are examples of the wide variety of options that cardiologists can apply to evaluate the symptoms. The gold standard for the diagnosis of coronary disease is a coronary angiogram or a computed tomography angiogram.

Differential diagnosis

All patients considered for SCS with refractory angina pectoris should have been seen by a cardiologist. In practice, patients who are eligible for SCS have often undergone comprehensive interventions, such as CABG and PTCA procedures. Patients with small vessel disease should be considered for SCS if medical treatment is unsatisfactory. The differential diagnosis includes but is not limited to[5]:

- Pulmonary disorders: pulmonary hypertension, pulmonary embolism, pleuritis, pneumothorax, and pneumonia.
- Nonischemic cardiac disease, mitral valve prolapse, and cardiac syndrome X.
- Gastrointestinal disorders: peptic ulcer, pancreatitis, esophageal spasms, esophageal reflux, cholecystitis, and cholelithiasis.
- Musculoskeletal related: costochondritis, Tietze's syndrome, thoracic trauma, cervical arthritis with or without radiculopathy, myositis, and cancer.
- Spinal cord injury and thoracic radiculopathy.
- Acute aortic dissection.
- Herpes zoster with post-herpetic neuralgia.
- Panic disorder.

Treatment options

Conservative management

All therapies for (refractory) angina pectoris aim to improve the myocardial ischemia by means of either the reduction of oxygen demand (β blockers, calcium channel blockers) or the increase of oxygen supply (nitrates, revascularization procedures, coronary angioplasty, or CABG). In addition, the patients are often treated with anticholesterol drugs and platelet aggregation inhibitors.

Interventional management

Spinal cord stimulation

A therapy that has anti-anginal effects, enhances the quality of life of patients with refractory angina pectoris, and is not harmful is a valuable treatment. An additional argument is that patients in this category show an annual mortality between 5% and 8%.[1] The population that should be treated includes patients who experience substantial limitations because of their angina pectoris despite exhaustive conservative and surgical intervention.

The mechanism of action of SCS remains as yet unsolved. The obtained pain reduction is related to the increased release of inhibitory neuropeptides such as GABA, dopamine, and glycine, and a reduced release of stimulating neuropeptides such as substance P and acetylcholine.[6,7]

It has recently been suggested that the effects of SCS in angina pectoris are in part attributed to the protection of the myocardium and the normalization of the intrinsic nerve system of the heart muscle.[8] Studies have shown that patients treated with SCS have less angina symptoms, a lower use of short-acting nitrates, and an improved exercise tolerance.[9,10] Moreover, clear anti-ischemic effects have been demonstrated, such as an increased exercise time without a deterioration of the myocardial symptoms and an increased tolerance for arterial pacing. The reduced myocardial ischemia and reduced myocardial oxygen consumption (MVO_2) result in delayed angina pectoris symptoms.[11,12]

SCS in patients with refractory angina pectoris results in reduced attacks that may be caused by the increased angina pectoris threshold as a result of the reduced MVO_2 and possibly the redistribution of the coronary blood flow.

It has also been suggested that angiogenesis would take place under the influence of SCS.[13] Redistribution of the myocardial blood flow has been demonstrated in three studies,[11,12,14] and it is proposed that some of the redistribution may be because of the formation of collaterals. Also, there are a number of studies that demonstrate that SCS does not mask acute myocardial infarction.[15–17]

Efficacy of spinal cord stimulation treatment

The efficacy of the treatment has been investigated in two prospective, randomized studies.[9,10] The first study was a prospective, randomized clinical study in 17 patients conducted between 1990 and 1994. One group was implanted immediately after inclusion. The other group was implanted after a period of 8 weeks. Inclusion criteria of both studies were: (1) angina pectoris, (2) coronary angiogram in which coronary angioplasty or CABG was no longer an option, (3) New York Heart Association classification 3 or 4, (4) an exercise test with reversible ischemia, and (5) optimal pharmacological treatment for at least 1 month. The results demonstrated that the exercise capacity in the SCS group was better than in the control group and that the quality of life variables in both groups were better after 12 months compared with baseline.

Mannheimer et al.'s Electrical Stimulation versus coronary artery BYpass surgery in severe angina pectoris study[9] was a prospective, randomized study in 104 patients. The inclusion criteria were patients with angina pectoris refractory to pharmacological treatment in cases with no proven benefit from CABG and with an increased risk of surgical complications. Group I, consisting of 51 patients, was treated with CABG, and group 2, consisting of 53 patients, received SCS. This study had a remarkably long follow-up of 5 years.[18] The results of this study showed improvement of symptoms in both groups after 1 year. There was reduced myocardial ischemia, but only in the CABG surgery group. The mortality in the CABG group was higher than in the spinal cord stimulation group (seven and one cases of death, respectively). It should be mentioned that three patients died before their operation took place.With respect to morbidity, slightly more cerebrovascular accidents were reported in the CABG group. The long-term results demonstrated an improvement in anginal symptoms and of the quality of life in both groups. A prospective Italian publication of spinal cord stimulation in 104 patients with severe refractory angina showed a significant improvement of angina symptoms in 73% of the patients after a 13.2-month follow-up.[19] Based on the above studies of efficacy, it can be concluded that SCS can be considered an alternative to surgical intervention in a select patient population. SCS may also be a viable option in patients in whom surgery is not possible.

The indications for SCS in angina pectoris are controversial. An open-label, randomized study compared the efficacy of SCS to percutaneous myocardial laser revascularization. In this study, two groups of 30 patients each were followed for 1 year. Both groups demonstrated improved pain control and improved exercise tolerance. However, no significant difference of efficacy was observed between the groups.[20] Critics point out that the available randomized controlled trials are rather dated (10 to 14 years old). During that time, it is possible that the improvement in the anticholesterol drugs or anti-anginal drugs may have made SCS for angina obsolete. Also, the quality of percutaneous angioplasty has clearly improved, which makes the comparative therapy less definitive. A recent cohort study shows that this therapy may have good results on a longer term as well.[21] It can be concluded that there is a need for a new prospective, randomized study.

Complications of interventional management

The complications of SCS treatment are limited to minor complications in approximately 6.8% of the patients receiving the treatment and include lead migrations, electrode fractures, battery failure, and subcutaneous infection.[1,10,18,22]

Major complications have not been described in previously published studies. There are, of course, absolute contraindications for this treatment, including implantable cardioverter defibrillator pacemaker, irreversible bleeding diathesis, neuraxial malignancy, or cognitive disorders, that do not allow the patient to operate the spinal cord stimulator.

Table 24.1. Summary of the evidence for interventional management of chronic refractory angina pectoris.

Technique	Evaluation
Spinal cord stimulation	2 B+

Evidence for interventional management

The summary of the evidence for the interventional management for chronic refractory angina pectoris is given in Table 24.1.

Recommendations

Based on the present literature, SCS is recommended in patients with chronic refractory angina pectoris that does not respond to conventional therapy who are referred by a cardiologist.

Clinical practice algorithm

Figure 24.1 represents the treatment algorithm for refractory angina pectoris based on the available evidence.

Technique(s)

The intervention takes place under strictly sterile conditions and antibiotic prophylaxis, eg, 1,000 mg of a cephalosporin intravenously. The patient is placed in a prone position on an operating table suitable for X-ray screening. The T8–T9 vertebral level is identified by means of a C-arm. A Tuohy needle is inserted under X-ray guidance to find the epidural space, and a four-contact or eight-contact electrode array is placed with its cephalad tip at the T2–T3 level left of midline. Subsequently, test stimulations are performed; the test stimulations should overlap the areas that are painful during angina attacks. The electrode is normally located in the T1–T4 area. When the correct level has been found, the lead is fixated, and the pacemaker is inserted in the left or right buttock, or in the upper abdomen. The electrical continuity is then restored via an extension lead. The patient is hospitalized and treated with antibiotics for 24 hours. The patient can be discharged the following day. The treatment does not include a period of test stimulation. The system is implanted directly.

Summary

Angina pectoris is termed refractory if conventional treatment fails.

In case of persisting symptoms, spinal cord stimulation can be recommended after extensive multidisciplinary evaluation.

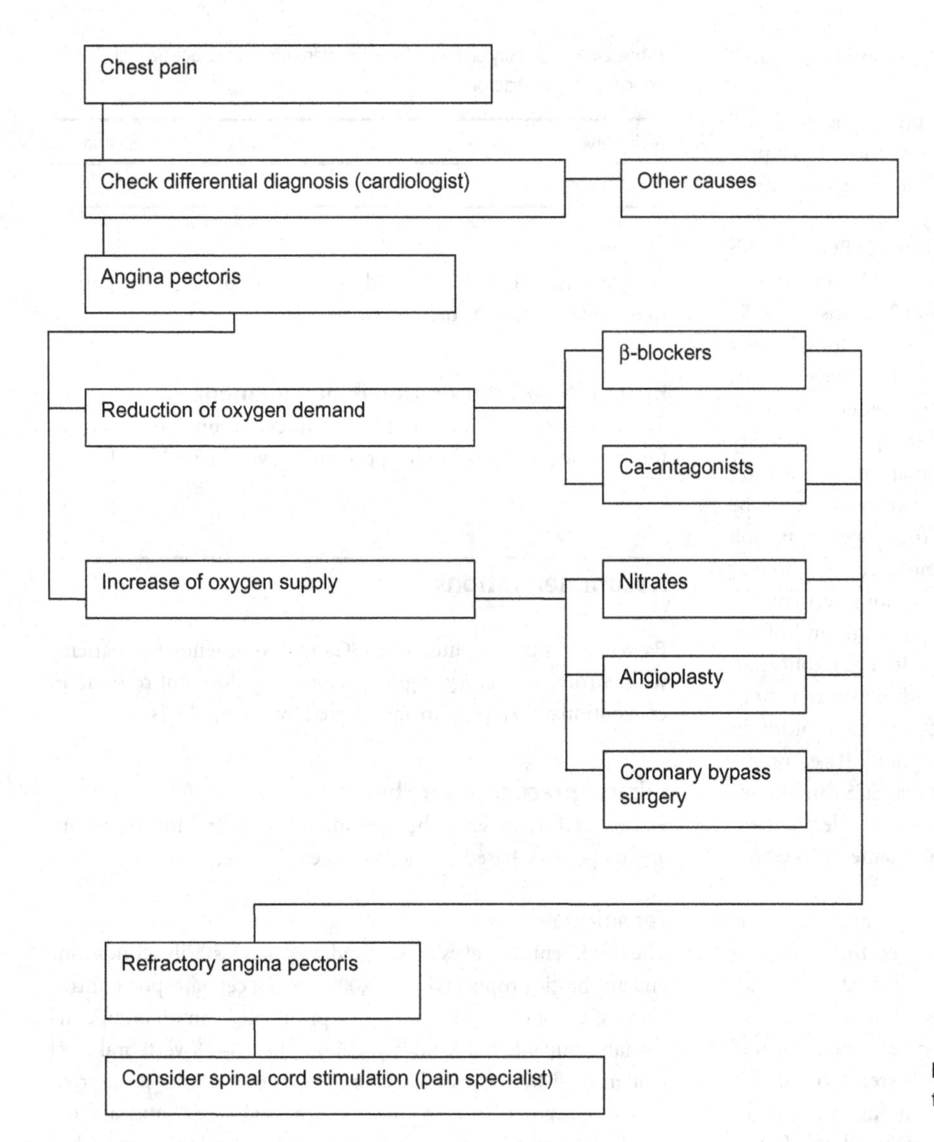

Figure 24.1. Clinical practice algorithm for the treatment of refractory angina pectoris.

References

1. TenVaarwerk IA, Jessurun GA, DeJongste MJ, et al. Clinical outcome of patients treated with spinal cord stimulation for therapeutically refractory angina pectoris. TheWorking Group on Neurocardiology. *Heart.* 1999;82:82–88.
2. Schoebel FC, Frazier OH, Jessurun GA, et al. Refractory angina pectoris in end-stage coronary artery disease: evolving therapeutic concepts. *Am Heart J.* 1997;134:587–602.
3. Mannheimer C, Camici P, Chester MR, et al. The problem of chronic refractory angina; report from the ESC Joint Study Group on the Treatment of Refractory Angina. *Eur Heart J.* 2002;23:355–370.
4. Murphy DF, Giles KE. Dorsal column stimulation for pain relief from intractable angina pectoris. *Pain.* 1987;28:365–368.
5. Ferri F. Angina pectoris. In: Ferri F, ed. *Ferri's Clinical Advisor 2008: Instant Diagnosis and Treatment.* Vol. ed. Philadelphia, PA: Mosby Elsevier; 2008.
6. Meyerson BA, Linderoth B. Mechanisms of spinal cord stimulation in neuropathic pain. *Neurol Res.* 2000;22:285–292.
7. Woolf CJ, Doubell TP. The pathophysiology of chronic pain—increased sensitivity to low threshold A beta-fibre inputs. *Curr Opin Neurobiol.* 1994;4:525–534.
8. Wu M, Linderoth B, Foreman RD. Putative mechanisms behind effects of spinal cord stimulation on vascular diseases: a review of experimental studies. *Auton Neurosci.* 2008;138:9–23.
9. Mannheimer C, Eliasson T, Augustinsson LE, et al. Electrical stimulation versus coronary artery bypass surgery in severe angina pectoris: the ESBY study. *Circulation.* 1998;97:1157–1163.
10. de Jongste MJ, Hautvast RW, Hillege HL, Lie KI. Efficacy of spinal cord stimulation as adjuvant therapy for intractable angina pectoris: a prospective, randomized clinical study. Working Group on Neurocardiology. *J Am Coll Cardiol.* 1994;23:1592–1597.
11. Mannheimer C, Eliasson T, Andersson B, et al. Effects of spinal cord stimulation in angina pectoris induced by pacing and possible mechanisms of action. *BMJ.* 1993;307:477–480.
12. Hautvast RW, Blanksma PK, DeJongste MJ, et al. Effect of spinal cord stimulation on myocardial blood flow assessed by positron emission tomography in patients with refractory angina pectoris. *Am J Cardiol.* 1996;77:462–467.

13. Egginton S, Hudlicka O. Selective long-term electrical stimulation of fast glycolytic fibres increases capillary supply but not oxidative enzyme activity in rat skeletal muscles. *Exp Physiol.* 2000;85:567–573.
14. Mobilia G, Zuin G, Zanco P, et al. [Effects of spinal cord stimulation on regional myocardial blood flow in patients with refractory angina. A positron emission tomography study]. *G Ital Cardiol.* 1998;28:1113–1119.
15. Sanderson JE, Ibrahim B, Waterhouse D, Palmer RB. Spinal electrical stimulation for intractable angina—long-term clinical outcome and safety. *Eur Heart J.* 1994;15:810–814.
16. Jessurun GA, Ten Vaarwerk IA, DeJongste MJ, Tio RA, Staal MJ. Sequelae of spinal cord stimulation for refractory angina pectoris. Reliability and safety profile of long-term clinical application. *Coron Artery Dis.* 1997;8:33–38.
17. Greco S, Auriti A, Fiume D, et al. Spinal cord stimulation for the treatment of refractory angina pectoris: a two-year follow-up. *Pacing Clin Electrophysiol.* 1999;22:26–32.
18. Ekre O, Eliasson T, Norrsell H, Wahrborg P, Mannheimer C. Long-term effects of spinal cord stimulation and coronary artery bypass grafting on quality of life and survival in the ESBY study. *Eur Heart J.* 2002;23:1938–1945.
19. Di Pede F, Lanza GA, Zuin G, et al. Immediate and long-term clinical outcome after spinal cord stimulation for refractory stable angina pectoris. *Am J Cardiol.* 2003;91:951–955.
20. McNab D, Khan SN, Sharples LD, et al. An open label, single-centre, randomized trial of spinal cord stimulation vs. percutaneous myocardial laser revascularization in patients with refractory angina pectoris: the SPiRiT trial. *Eur Heart J.* 2006;27:1048–1053.
21. de Vries J, Dejongste MJ, Durenkamp A, Zijlstra F, Staal MJ. The sustained benefits of long-term neurostimulation in patients with refractory chest pain and normal coronary arteries. *Eur J Pain.* 2007;11:360–365.
22. DeJongste MJ. Spinal cord stimulation for ischemic heart disease. *Neurol Res.* 2000;22:293–298.

25 Ischemic Pain in the Extremities and Raynaud's Phenomenon

Jacques Devulder, Hans van Suijlekom, Robert van Dongen, Sudhir Diwan, Nagy Mekhail, Maarten van Kleef and Frank Huygen

Introduction

Pain takes a central position in a varied group of disorders, due to insufficient blood supply to the extremities. It results in ischemia of the peripheral tissues, which causes pain and often functional limitation in the patient. Pain is a signal indicating a serious problem. Two important groups of disorders can be distinguished: critical vascular disease[1] and the Raynaud's phenomenon.[2–4] The latter can be subdivided into a primary and a secondary type.[2,3] The context and the cause of each of these three groups is different, which means that good diagnostics are essential to identify and influence the prognosis.

Epidemiology

Since there are two subgroups, the incidence and epidemiology of these groups is also different.

Critical ischemic vascular disease is most common in patients over 55 years old as a result of arterial vascular disease. The annual incidence is 0.25 to 0.45 patients per 1,000 population. The disease initially presents as vague pain in the extremities, but ends in necrosis and amputation of the extremity in the course of 5 years.

Raynaud's phenomenon occurs frequently in our society with an incidence of 3% to 21%.

There is a primary form, also termed Raynaud's disease, in which no underlying cause for the symptoms can be found. The secondary form, indicated with the general term Raynaud's syndrome, does have an underlying cause. It is usually associated with systemic pathology, in particular rheumatic pathology.

The main pathophysiology is impaired perfusion of the peripheral parts of the extremities. Initially, it manifests itself as white discoloration of the fingers or toes and later as blue discoloration leading to ulcers. The most important diseases to consider include systemic diseases such as generalized sclerosis and scleroderma. In 90% of the cases with these diseases, Raynaud's phenomenon is the first symptom. Thromboangiitis obliterans or Buerger's disease[5] can also be classified under secondary Raynaud's. The age at onset is usually under 45 years. It is an immune-mediated arteritis of which the pathology is not fully known, but smoking or smoke cessation can seriously affect the symptomatology. The incidence of the diseases varies considerably throughout the world. In the U.S. and Europe, the incidence is 0.5% to 15%, whereas the incidence mounts to 60% in some Asian countries. It is not clear how this large difference can be explained; it may be related to smoking and the type of tobacco used.

Etiology

As indicated above, the etiology of the diseases is different.

Critical ischemic disease is often caused by arteriosclerosis due to hypertension or diabetes. Prevention by means of proper health hygiene is important and can influence the incidence and severity as well as the prognosis.

Primary Raynaud's is idiopathic and will be diagnosed as such if underlying systemic pathology has been excluded.

Secondary Raynaud's is often a manifestation of a systemic disease. It is essential to try to establish a diagnosis as soon as possible in order to influence the evolution of the disease. A sclerotic disease can indeed have a large impact on the functioning of vital organs such as the lungs, liver, or kidneys. Because secondary Raynaud's also occurs in other disorders such as Buerger's disease or even as an expression of a paraneoplastic phenomenon, these should always be considered. In some cases, it can be an adverse effect of chemotherapeutics.[6]

Evidence-Based Interventional Pain Medicine: According to Clinical Diagnoses, First Edition. Edited by Jan Van Zundert, Jacob Patijn, Craig T. Hartrick, Arno Lataster, Frank J.P.M Huygen, Nagy Mekhail, Maarten van Kleef.

Table 25.1. Differences between primary and secondary Raynaud's phenomenon.

	Primary	Secondary
Incidence	3% to 5%	0.2%
In combination with other diseases	No	Yes
Associated with antibodies	No	Often
Dilated capillaries in nail bed	No	Often
Familial predisposition	Yes	Yes
Connective tissue disorders in family	Yes	Yes
Medicinal treatment necessary	Rarely	Often
Complications	No, rarely	Yes
Improves after some time	Yes, often	Sometimes

From Pope JE[9] Reprinted by permission of the publisher.

Buerger's disease appears to be an immune-mediated pathology, occurring both in men and in women. The symptoms already present at an early age, but are predominantly determined by smoking behavior. The first step in the treatment is therefore to refrain from tobacco use.

Table 25.1 gives an overview of the differences between primary and secondary Raynaud's phenomenon, based on a recent publication by Pope.[7]

Pathophysiology

The exact pathophysiological mechanism remains as yet largely unclear. However, it has been shown that the physiological vasoconstriction on noradrenaline is enhanced by cold and that there is an increased sensitivity to α_2-agonists and serotonin. The vasoconstrictive endothelin-1 would also be involved, and the Calcitonin Gene Related Peptide (CGRP) and Cyclooxygenase supposedly play a (modulating) role.[8]

The primary or idiopathic form (Raynaud's disease) often presents without an apparent cause and has a favorable course over time. In case of the secondary form (Raynaud's syndrome), there is often a disorder of the connective tissue, collagen or a rheumatic disease, often with autoimmune features (scleroderma, Sjögren's disease, rheumatoid arthritis, systemic lupus erythematosus, polymyositis) or a peripheral vascular disease (thromboangiitis obliterans or Buerger's disease). In rare cases, it occurs in combination with a malignancy or chemotherapy (cisplatinum, bleomycin, and vincristine).

Diagnosis

History

The clinical history will mainly include pain in the extremities. In case of critical ischemic disease due to arteriosclerosis, patients often indicate evolution of nonspecific pain in the extremities while walking that disappears at rest. The first symptom is usually intermittent claudication followed by an increasingly serious symptomatology over the years. Eventually, slow-healing ulcers will develop.

Critical ischemic disease predominantly occurs in the older population. This is in contrast to Buerger's disease in which the first symptoms are also atypical pain with eventual discoloration and ulceration. Patients with Raynaud's phenomenon mostly complain of pain in the distal parts of extremities, often accompanied by white discoloration of the extremities. At a later stage, the discoloration darkens and ulcers may eventually develop.

Physical examination

Ischemic pain is usually accompanied by a discoloration of the extremities. This is mostly a white discoloration of the distal parts of extremities, but it may change to a dark blue, color. Also important is that there are no arterial pulsations in the affected area. The extremity will feel colder and may show skin lesions that heal very poorly in a later stage. The distal peripheral parts may show a tendency to necrosis.

General examination to evaluate the patient's health (weight loss, malignancy) is relevant. The blood pressure should be measured and examination focusing on disorders of the connective tissues or on peripheral vascular disease should be carried out. The hands and feet should be inspected (wounds, ulcers); presence of dilated capillaries in the nail bed is also important.

Additional tests

Additional laboratory testing (sedimentation, antibodies, renal function) focusing on autoimmune disorders can best be performed by an internist/rheumatologist.

In case of critical ischemic vascular disease, the imaging of the coronary arteries will be important, because it provides information about the prognosis and about whether surgical intervention could be useful. Imaging is less relevant in cases of Buerger's disease and Raynaud's phenomenon; clinical and laboratory examination will provide sufficient information to make the diagnosis.

Once the diagnosis has been established, the evolution can be followed by means of capillaroscopy, which determines both the number of capillaries and the rate of red blood cell circulation. The determination of the transcutaneous oxygen saturation is also a parameter indicating the severity of the disease; it can also be used to demonstrate improvement in the microcirculation resulting from particular treatments.

Differential diagnosis

In cases of secondary Raynaud's especially, it is important to demonstrate or exclude concomitant disorders. Severe vascular disease may lead to organ damage. Medicinal therapy is often indicated. The primary form may resemble acrocyanosis (blue discoloration of the nails) and primary livedo reticularis (red-blue discolored skin in a reticular pattern); both are caused by reduced perfusion of the skin and are enhanced by cold exposure and emotional stress.

Table 25.2. Classification of perfusion disorders in peripheral arterial vascular disease according to Fontaine.

Stage I	No symptoms (sufficient peripheral circulation)
Stage II	Pain upon exertion, intermittent claudication
IIa	ability to walk >100 m
IIb	ability to walk <100 m
Stage III	Pain at rest in the extremity concerned and in the supine position due to a poor muscle perfusion. The pain often temporarily decreases if the leg is dependent
Stage IV	Trophic disorders such as necrosis/gangrene

Treatment options

Conservative management for ischemic vascular disease

Patients with pain due to a vascular disease initially receive conservative and pharmacological therapy that aims at treating the underlying cause. If the symptoms persist, it may be decided to perform vascular surgery. The patient group discussed in this chapter concerns inoperable, vascular patients with pain at rest and/or ulcers (Fontaine III en IV)[9] (Table 25.2).

Interventional management for ischemic vascular disease

The treatment of these patients is aimed at pain reduction and cure of the ulcers in order to prevent amputation. The literature mentions two methods:

1 Sympathectomy
2 Spinal cord stimulation

Sympathectomy

Sympathectomy primarily has a vasodilatatory effect on the collateral circulation resulting from a reduced sympathetic tone. Improved oxygenation of the tissues leads to less tissue damage, which results in decreased pain and increased healing of the ulcers. Pain reduction also occurs due to the interruption of sympathetic nociceptive interaction.

Three randomized studies were reported in the literature. Only Cross and Cotton[10] found significant pain reduction in the group treated with chemical lumbar sympathectomy compared to the control group (bupivacaine injection) (66.7% vs. 23.5%), but no changes in the anklebrachial index. The two other randomized controlled trials (RCTs) did not show any objective advantages.[11,12]

Over the years, however, several cohort studies have been conducted examining the effect of sympathectomy, either surgical or chemical. Sanni et al.[13] concluded in their review that although the RCTs did not support its use, many cohort studies have shown a positive effect of sympathectomy in patients with critical ischemic vascular disease. A retrospective study by Repealer van Driel et al.,[14] including 60 successive surgical lumbar sympathectomies, showed good results (no rest pain, healing of ulcers and no major amputations) in 48% of the patients after 6 months.

Keane[15] performed lumbar chemical sympathectomy using phenol 6% under X-ray guidance in 132 patients with critical ischemic vascular disease. Favorable results (no rest pain, warm extremity, and no amputation) were obtained in 52% of the patients after a follow-up of 16 months. Mashiah[16] studied 373 patients with critical ischemic vascular disease who were treated with lumbar chemical sympathectomy. Success (no pain, healing of ulcers after 6 to 12 months and no amputation) was achieved in 58.7% of the patients. The amputation ratio was 20% and the mortality was 9%. Although the effect of sympathectomy in critical ischemic vascular disease is not consistent, several studies have shown a trend toward better pain reduction and ulcer healing, which justifies its consideration.

Spinal cord stimulation

Spinal cord stimulation (SCS) has been used to treat a variety of chronic pain syndromes since 1967. The effect of SCS is probably based on several mechanism of action.[17] In 1996, Jivegard et al.[18] published a randomized study on the effect of SCS in 51 patients with critical ischemic vascular disease with a follow-up of 18 months. He concluded that SCS resulted in better pain reduction than treatment with analgesics, but there was no significant difference in amputation rates between both groups. A subgroup analysis in patients without arterial hypertension did show a significant difference in amputation percentages.

A Belgian national study by Suy et al.[19] showed no significant difference in amputation percentages, although there was a tendency favoring fewer amputations in the group receiving SCS. A randomized study by Klomp et al.[20] including 120 patients with critical ischemic vascular disease showed that SCS with pharmacological treatment was not significantly better with respect to amputation scores at 2-year follow-up than the group receiving pharmacological treatment alone. In 2001, the same research group published the results of a subgroup in whom the difference in transcutaneous pO_2 between a lying and a sitting position was >15 mm Hg, and who showed a significant amputation reduction.[21] Several nonrandomized studies have demonstrated a significantly lower amputation percentage in SCS groups.[1,22–24]

A Cochrane Review of 2005 concluded that SCS in critical ischemic vascular disease: (1) leads to fewer amputations; (2) provides better pain relief; and (3) restores more patients to Fontaine stage II.[1] Patients receiving conservative treatment exhibited more adverse effects due to medication, including: (1) gastrointestinal hemorrhage; (2) nausea; and (3) dizziness. It should be noted that SCS also is associated with complications including implantation problems, as well as additional intervention due to lead migration and infection. SCS is more expensive: 36,500 Euros (SCS) vs. 28,600 Euros (conservative).

Spinal cord stimulation may reduce amputation rate and pain in selected patients with critical ischemic vascular disease that is refractory to conservative and minimally invasive pain treatment.

Table 25.3. Summary of the evidence for interventional management for ischemic vascular disease.

Technique	Evaluation
Sympathectomy	2B±
Spinal cord stimulation	2B±

Complications of interventional management for ischemic vascular disease

Complications of sympathectomy and SCS are described in the chapter, "Complex Regional Pain Syndrome (CRPS)."[25]

Evidence for interventional management for ischemic vascular disease

The summary of the evidence for the interventional management of extremity pain due to vascular disease is given in Table 25.3.

Recommendations for ischemic vascular disease

A sympathetic nerve block can be considered in patients with critical ischemic vascular disease after extensive conservative treatment, preferably in the context of a study. If this has insufficient effect, SCS can be considered in a selected patient group. In view of the degree of invasiveness and the costs involved, this treatment should preferably be applied in the context of a study, with transcutaneous pO_2 measurements recommended.

Clinical practice algorithm for ischemic vascular disease

Figure 25.1 represents the treatment algorithm for ischemic vascular disease.

Technique(s)

We refer to the chapter on "CRPS" for the techniques.[25]

Conservative management for raynaud's phenomenon

The treatment of the primary form of Raynaud's phenomenon is usually conservative and not pharmacological. In case of primary Raynaud's, it is generally sufficient to inform the patient well and advise them to avoid provoking factors by wearing warm clothes, stopping smoking, taking sufficient exercise and avoiding vasoconstrictive medication. If pharmacological treatment is required, the vasodilators nifedipine (Ca-antagonist) and prazosin (α_1-blocker) have been studied most, but their effects have been disappointing.[2,3] The main problems encountered with these drugs are the adverse effects and the loss of long-term efficacy.

The treatment of secondary Raynaud's is initially aimed at the underlying disease. Figure 25.2 presents an algorithm for the conventional treatment of Raynaud's disease.

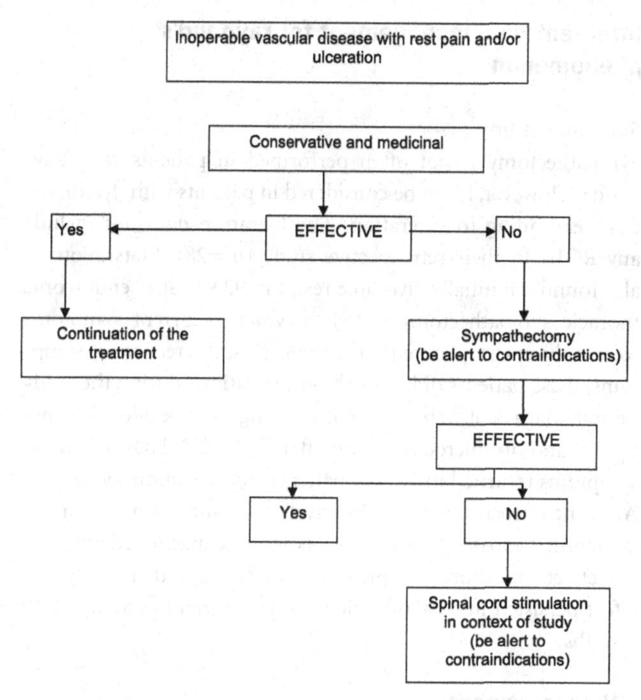

Figure 25.1. Clinical practice algorithm for the treatment of critical ischemic vascular disease.

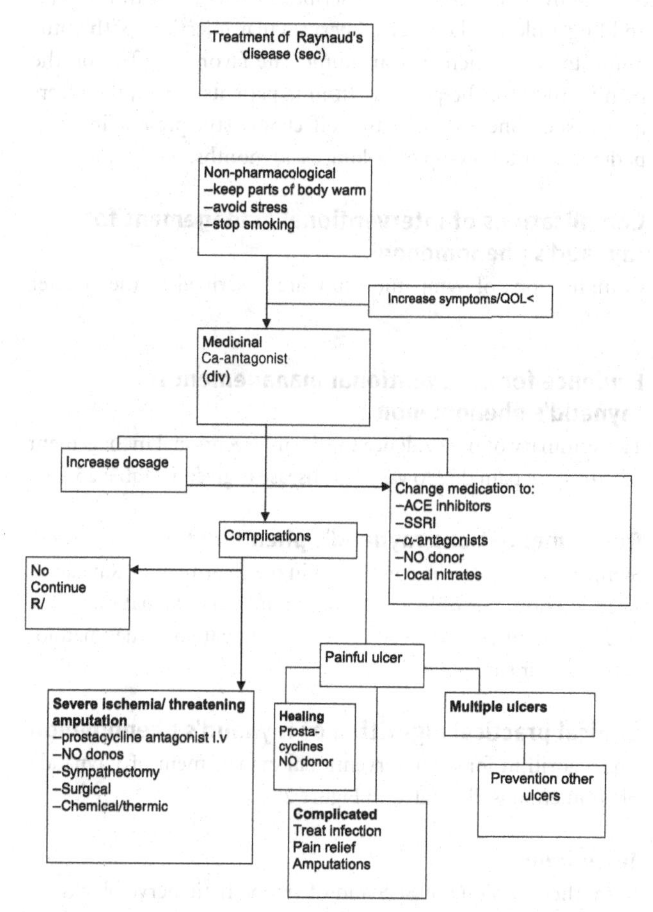

Figure 25.2. Clinical practice algorithm for the conventional treatment of secondary Raynaud's disease.

Interventional management for raynaud's phenomenon

Sympathectomy

Sympathectomy is not often performed in patients with Raynaud's. However, it can be considered in patients with dystrophic changes leading to ulceration. The literature does not include any RCTs. In their retrospective study ($n = 28$), Matsumoto et al.[26] found an initially favorable result in 92.9% after endoscopic thoracic sympathectomy (ETS); however, recurrent symptoms were subsequently noted in 82.1%. Despite recurrent symptoms, these patients did not exhibit ulcerations during the study period. Maga et al.[27] showed a long-lasting positive effect (follow-up 5 years) on microcirculation after ETS (Th2-Th4). Although symptoms returned in 28% of patients, no ulcerations were seen. A recent retrospective ($n = 34$) study by Thune et al.[28] demonstrated that most patients (83%) experience an immediate positive effect after thoracoscopic sympathectomy. In their study, this effect persisted in 33% of patients after a mean follow-up of 40 months.

Other treatments

Botulinum toxin a injections

A study by Van Beek et al.[29] describes 11 patients with rest pain and finger ulcers who received perivascular injections with botulinum toxin A. There was an immediate favorable effect on the pain in 100% of the patients. In nine patients (82%), the ulcers healed spontaneously and this effect was still present in these patients after follow-up of as long as 30 months.

Complications of interventional management for raynaud's phenomenon

Complications of sympathectomy are described in the chapter "CRPS."[25]

Evidence for interventional management for raynaud's phenomenon

The summary of the evidence for the interventional management of extremity pain due to vascular disease is given in Table 25.4.

Recommendations raynaud's phenomenon

Sympathectomy can be considered in the treatment of Raynaud's phenomenon, but only after multidisciplinary evaluation of the patient and in close consultation with the patient's rheumatologist, vascular surgeon or internist.

Clinical practical algorithm of raynaud's phenomenon

The algorithm for the interventional management of Raynaud's phenomenon is illustrated in Figure 25.3.

Technique

Both, the technique of SCS and of sympathetic nerve blocks are described in the chapter on CRPS.[25]

Table 25.4. Summary of the evidence for interventional management for Raynaud's phenomenon.

Technique	Evaluation
Sympathectomy	2C+

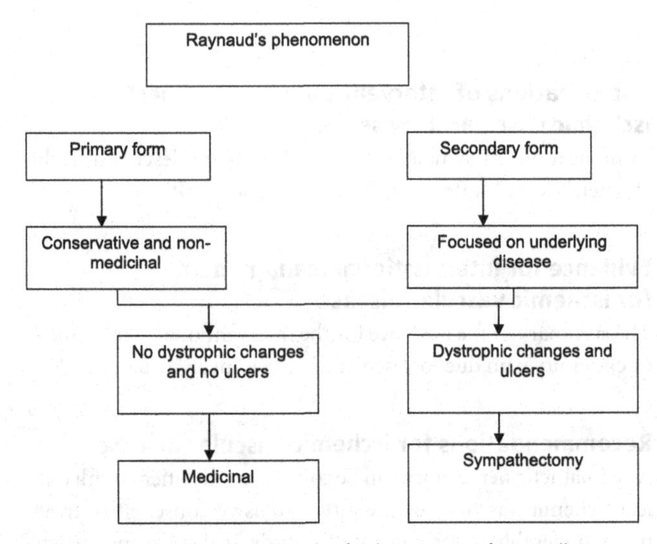

Figure 25.3. Clinical practice algorithm for the treatment of Raynaud's phenomenon.

Summary

Patients with pain due to *critical ischemic vascular disease* should first receive conservative and medicinal treatment directed at the underlying cause. A sympathetic nerve block can be considered in inoperable vascular patients with refractory rest pain and/or ulcers.

Considering the degree of invasiveness, SCS can be considered, preferably in the context of a study.

Treatment of the primary form of *Raynaud's* is generally conservative and nonmedicinal.

Treatment of secondary Raynaud's phenomenon is initially aimed at the underlying cause.

Sympathectomy can be considered in patients with refractory pain after extensive multidisciplinary evaluation and in consultation with the patient's rheumatologist, vascular surgeon or internist.

References

1. Ubbink DT, Vermeulen H. Spinal cord stimulation for non-reconstructable chronic critical leg ischaemia. *Cochrane Database Syst Rev.* 2005;3:CD004001.
2. Block JA, Sequeira W. Raynaud's phenomenon. *Lancet.* 2001;357: 2042–2048.

3. Wigley FM. Clinical practice. Raynaud's Phenomenon. *N Engl J Med.* 2002;347:1001–1008.
4. Carpentier P, Sotger B, Poensin D, Maricq H. Incidence and natural history of Raynaud's phenomenon: a long-term follow-up (14 years) of a random sample from the general population. *J Vasc Surg.* 2006;44:1023–1028.
5. Mills JL Sr. Buerger's disease in the 21st century: diagnosis, clinical features, and therapy. *Semin Vasc Surg.* 2003;16:179–189.
6. Ting J, Fukshandsky M, Burton A. Treatment of refractory ischemic pain from chemotherapy-induced Taynaud's syndrome with spinal cord stimulation. *Pain Practice.* 2007;7(2):143–146.
7. Pope JE. The diagnosis and treatment of Raynaud's phenomenon: a practical approach. *Drugs.* 2007;67:517–525.
8. Cooke JP, Marshall JM. Mechanisms of Raynaud's disease. *Vasc Med.* 2005;10:293–307.
9. Fontaine R, Kim M, Kieny R. [Surgical treatment of peripheral circulation disorders.]. *Helv Chir Acta.* 1954;21:499–533.
10. Cross FW, Cotton LT. Chemical lumbar sympathectomy for ischemic rest pain. A randomized, prospective controlled clinical trial. *Am J Surg.* 1985;150:341–345.
11. Barnes RW, Baker WH, Shanik G, et al. Value of concomitant sympathectomy in aortoiliac reconstruction. Results of a prospective, randomized study. *Arch Surg.* 1977;112:1325–1330.
12. Fyfe T, Quin RO. Phenol sympathectomy in the treatment of intermittent claudication: a controlled clinical trail. *Br J Surg.* 1975;62:68–71.
13. Sanni A, Hamid A, Dunning J. Is sympathectomy of benefit in critical leg ischaemia not amenable to revascularisation? *Interact Cardiovasc Thorac Surg.* 2005;4:478–483.
14. Repealer van Driel O, Van Bockel J, Van Schilfgarde R. Lumbar sympathectomy for severe lower limb ischaemia: results and analysis of factors influencing outcome. *J Cardiovasc Surg.* 1998;29:310–314.
15. Keane FB. Phenol lumbar sympathectomy for severe arterial occlusive disease in the elderly. *Br J Surg.* 1977;64:519–521.
16. Mashiah A, Soroker D, Pasik S, Mashiah T. Phenol lumbar sympathetic block in diabetic lower limb ischemia. *J Cardiovasc Risk.* 1995;2:467–469.
17. Barendse GA, Köke A, Kemler M. Neuromodulatie en TENS. In: Van Kleef M, Weber W, Winter F, Zuurmond W, eds. *Handboek pijnbestrijding, Vol. ed.* Leusden, Nederland: De Tijdstroom; 2000: 279–285.
18. Jivegard LE, Augustinsson LE, Holm J, Risberg B, Ortenwall P. Effects of spinal cord stimulation (SCS) in patients with inoperable severe lower limb ischaemia: a prospective randomised controlled study. *Eur J Vasc Endovasc Surg.* 1995;9:421–425.
19. Suy R, Gybels J, Van DH, Martin D, Van MR, Delaporte C. Spinal cord stimulation for ischaemic rest pain. The Belgian randomized study. In: Horschs S, Claeys L, eds. *Spinal cord Stimulation: An Innovative Method in the Treatment of PVD, Vol. ed.* Darmstadt: Steinhoff; 1994: 197–202.
20. Klomp HM, Spincemaille GH, Steyerberg EW, Habbema JD, van Urk H. Spinal-cord stimulation in critical limb ischaemia: a randomised trial. ESES Study Group. *Lancet.* 1999;353:1040–1044.
21. Spincemaille GH, de Vet HC, Ubbink DT, Jacobs MJ. The results of spinal cord stimulation in critical limb ischaemia: a review. *Eur J Vasc Endovasc Surg.* 2001;21:99–105.
22. Amann W, Berg P, Gersbach P, Gamain J, Raphael JH, Ubbink DT. Spinal cord stimulation in the treatment of non-reconstructable stable critical leg ischaemia: results of the European Peripheral Vascular Disease Outcome Study (SCS-EPOS). *Eur J Vasc Endovasc Surg.* 2003;26:280–286.
23. Augustinsson LE, Carlsson CA, Holm J, Jivegard L. Epidural electrical stimulation in severe limb ischemia. Pain relief, increased blood flow, and a possible limb-saving effect. *Ann Surg.* 1985;202:104–110.
24. Broseta J, Barbera J, de Vera JA, et al. Spinal cord stimulation in peripheral arterial disease. A cooperative study. *J Neurosurg.* 1986;64:71–80.
25. van Eijs F, Stanton-Hicks M, Van Zundert J, et al. 16. Complex regional pain syndrome. *Pain Pract.* 2011; 11:70–87.
26. Matsumoto Y, Ueyama T, Endo T, et al. Endoscopic thoracic sympathicotomy for Raynaud's phenomenon. *J Vasc Surg.* 2002;36:57–61.
27. Maga P, Kuzdzal J, Nizankowski R, Szczeklik A, Sladek K. Long-term effects of thoracic sympathectomy on microcirculation in the hands of patients with primary Raynaud disease. *J Thorac Cardiovasc Surg.* 2007;133:1428–1433.
28. Thune TH, Ladegaard L, Licht PB. Thoracoscopic sympathectomy for Raynaud's phenomenon–a long term follow-up study. *Eur J Vasc Endovasc Surg.* 2006;32:198–202.
29. Van Beek AL, Lim PK, Gear AJ, Pritzker MR. Management of vasospastic disorders with botulinum toxin A. *Plast Reconstr Surg.* 2007;119:217–226.

26 Pain in Chronic Pancreatitis

Martine Puylaert, Leonardo Kapural, Jan Van Zundert, Dirk Peek, Arno Lataster, Nagy Mekhail, Maarten van Kleef and Yolande C. A. Keulemans

Introduction

The pancreas consists of acini, islets of Langerhans, and ducts. Acini are units of approximately 20 acinar cells with a few centroacinar cells. Several pancreatic enzymes are produced in the acinar cells: amylase in an active form, lipases, nucleases, and proteolytic enzymes (trypsins) in an inactive form. The centroacinar cells produce bicarbonate. The A cells in the islets of Langerhans produce glucagon and the B cells insulin. The regulation of the pancreas is controlled by hormones and the autonomic (sympathetic and parasympathetic) nervous system. The hormone cholecystokinin (CCK) is released from special intestinal cells and has a stimulating effect on the exocrine function of the pancreas. The release of CCK is stimulated by CCK-releasing peptide, a protein that is intraluminally active and denatured by trypsin.

Innervation of the pancreas consists of sympathetic fibers from the nervi splanchnici and parasympathetic fibers from the nervi vagi. The intrapancreatic acinar plexus contains both sympathetic and parasympathetic fibers. Parasympathetic fibers stimulate exocrine as well as endocrine secretion. Sympathetic fibers mainly have an inhibiting effect on this release. A rich sensory network is located in the pancreas around the acinar cells.[1–3]

Chronic pancreatitis is defined as a progressive inflammatory response of the pancreas that leads to irreversible morphological changes of the parenchyma (fibrosis, loss of acini and islets of Langerhans, and the formation of pancreatic stones), as well as the pancreatic duct (stenosis and pancreatic stones).

In contrast to acute pancreatitis, in which the acute inflammatory damage is transient, chronic pancreatitis involves a progressive process. Although these two clinical pictures may overlap (recurrent episodes of acute pancreatitis may lead to chronic pancreatitis), they each have a different pathological picture, etiology, and course.[4]

Also in contrast to acute pancreatitis, which involves a neutrophilic inflammatory reaction, chronic pancreatitis is characterized by mononuclear infiltration and fibrosis. Fibrosing of the parenchyma accompanied by the loss of acini and islets of Langerhans eventually leads to loss of function. This functional loss can be both exocrine (resulting in lipase deficiency with steatorrhea, diarrhea, and weight loss) and endocrine (causing diabetes mellitus [DM] in case of insulin deficiency). This functional loss only occurs when 90% of the acini or islets of Langerhans are lost, respectively. Moreover, the fibrosing process can lead to strictures in the structures next to the pancreas, such as the duodenum, ductus choledochus, and colon. Fibrosis around the vena lienalis can cause thrombosis of this vein, eventually resulting in hemorrhages from gastric (fundal) varices. Morphological changes of the ductus pancreaticus may lead to a rupture resulting in pseudocysts, ascites, and fistulas. Two to three per cent of the patients with chronic pancreatitis ultimately develop a pancreatic carcinoma. The most common symptoms, however, are exocrine pancreatic insufficiency and pain.[5–8]

Epidemiology

The incidence of chronic pancreatitis in the Western world amounts to 10/100,000. It is more common in men (3:1), and presents mostly between ages 40 and 50. Chronic pancreatitis cannot be cured. Ten years after the disorder has been diagnosed, 30% of the patients will have died. Death rarely results from multiple organ failure or sepsis in case of an acute exacerbation, surgical complications or late complications of DM. It is more likely that premature death is caused by the patient's lifestyle. These patients have an increased risk to develop lung cancer or esophageal cancer as a result of nicotine and alcohol abuse. In addition, they have an increased risk of cardiovascular disease and alcohol-related accidents. Finally, these patients have an increased risk to develop a pancreatic carcinoma.[9–11]

Evidence-Based Interventional Pain Medicine: According to Clinical Diagnoses, First Edition. Edited by Jan Van Zundert, Jacob Patijn, Craig T. Hartrick, Arno Lataster, Frank J.P.M Huygen, Nagy Mekhail, Maarten van Kleef.

Table 26.1. Possible etiologies of chronic pancreatitis.

Etiologies
Alcoholic pancreatitis
Hereditary pancreatitis
Autoimmune pancreatitis
Metabolic pancreatitis (hypercalcemia, hyperlipidemia)
Tropical pancreatitis
Idiopathic pancreatitis

Etiology

Chronic pancreatitis is associated with (excessive) alcohol use in 70% to 80% of the patients. The mechanism of how alcohol causes pancreatitis is not yet clear. A large number of alcoholics do not develop pancreatitis, so a genetic factor may also be involved. It has been difficult to unravel the mechanism that causes alcohol-associated pancreatitis because there is no animal model in which the symptoms can be reproduced to simulate human alcoholic pancreatitis. It has been possible, however, to use animal models to show that alcohol increases the severity of pancreatitis that has been induced in another way.[12]

Alcohol does not play a role in 30% of the patients. In approximately half of these patients, the etiology can be established (Table 26.1); the other patients are considered to have idiopathic chronic pancreatitis.[13]

Pain is one of the most important symptoms of chronic pancreatitis. The pathogenesis of this pain can only partly be explained and it is therefore often difficult to treat this symptom. Pain in pancreatitis may be caused by different mechanisms.

1 Nociceptive pain
2 Neuropathic pain
3 Neurogenic inflammation

Nociceptive pain occurs after the activation of primary afferent neurons that respond to a chemical or mechanical stimuli. The pain is proportional to the degree of stimulation. Chronic pancreatitis involves inflammatory infiltration of sensory nerves. In human and animal models with chronic pancreatitis, perineural infiltrates are found with a high percentage of eosinophils in which the degree of infiltrative disorder correlates with the severity of the pain.[14] In the presence of inflammation, ischemia, increased pressure and release of, for instance, bradykinins, prostaglandins and substance P, nociceptors are activated, generating action potentials, and nociceptive pain thus develops.[15]

One theory argues that high pressure in the ductus pancreaticus leads to pain due to obstruction. Obstruction of the ductus pancreaticus can cause an "overpressure" proximally. This explanation of the pain is the basis for endoscopic and surgical drainage procedures. In 1970, an article was published about a patient in whom pain could be induced by injecting salt solutions in a drainage catheter located in a pancreatic fistula.[16]

Subsequently, several studies into overpressure in the ductus pancreaticus were carried out (preoperatively and during endoscopic retrograde cholangio pancreatography with manometry of the ductus pancreaticus), which showed inconsistent results. There are three studies in which the pressure in the pancreatic parenchyma was determined before surgery or partial pancreatic resection. Although higher pressures were found in the patients' parenchyma and the pressures were lower after the procedure, there was no consistent correlation with the pain.[17–19]

Other factors that may cause nociceptive pain in chronic pancreatitis include: obstruction of the duodenum or ductus choledochus, infiltration of the retroperitoneum, pseudocyst formation with compression of the surrounding organs, obstruction of the ductus pancreaticus due to fibrosis/stones/protein plugs, pancreatic ischemia due to atherosclerosis, gastric or duodenal ulcers, and meteorism due to malabsorption.[20,21]

Neuropathic pain involves a change of the sensory nerves or the central nervous system itself. This change or damage is caused by (but is not dependent on for perpetuation) nociceptive activation. It has been shown that changes occur in the neurons innervating the pancreas that are located in the ganglia spinalia (dorsal root ganglia).[22] Patients with chronic pancreatitis appear to show generalized hyperalgesia, possibly based on deep sensitization.[23]

Neurogenic inflammation is another proposed mechanism for pain. Cell death and tissue inflammation cause changes in the pH and the release of ions and inflammatory products such as cytokines and ATP. These inflammatory substances have direct as well as indirect effects on the nerve fibers and their ganglia once neuropathic pain develops. Neurogenic inflammation itself induces the production and increased release of neuropeptides, which then reinforces the inflammatory reaction in the tissues.[24]

Diagnosis

History

Patients with chronic pancreatitis can be free of pain for long periods of time (acute pancreatitis is always painful). This occurs in 20% of the patients with chronic pancreatitis and exocrine pancreatic insufficiency. These patients mainly suffer from diarrhea, foul-smelling stools that are difficult to flush (floating) and weight loss. Steatorrhea may lead to deficiencies of fat-soluble vitamins (A, D, E, and K) and vitamin B12. Also, chronic pancreatitis can cause insulindependent DM. This usually occurs later in the course of the disease. The risk of developing early DM appears to be increased in patients with a positive family history for DM and in patients with chronic pancreatitis and multiple pancreatic calcifications upon imaging. As the production of glucagon is disturbed in chronic pancreatitis, this form of DM includes a higher risk of hypoglycemia. Diabetic ketoacidosis and nephropathy are rare, but neuropathy and retinopathy are very common.[6,25,26]

Patients with pain typically complain of epigastric pain that radiates through to the back. The pain may deteriorate 20 to 30 minutes after a meal and is often accompanied by nausea and vomiting. Two patterns of symptoms are described in patients with alcoholic chronic pancreatitis. Type I is pain presenting in episodes of one to several weeks duration with pain-free intervals that can last for months or years. Type II is persistent pain with exacerbations requiring hospitalization.[27]

Physical examination

Physical examination usually does not reveal more than pain with pressure applied to the epigastrium.

Fever or a palpable mass suggests a complicated course of chronic pancreatitis (pseudocyst).

Additional tests

Because the pancreas is not encapsulated, acute pancreatitis can spread rapidly in a normal pancreas from parenchymal edema via surrounding fat (fat necrosis) to the retroperitoneal areas. In case of a chronically inflamed pancreas, a possible additional acute inflammatory component may be limited to a small area due to fibrosis of the pancreas. Therefore, routine laboratory examination does not play an important role in the diagnosis of chronic pancreatitis because amylase, lipase, and inflammatory parameters can be completely normal or only slightly elevated.[28]

A decreased exocrine function due to chronic inflammation can be demonstrated by means of a determination of elastase and fecal fat excretion. Glucose/HbA1c determination can be used to assess the endocrine pancreatic function. In case of chronic pancreatitis, the exocrine function is usually affected sooner and more severely than the endocrine function.[29]

Imaging techniques that may contribute to the diagnosis of chronic pancreatitis include: ultrasound, CT, MRI, and endoscopic ultrasound (EUS). The diagnosis is established by means of imaging and functional evaluation. Ultrasound and CT can be used to demonstrate abnormalities in the pancreatic parenchyma, such as calcifications, pseudocysts, and tumors. Magnetic resonance cholangio pancreatography examination can show abnormalities in the ductus pancreaticus, such as strictures, dilatations, and intraductal concrements. If the diagnosis of pancreatitis is doubted, EUS can be used to perform a puncture of the focal lesions or cysts to exclude malignancies.[30–34]

Differential diagnosis

1. Pancreatic carcinoma
2. Peptic ulcer
3. Symptomatic gallstone disease
4. Irritable bowel syndrome

Treatment options

Conservative management

Causal treatment

The following symptoms and complications of chronic pancreatitis should be treated first.[35–37]

- Pseudocysts, if they are causing pain because of their location or if their size increases. Treatment: endoscopic, radiological or surgical drainage.
- Obstruction of the ductus choledochus. Treatment: endoscopic stenting or surgical choledochoenterostomy.
- Duodenal obstruction with passage problems. Treatment: gastrojejunostomy.

The initial treatment of pain in chronic pancreatitis consists first of all of lifestyle adjustments and analgesics.

Lifestyle adjustments

In view of the association between alcohol abuse and pancreatitis, total abstinence from alcohol is recommended (also in patients with chronic pancreatitis in whom another etiology has been found). This may result in pain reduction, and in better survival-rates.[6,38,39] However, there are no prospective randomized studies or systematic reviews that prove this assertion.

Analgesics

All treatment guidelines for pain in chronic pancreatitis follow the 3-step ladder of the World Health Organization for the treatment of chronic pain.

The treatment should start with monotherapy. If this has insufficient effect, a combination therapy can be applied. Peripherally acting medication is then combined with centrally acting medication.

The first step in cases of limited-to-mild pain consists of nonopioid analgesics. The second step is applied in cases of mild-to-moderate pain and combines a nonopioid analgesic with a weak opioid. Titration is performed until the result is satisfactory. In cases of severe pain, a strong opioid such as morphine is prescribed (Step 3). The three steps can be combined with co-analgesics: an antiepileptic or a tricyclic antidepressant drug.

There are no randomized studies that compare the efficacy of the analgesics mentioned above for the treatment of pain in chronic pancreatitis. It is important to prescribe long-acting instead of short-acting morphinomimetics because of the tendency of this patient group to become addicted. It is also essential to register the effect of pain medication, for example by means of the visual analog score. The pain medication should preferably be prescribed by only one doctor to monitor the effect and reduce the risk of doctor-shopping behavior and addiction.

Paracetamol

Paracetamol (acetaminophen) is the pain medication of first choice. It has good analgesic and antipyretic properties and few side effects, especially no gastrointestinal side effects in the recommended dosage. However, paracetamol does not have any activity on cyclooxygenase (COX) and thus no anti-inflammatory activity.

Nonsteroidal anti-inflammatory drugs

The mechanisms of pain in chronic pancreatitis described above (nociceptive pain, neuropathic pain, and neurogenic inflammation) justify the prescription of antiinflammatory analgesics. Nonsteroidal anti-inflammatory drugs (NSAIDs), compared to the prototype aspirin, exert COX-1 and COX-2-inhibiting activity in varying degrees. Therefore, they possess a pain-relieving, antipyretic as well as anti-inflammatory activity. NSAIDs are therefore considered the first choice for nociceptive pain. Theoretically, NSAIDs can also play a positive role in reducing neurogenic inflammation.

However, the possible advantages of NSAIDs should be weighed against the disadvantages compared to, for instance, paracetamol. The side effects of NSAIDs vary from dyspepsia and skin disorders to gastric ulcerations and renal toxicity. Renal toxicity depends especially on the glomerular filtration rate. This implies that patients with renal disorders, liver cirrhosis and heart failure have an increased risk of nephrotoxicity. Risk factors for gastrointestinal side effects include: advanced age, liver cirrhosis, and additional factors that influence coagulation. If NSAIDs are chronically prescribed, it is generally recommended to add a proton pump inhibitor to the therapy.

Selective COX-2 inhibitors

Recent data show overexpression of COX-2 in chronic pancreatitis.[40] The contribution of COX-1 inhibitors should not be underestimated in the treatment of pronociceptive factors such as prostaglandins as part of the treatment of chronic pancreatitis. Moreover, long-term use of selective COX-2 inhibitors presumably increases the risk of cardiac disease, and they are therefore not indicated in the treatment of chronic pancreatitis. There are case reports that suggest COX-2 inhibitors induce flares of acute pancreatitis.

Opioids

If NSAIDs do not result in sufficient pain relief, opioids can be prescribed. Long-acting preparations are preferred. If necessary, a fast-acting morphine preparation can be prescribed. Nausea and vomiting may occur when these preparations are started, but the side effects will soon disappear and can be treated with low doses of a centrally acting antiemetic or haloperidol. In cases of constipation caused by medication, laxatives can be added to the therapy. Opioids therapy might be controversial in chronic pancreatitis patients as there is often a coincidence with addiction.

Opioids are active by binding to one of the known opioid receptors (mu, kappa, and delta). Opioid receptors are also present in the sphincter of Oddi. The sphincter of Oddi is a muscular valve in the duodenal wall that controls the release of bile and pancreatic juice, which is influenced by the hormone CCK. There is a tonic rest pressure as well as phasic antegrade contractions in this sphincter. Opioids result in an increase of the contraction frequency, amplitude and rest pressure. As this effect can only partly be counteracted by naloxone (μ-antagonist), it is likely that the effect of morphine on the sphincter of Oddi is mediated by several opioid receptors. The degree to which various morphinomimetics influence the pressure in the sphincter of Oddi has been studied. The results vary, partly also because different manometric techniques were used. From the different studies, it can be concluded that all opioids cause an increase of the sphincter pressure. However, there are no studies that justify the conclusion that increased pressure of the sphincter of Oddi has an effect on the development or deterioration of acute or chronic pancreatitis.[41–44]

Patients with chronic pancreatitis often suffer from depression due to their chronic pain symptoms. Tricyclic antidepressants have an effect on neuropathic pain as well as on depressive symptoms and can therefore contribute substantially to the treatment of pain in chronic pancreatitis.

Anticonvulsive drugs, gabapentin in particular, appear to be effective in the treatment of neuropathic pain in DM. Gabapentin is now frequently prescribed in cases of chronic pain in pancreatitis.[44]

Interventional management

- Anesthesiological: radiofrequency (RF) treatment of the nervi splanchnici and spinal cord stimulation (SCS).
- Endoscopic: stenting, stone extraction possibly in combination with lithotripsy.
- Surgical.

Anesthesiological pain treatment

Relevant anatomy

The sympathetic innervation of the abdominal organs starts from the anterolateral horn in the spinal cord. Preganglionar (preganglionic) fibers of Th5 to Th12 leave the spinal column after merging with the ramus ventralis. Together with these communicating rami they course in the direction of the truncus sympathicus (sympathetic chain). The fibers do not form synapses in the sympathetic chain, but run through it. The formation of synapses occurs more peripheral to the level of the ganglia: ganglion coeliacum, ganglion aorticorenale, ganglion mesentericum superius.

Preganglionar nerves confluence into three nervi splanchnici (major, minor, imus) that course along the paravertebral border (Table 26.2).

Just below the level of the crus of the diaphragm, the nervi splanchnici confluence with the vagal preganglionar parasympathetic fibers, sensory fibers of the nervus phrenicus, and postganglionar sympathetic fibers to the plexus coeliacus that are draped around the aorta abdominalis, especially at the anterior side. Figure 26.1 provides an image of the innervation of abdominal organs.

The nervi splanchnici are localized in a narrow pyramid of which the medial edge is formed by the lateral border of the vertebra, the lateral edge by the medial pleura and the crus of the diaphragm forms the basis of the triangle. The anterior side is formed by the posterior wall of the mediastinum and the

Table 26.2. Nervi splanchnici and preganglionair fiber level.

Nervus splanchnicus division	Preganglionar fiber level
Nervus splanchnicus major	Th5 to Th9
Nervus splanchnicus minor	Th10 to Th11
Nervus splanchnicus imus	Th11 to Th12

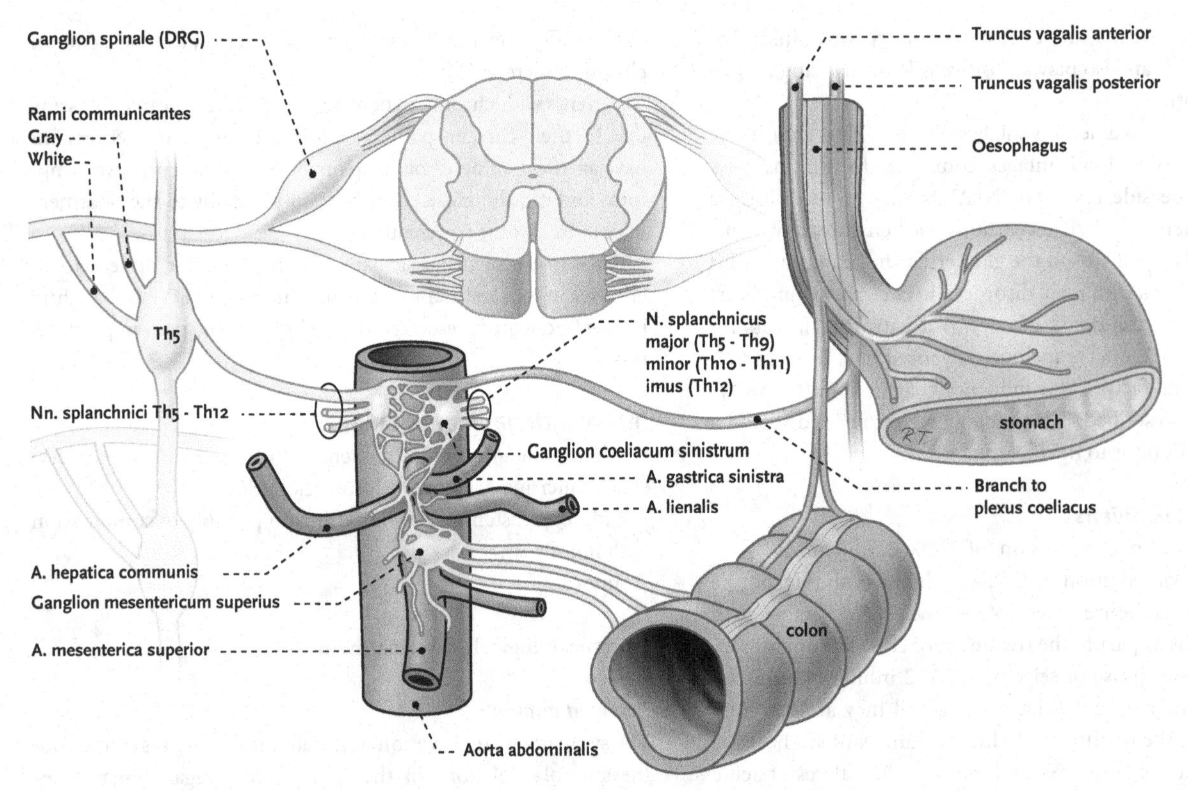

Figure 26.1. Innervation of the abdominal organs. Illustration: Rogier Trompert, Medical Art, www.medical-art.nl.

posterior wall by the attachment of the pleura parietalis on the lateral wall of the vertebrae.

Nervus splanchnicus block

The specific anatomy in which the nervi splanchnici are located in a narrow compartment allows a targeted denervation. The use of neurolytic agents—in patients with nonmalignant pain—has gradually been abandoned because of possible complications. RF thermolesioning, in which denervation only takes place at the tip of the electrode, seems more suitable for this indication.

The use of RF nervus splanchnicus treatment has been described in two patient series.[45,46] Raj et al.[45] reported on 107 patients who underwent RF treatment of the nervi splanchnici as a treatment of upper abdominal pain. The involvement of the nervi splanchnici was confirmed by means of a diagnostic block with a local anesthetic. Seventy-three patients were followed prospectively. Thirty-eight patients only received a block with a local anesthetic and 31 received RF treatment. In both groups, a pain relief of >50% was found in 40% of the patients.

Garcea et al.[46] described 10 patients who underwent RF nervus splanchnicus denervation as a treatment of chronic pancreatitis with a mean follow-up of 18 months (12 to 24 months). A significant pain reduction was observed, accompanied by a clear decrease in the need for opiates and acute hospitalization. Moreover, the parameters of the quality of life improved as well.

Spinal cord stimulation

The use of SCS to treat visceral pain was initially described in case reports.[47–52] A recent publication of a retrospective review of 35 patients who received a trial with SCS reported that 30 patients experienced ≥50% pain relief at the end of the trial.[53] In the 28 patients who received a permanent implant, one was lost to follow-up and five had the lead and generator removed for various reasons. Nineteen of the 22 patients were followed for more than 1 year. Over the complete evaluation period pain scores and opioid use remained low, suggesting that SCS for chronic abdominal pain of various causes may provide consistent long-term improvements. A national survey on SCS for chronic abdominal pain that followed this retrospective study included 76 case reports and its results were consistent in technical aspects of SCS implantation, as well as the opioid use and pain score improvements.[53,54] Both studies described SCS leads positioned with their tips mostly at the level of Th5 corpus vertebrae. Pain relief exceeded 50% in most of the patients and long-term opioid use decreased by more than two-thirds.[53,54] Another interesting feature noted in both studies is the presence of the large treated population of the patients with severe chronic pancreatitis.[53,54] There were 26 of 35 patients in a retrospective, and 26 of 70 patients in survey study who had diagnosis of chronic pancreatitis. Analyzed effects of SCS in this subgroup of the patients helped to conclude that the improvements in opioid use and pain scores were similar to those of patients with other sources of their chronic visceral abdominal pain.

Complications of interventional management

Complications of RF nervus splanchnicus block

The data available are insufficient to provide information about the incidence of complications. No major complications have been reported. Taking the information about neurolytic blocks into account, RF treatment can also induce postprocedural neuritis. This usually disappears within a few weeks and should be treated with medication. Hypotension and diarrhea may occur shortly after the intervention, but can be treated easily. As in all procedures at thoracic level, one should be alert to possible pneumothorax. A control radiograph of the thorax should therefore be made no more than 1 hour after the procedure. The patient may report a subjective feeling of dyspnea, which is attributed to a high position of the diaphragm, caused by the anesthetization of the nervus phrenicus.

Ductus thoracicus injury: upon aspiration a yellowish, turbid fluid is noted.

Intradiscal and intravascular injection: this should always be verified with a contrast.

Paresthesia: when contacting lumbar or thoracic roots.

Complications of SCS

The main complications of SCS are migration and breakage of the electrode. Additionally, infection is possible, which includes anything from local cellulites to epidural abscess.

Evidence for interventional management

The summary of the evidence for the interventional management of chronic pancreatitis is given in Table 26.3.

Table 26.3. Summary of the evidence for interventional management of pain due to chronic pancreatitis.

Technique	Assessment
Radiofrequency nervus splanchnicus block	2 C+
Spinal cord stimulation	2 C+

Recommendations

Radiofrequency (RF) nervus splanchnicus block can be considered in patients with chronic pancreatitis that is refractory to conventional treatment.

Spinal cord stimulation can be applied in the context of studies in patients with symptoms that cannot be treated by means of RF nervus splanchnicus block.

Clinical practice algorithm

Figure 26.2 represents the treatment algorithm for painful chronic pancreatitis based on the available evidence.

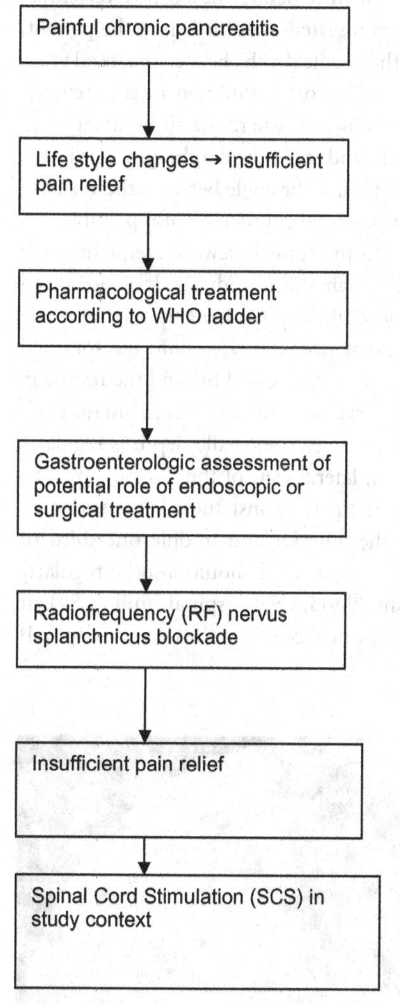

Figure 26.2. Clinical practice algorithm for the treatment of chronic pancreatitis.

Technique(s)

Percutaneous RF nervus splanchnicus treatment

The intervention is performed under X-ray guidance. The patient is placed in prone position on a translucent table with a pillow underneath the abdomen to reduce lumbar lordosis. Prior to the procedure, an intravenous infusion line is placed and an ECG and saturation monitoring are installed. Also, the patient is provided with 3 L/minute O_2 via nasal cannula. The procedure takes place under sedation with propofol or remifentanyl and spontaneous respiration.

Th12 and L1 are identified in a posteroanterior position and the vertebral endplates are aligned. The C-arm is rotated 5° to 10° to the side to be treated. The patient is asked to breathe in and out deeply. The attachment of the diaphragm is identified at mid-Th12 level. The needle placement site is located where the rib is attached to vertebrae Th11 and Th12, and above the diaphragm. The entry site is marked with a pen. The skin and the deeper layers are infiltrated with 5 mL of a local anesthetic (eg, lidocaine 2%) with a 22-G needle.

The treatment is performed with a 10- to 15-cm 22-G blunt or sharp curved needle with an active tip of 10 mm. As these patients are often very lean, a 10-cm needle is usually of sufficient length. The direction of the curve is visualized by a red dot at the hub of the needle. If a curved blunt needle is used, an intravenous 14-G catheter (as an introducer) is first inserted in perfect *tunnel view* aiming for a needle position just beside the corpus vertebrae. When the catheter has been inserted two-thirds into the patient, the stylet is removed and the needle depth checked in lateral view. The needle must stay posterior to the foramen intervertebrale. The needle placement site is located where the rib is attached to the vertebrae Th11 abd Th12 and above the diaphragm. The infracostal appraoch is preferred but if the angle between the vertebra and the rib is too sharp, supracostal approach is also possible.

The C-arm is returned to the tunnel view. Subsequently, the RF cannula is inserted through the introducer. It is advanced maintaining the tunnel view. Initially, the bent tip of the needle is turned outwards to prevent needle passage into the foramen intervertebrale. Once the needle has passed beyond the foramen, it is turned such that the curve faces medially to maintain close contact with the corpus vertebrae. The needle depth is regularly monitored (every 0.5 cm) in lateral view of the fluoroscopy. The final position of the needle tip is against the corpus vertebrae at the junction between the anterior and middle one-third of the vertebra (Figures 26.3 and 26.4). It should also be regularly checked as to whether any blood, cerebrospinal fluid (CSF) or chyle appears from the needle depending on the catheter depth. If any CSF or chyle is noticed, the procedure should be discontinued and a new session can be considered a few days later.

One milliliter of nonionic, non-neurotoxic contrast fluid (iohexol) is injected. The needle is located in posteroanterior view just over the lateral vertebral edge. The contrast should show an overlapping sausage-shaped image between the thoracic vertebrae over the lateral vertebral edge. The contrast fluid will fan out in case of an intrapleural location.

Initially, a diagnostic block will be performed by injecting bupivacaine 0.5% 3 mL (up to 5 mL). Higher volumes result in an increased incidence of false-positive blocks. This can also lead to additional anesthesia of the nervus phrenicus, which may cause an elevation of the diaphragm with secondary respiratory problems.

If the diagnostic block had positive results, RF treatment can be performed at a second session. The needle is positioned at the same location under fluoroscopic control. Once a good location is verified in tunnel and lateral view, the needle position is then also checked by electrical stimulation.

The RF device is connected to the needle and a grounding plate applied to the patient. The impedance should be lower than 250 Ω. The patient will feel a vibrating epigastric sensation at 50 Hz and a threshold of <1 V. If the electrical sensation is noted in the intercostal area, the needle should be moved further ventral. In addition, motor stimulation is applied at 2 Hz, focusing mainly on intercostal stimulation. Normally, no stimulation is felt.

If the test results are positive, local anesthetics are administered (2 to 3 mL of lidocaine 2% or bupivacaine 0.5%). The RF treatment can be carried out after several minutes. The needle position

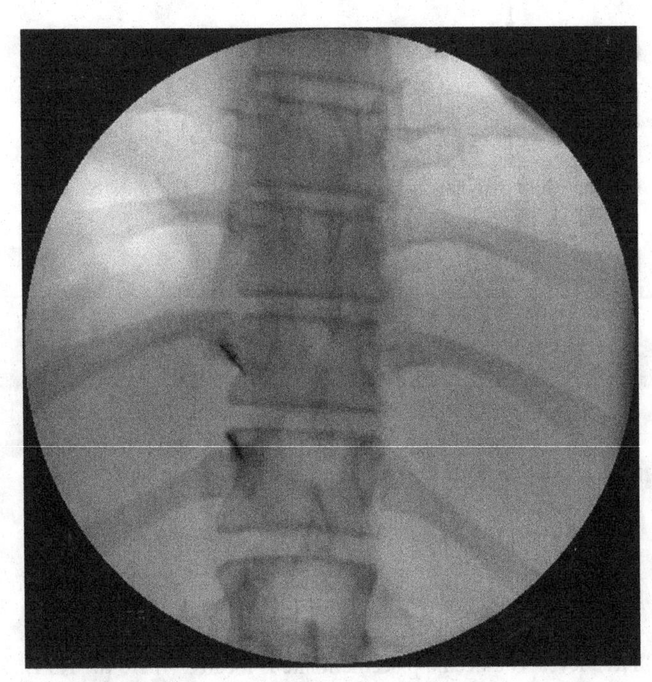

Figure 26.3. Radiofrequency nervus splanchnicus block at Th11 and T12 level: anterioposterior view.

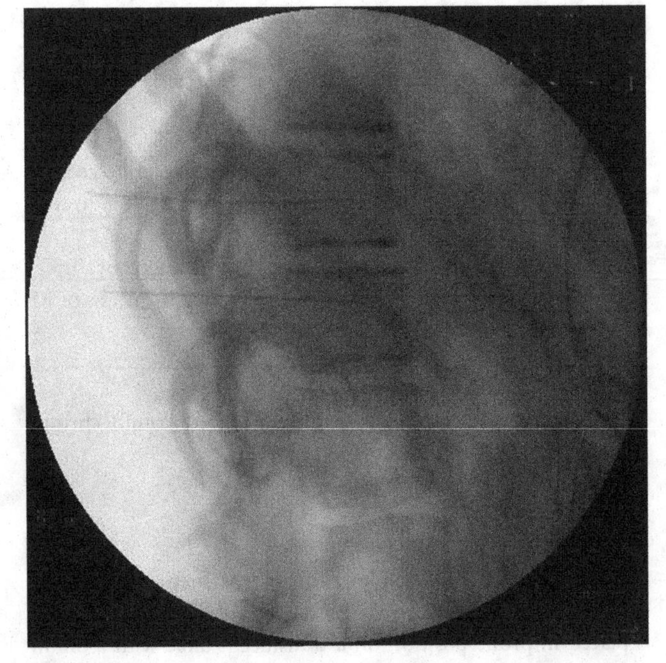

Figure 26.4. Radiofrequency nervus splanchnicus block at Th11 and T12 level: lateral image.

is monitored in the lateral view. For each level, the treatment consists of three 90-second cycles at 80°C. The needle is first turned with its curve in cranial direction, then neutral, and finally in caudal direction as a maximum area can thus be treated.

Spinal cord stimulation

The technique for SCS is described in the chapter on CRPS of this series.[55]

Other treatment options

Endoscopy

It is possible to bypass endoscopic obstructions of the ductus pancreaticus due to stones or stenosis. It is important in this respect to realize that no correlation has been shown between pain and the presence of intraductal stones nor are there any guidelines stipulating which degree of obstruction justifies or requires endoscopic intervention. Three recent studies into the effect of pancreatic stenting, either alone or combined with lithotripsy and/or sphincterotomy, showed a decrease of the pain[56,57] or no effect.[58] The effect of therapy on pain is often good in the short term, but soon decreases. Five years after endoscopic treatment, only 14% of the patients are still free of pain.[59] In recent literature, a block of the plexus coeliacus via EUS is increasingly used for cancer pain but also for pancreatitis.

Two reviews on endoscopic US-guided plexus coeliacus neurolysis (celiac plexus neurolysis [CPN]) in pancreatic cancer as well as chronic pancreatitis patients were published recently.[60,61]

Local anesthetics alone or in combination with steroids are injected. In a few cases, alcohol was injected. These studies have had a short effect and short follow-up periods, except for the study of Gress et al.[62] Endoscopic US-guided CPN is often described as safe. Diarrhea and hypotension are minor and transient side effects. Also empyema has been described. Recently a case report of infarction of the spleen, pancreas, and gastric antrum was published.[63] An ischemic injury occurred due to diffusion of ethanol into the truncus coeliacus with subsequent arterial vasospasm. Paraplegia, a rare but well-established adverse side effect of CPN, is thought to be secondary to diffusion of the neuroablative alcohol into the arteries supplying the spinal cord.[1–3]

Surgery

Pain can be treated by means of various techniques involving drainage (Puestow procedure) or resection (pancreaticoduodenectomy, total pancreatectomy with autotransplantation of the islets of Langerhans) or a combination of both (Frey procedure). Drainage procedures are intended to reduce pain by decompression of the ductus pancreaticus. The theory behind pain relief due to resection is that inflammatory activity causes pain as a result of qualitative and quantitative changes of the nerve fibers. Two recent randomized studies show that these surgical procedures lead to better results.[59,64] The percentage of patients who are free of pain after 5 years is 40%.

Other treatments

The results of the treatments discussed below (pancreatic enzyme supplementation, octreotide, and antioxidants) are not unambiguously proven in randomized studies.

Enzyme supplementation

The assumed mechanism of action of pancreatic enzymes with respect to pain relief reflects the role they play in the negative feedback of the pancreatic exocrine function. A CCK-releasing peptide is released in the duodenum and denaturized by trypsin. In patients with chronic pancreatitis, there is a reduced release of this trypsin, a reduced breakdown of CCK-releasing peptides with increases in pancreatic enzymes and flow in the ductus pancreaticus resulting in pain. Oral pancreatic enzymes lead to an increased breakdown of CCK-releasing peptides.

Two old studies show that treatment with pancreatic enzymes actually does lead to pain reduction.[65,66] The best response was obtained in young women with idiopathic chronic pancreatitis without steatorrhea. Four other studies found no effect of enzyme preparation on pain. Meta-analysis of these six randomized, double-blind placebo-controlled studies did not show a relevant, significant effect of treatment with enzyme preparations.[67] Strikingly though, the two studies showing an effect of pancreatic enzymes used nonenteric-coated preparations whereas the other four studies used enteric-coated preparations.

Octreotide

Octreotide—a somatostatin-analog with a prolonged half-life, stronger action, and the option to be administered subcutaneously—has been investigated for its efficacy in chronic pancreatitis. Octreotide inhibits exocrine pancreatic function. However, these studies could not establish a significant effect on pain reduction.[44]

Antioxidants

Lower plasma levels of several antioxidants (eg, selenium, vitamin A, vitamin E, and beta carotene) have been demonstrated in patients with chronic pancreatitis. There was a lower expression of antioxidants in the pancreatic tissue of patients with chronic pancreatitis than in healthy pancreatic tissue. Lower antioxidant levels may activate oxygen radicals, which may cause metabolic changes resulting in pancreatic ischemia. Oxidative stress is one of the assumed causes of pain produced by chronic pancreatitis. Two studies achieve pain reduction with dietary supplements containing antioxidants.[44,68]

Allopurinol, which reduces the formation of oxygen radicals by inhibiting xanthineoxidase, has been investigated in a crossover double-blind study in 13 patients with chronic pancreatitis. Allopurinol was proven to be ineffective. However, another study in which allopurinol was combined with intramuscular pethidine showed a significantly better effect compared to treatment with pethidine alone.[69,70]

Summary

Chronic pancreatitis is a progressive inflammatory reaction of the pancreas that causes irreversible morphological changes of the parenchyma (fibrosis, loss of acini and islets of Langerhans, and pancreatic stone formation) as well as the ductus pancreaticus (stenosis).

Pain in chronic pancreatitis requires a multidisciplinary approach, in which lifestyle changes are essential.

If the patient suffers from pseudocysts, obstruction of the ductus choledochus or the duodenum, this should be treated first.

Treatment with pancreatic enzyme supplementation, octreotide, and antioxidants can be considered, but results have not been proven unambiguously in randomized studies.

The use of analgesic medication generally, and opioids in particular, should be accompanied by evaluation of the degree of addiction and, if indicated, close supervision.

Radiofrequency treatment of the nervi splanchnici can be considered in patients with pain that is refractory to conservative treatment.

References

1. Morisset J. Negative control of human pancreatic secretion: physiological mechanisms and factors. *Pancreas.* 2008;37:1–12.
2. Bockman D. Nerves in the pancreas: what are they for? *Am J Surg.* 2007;1997:S61–S64.
3. Salvioli B, Bovara M, Barbara G, et al. Neurology and neuropathology of the pancreatic innervation. *JOP.* 2002;3:26–33.
4. Mariani A, Testoni PA. Is acute recurrent pancreatitis a chronic disease? *World J Gastroenterol.* 2008;14:995–998.
5. Ammann RW, Akovbiantz A, Largiader F, Schueler G. Course and outcome of chronic pancreatitis. Longitudinal study of a mixed medical-surgical series of 245 patients. *Gastroenterology.* 1984;86:820–828.
6. Lankisch PG, Lohr-Happe A, Otto J, Creutzfeldt W. Natural course in chronic pancreatitis. Pain, exocrine and endocrine pancreatic insufficiency and prognosis of the disease. *Digestion.* 1993;54: 148–155.
7. Lowenfels AB, Maisonneuve P, Cavallini G, et al. Pancreatitis and the risk of pancreatic cancer. International Pancreatitis Study Group. *N Engl J Med.* 1993;328:1433–1437.
8. Bornman PC, Marks IN, Girdwood AW, Berberat PO, Gulbinas A, Buchler MW. Pathogenesis of pain in chronic pancreatitis: ongoing enigma. *World J Surg.* 2003;27:1175–1182.
9. Hayakawa T, Kondo T, Shibata T, Sugimoto Y, Kitagawa M. Chronic alcoholism and evolution of pain and prognosis in chronic pancreatitis. *Dig Dis Sci.* 1989;34:33–38.
10. Ammann RW, Heitz PU, Kloppel G. Course of alcoholic chronic pancreatitis: a prospective clinicomorphological long-term study. *Gastroenterology.* 1996;111:224–231.
11. Behrman SW, Fowler ES. Pathophysiology of chronic pancreatitis. *Surg Clin North Am.* 2007;87:1309–1324, vii.
12. Apte MV, Pirola RC, Wilson JS. Molecular mechanisms of alcoholic pancreatitis. *Dig Dis.* 2005;23:232–240.
13. Lee JK, Enns R. Review of idiopathic pancreatitis. *World J Gastroenterol.* 2007;13:6296–6313.
14. Di Sebastiano P, Fink T, Weihe E, et al. Immune cell infiltration and growth-associated protein 43 expression correlate with pain in chronic pancreatitis. *Gastroenterology.* 1997;112:1648–1655.
15. Kawabata A, Matsunami M, Sekiguchi F. Gastrointestinal roles for proteinase-activated receptors in health and disease. *Br J Pharmacol.* 2008;153(suppl 1):S230–S240.
16. White TT, Bourde J. A new observation on human intraductal pancreatic pressure. *Surg Gynecol Obstet.* 1970;130:275–278.
17. Bradley EL III. Pancreatic duct pressure in chronic pancreatitis. *Am J Surg.* 1982;144:313–316.
18. Ebbehoj N, Borly L, Madsen P, Matzen P. Pancreatic tissue fluid pressure during drainage operations for chronic pancreatitis. *Scand J Gastroenterol.* 1990;25:1041–1045.
19. Manes G, Buchler M, Pieramico O, Di Sebastiano P, Malfertheiner P. Is increased pancreatic pressure related to pain in chronic pancreatitis? *Int J Pancreatol.* 1994;15:113–117.
20. Levy P, Lesur G, Belghiti J, Fekete F, Bernades P. Symptomatic duodenal stenosis in chronic pancreatitis: a study of 17 cases in a medical-surgical series of 306 patients. *Pancreas.* 1993;8:563–567.
21. Steer ML, Waxman I, Freedman S. Chronic pancreatitis. *N Engl J Med.* 1995;332:1482–1490.
22. Xu GY, Winston JH, Shenoy M, Yin H, Pasricha PJ. Enhanced excitability and suppression of A-type K+ current of pancreas-specific afferent neurons in a rat model of chronic pancreatitis. *Am J Physiol Gastrointest Liver Physiol.* 2006;291:G424–G431.
23. Buscher HC, Wilder-Smith OH, van Goor H. Chronic pancreatitis patients show hyperalgesia of central origin: a pilot study. *Eur J Pain.* 2006;10:363–370.
24. Vera-Portocarrero L, Westlund KN. Role of neurogenic inflammation in pancreatitis and pancreatic pain. *Neurosignals.* 2005;14:158–165.
25. Toskes PP, Hansell J, Cerda J, Deren JJ. Vitamin B 12 malabsorption in chronic pancreatic insufficiency. *N Engl J Med.* 1971;284:627–632.
26. Malka D, Hammel P, Sauvanet A, et al. Risk factors for diabetes mellitus in chronic pancreatitis. *Gastroenterology.* 2000;119:1324–1332.
27. Ammann RW, Muellhaupt B. The natural history of pain in alcoholic chronic pancreatitis. *Gastroenterology.* 1999;116:1132–1140.
28. Niederau C, Grendell JH. Diagnosis of chronic pancreatitis. *Gastroenterology.* 1985;88:1973–1995.
29. Lieb JG II, Draganov PV. Pancreatic function testing: here to stay for the 21st century. *World J Gastroenterol.* 2008;14:3149–3158.
30. Bozkurt T, Braun U, Leferink S, Gilly G, Lux G. Comparison of pancreatic morphology and exocrine functional impairment in patients with chronic pancreatitis. *Gut.* 1994;35:1132–1136.
31. Kahl S, Glasbrenner B, Leodolter A, Pross M, Schulz HU, Malfertheiner P. EUS in the diagnosis of early chronic pancreatitis: a prospective follow-up study. *Gastrointest Endosc.* 2002;55:507–511.
32. Graziani R, Tapparelli M, Malago R, et al. The various imaging aspects of chronic pancreatitis. *JOP.* 2005;6:73–88.
33. Kim DH, Pickhardt PJ. Radiologic assessment of acute and chronic pancreatitis. *Surg Clin North Am.* 2007;87:1341–1358, viii.
34. Wallace MB. Imaging the pancreas: into the deep. *Gastroenterology.* 2007;132:484–487.
35. Andren-Sandberg A, Dervenis C. Pancreatic pseudocysts in the 21st century. Part I: classification, pathophysiology, anatomic considerations and treatment. *JOP.* 2004;5:8–24.
36. Warshaw AL, Schapiro RH, Ferrucci JT Jr, Galdabini JJ. Persistent obstructive jaundice, cholangitis, and biliary cirrhosis due to

common bile duct stenosis in chronic pancreatitis. *Gastroenterology.* 1976;70:562–567.
37. Sonnenday C, Yeo CJ. Open gastrojejunostomy. *Oper Tech Gen Surg.* 2003;5:72–79.
38. Miyake H, Harada H, Kunichika K, Ochi K, Kimura I. Clinical course and prognosis of chronic pancreatitis. *Pancreas.* 1987;2: 378–385.
39. Layer P, Yamamoto H, Kalthoff L, Clain JE, Bakken LJ, DiMagno EP. The different courses of early- and lateonset idiopathic and alcoholic chronic pancreatitis. *Gastroenterology.* 1994;107:1481–1487.
40. Schlosser W, Schlosser S, Ramadani M, Gansauge F, Gansauge S, Beger HG. Cyclooxygenase-2 is overexpressed in chronic pancreatitis. *Pancreas.* 2002;25:26–30.
41. Radnay PA, Brodman E, Mankikar D, Duncalf D. The effect of equi-analgesic doses of fentanyl, morphine, meperidine and pentazocine on common bile duct pressure. *Anaesthesist.* 1980;29:26–29.
42. Helm JF, Venu RP, Geenen JE, et al. Effects of morphine on the human sphincter of Oddi. *Gut.* 1988;29:1402–1407.
43. van Voorthuizen T, Helmers JH, Tjoeng MM, Otten MH. [Meperidine (pethidine) outdated as analgesic in acute pancreatitis]. *Ned Tijdschr Geneeskd.* 2000;144:656–658.
44. Gachago C, Draganov PV. Pain management in chronic pancreatitis. *World J Gastroenterol.* 2008;14:3137–3148.
45. Prithvi Raj P, Sahinder B, Lowe M. Radiofrequency lesioning of splanchnic nerves. *Pain Pract.* 2002;2:241–247.
46. Garcea G, Thomasset S, Berry DP, Tordoff S. Percutaneous splanchnic nerve radiofrequency ablation for chronic abdominal pain. *ANZ J Surg.* 2005;75:640–644.
47. Tiede JM, Ghazi SM, Lamer TJ, Obray JB. The use of spinal cord stimulation in refractory abdominal visceral pain: case reports and literature review. *Pain Pract.* 2006;6:197–202.
48. Kapural L, Rakic M. Spinal cord stimulation for chronic visceral pain secondary to chronic non-alcoholic pancreatitis. *J Clin Gastroenterol.* 2008;42:750–751.
49. Ceballos A, Cabezudo L, Bovaira M, Fenollosa P, Moro B. Spinal cord stimulation: a possible therapeutic alternative for chronic mesenteric ischaemia. *Pain.* 2000;87:99–101.
50. Krames ES, Mousad D. Spinal cord stimulation reverses pain and diarrheal episodes of irritable bowel syndrome: a case report. *Neuromodulation.* 2004;7:82–88.
51. Khan I, Raza S, Khan E. Application of spinal cord stimulation for the treatment of abdominal visceral pain syndromes: case reports. *Neuromodulation.* 2005;8:14–27.
52. Kapural L. Proceedings from the 9th Annual Meeting of the North American Neuromodulation Society November 2005. Vol. 9, Neuromodulation: Technology at the Neural Interface, Whashington, DC; 2005;22, January 2006.
53. Kapural L, Nagem H, Tlucek H, Sessler DI. Spinal cord stimulation for chronic visceral abdominal pain. *Pain Med.* 2010;11:347–355.
54. Kapural L, Deer T, Yakovlev A, et al. Technical aspects of spinal cord stimulation for managing chronic visceral abdominal pain: the results from the national survey. *Pain Med.* 2010;11:685–691.
55. van Eijs F, Stanton-Hicks M, Van Zundert J, et al. Evidence-based interventional pain medicine according to clinical diagnoses. 16. Complex regional pain syndrome. *Pain Pract.* 2011;11:70–87.
56. Smits ME, Badiga SM, Rauws EA, Tytgat GN, Huibregtse K. Long-term results of pancreatic stents in chronic pancreatitis. *Gastrointest Endosc.* 1995;42:461–467.
57. Kozarek RA, Ball TJ, Patterson DJ, Brandabur JJ, Traverso LW, Raltz S. Endoscopic pancreatic duct sphincterotomy: indications, technique, and analysis of results. *Gastrointest Endosc.* 1994;40: 592–598.
58. Ashby K, Lo SK. The role of pancreatic stenting in obstructive ductal disorders other than pancreas divisum. *Gastrointest Endosc.* 1995;42:306–311.
59. Dite P, Ruzicka M, Zboril V, Novotny I. A prospective, randomized trial comparing endoscopic and surgical therapy for chronic pancreatitis. *Endoscopy.* 2003;35:553–558.
60. Kaufman M, Singh G, Das S, et al. Efficacy of endoscopic ultrasound-guided celiac plexus block and celiac plexus neurolysis for managing abdominal pain associated with chronic pancreatitis and pancreatic cancer. *J Clin Gastroenterol.* 2010;44:127–134.
61. Puli SR, Reddy JB, Bechtold ML, Antillon MR, Brugge WR. EUS-guided celiac plexus neurolysis for pain due to chronic pancreatitis or pancreatic cancer pain: a metaanalysis and systematic review. *Dig Dis Sci.* 2009;54:2330–2337.
62. Gress F, Schmitt C, Sherman S, Ciaccia D, Ikenberry S, Lehman G. Endoscopic ultrasound-guided celiac plexus block for managing abdominal pain associated with chronic pancreatitis: a prospective single center experience. *Am J Gastroenterol.* 2001;96: 409–416.
63. Ahmed HM, Friedman SE, Henriques HF, Berk BS. End-organ ischemia as an unforeseen complication of endoscopic-ultrasound-guided celiac plexus neurolysis. *Endoscopy.* 2009;41(suppl 2):E218–219.
64. Cahen DL, Gouma DJ, Nio Y, et al. Endoscopic versus surgical drainage of the pancreatic duct in chronic pancreatitis. *N Engl J Med.* 2007;356:676–684.
65. Slaff J, Jacobson D, Tillman CR, Curington C, Toskes P. Protease-specific suppression of pancreatic exocrine secretion. *Gastroenterology.* 1984;87:44–52.
66. Isaksson G, Ihse I. Pain reduction by an oral pancreatic enzyme preparation in chronic pancreatitis. *Dig Dis Sci.* 1983;28:97–102.
67. Brown A, Hughes M, Tenner S, Banks PA. Does pancreatic enzyme supplementation reduce pain in patients with chronic pancreatitis: a meta-analysis. *Am J Gastroenterol.* 1997;92:2032–2035.
68. Salim AS. Role of oxygen-derived free radical scavengers in the treatment of recurrent pain produced by chronic pancreatitis. A new approach. *Arch Surg.* 1991;126:1109–1114.
69. Banks PA, Hughes M, Ferrante M, Noordhoek EC, Ramagopal V, Slivka A. Does allopurinol reduce pain of chronic pancreatitis? *Int J Pancreatol.* 1997;22:171–176.
70. McCloy R. Chronic pancreatitis at Manchester, UK. Focus on antioxidant therapy. *Digestion.* 1998;59(suppl 4):36–48.

Index

Evidence-Based Interventional Pain Medicine: According to Clinical Diagnoses, First Edition. Edited by Jan Van Zundert, Jacob Patijn, Craig T. Hartrick, Arno Lataster, Frank J.P.M Huygen, Nagy Mekhail, Maarten van Kleef.

Printed in the United States
By Bookmasters